PSYCHOLOGY – SELECTED PAPERS

Edited by **Gina Rossi**

Psychology – Selected Papers
Edited by Gina Rossi

Published by InTech
Janeza Trdine 9, 51000 Rijeka, Croatia

Publishing Process Manager Masa Vidovic

Technical Editor Teodora Smiljanic

Cover Designer InTech Design Team

Additional hard copies can be obtained from orders@intechopen.com

Psychology – Selected Papers, Edited by Gina Rossi
p. cm.
ISBN 978-953-51-0587-9

For EU product safety concerns:
IN TECH d.o.o., Prolaz Marije Krucifikse Kozulić 3, 51000 Rijeka, Croatia,
info@intechopen.com or visit our website at intechopen.com.

Meet the editor

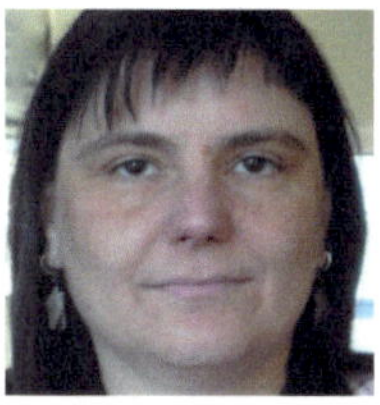

Professor Dr Gina Rossi obtained a PhD in Psychological Sciences at the Vrije Universiteit Brussel (VUB). She is currently Associate Professor at the VUB, where she teaches courses on personality psychology at the Faculty of Psychology and Educational Sciences (Personality Psychology I, Personality Psychology II, Capita Selecta Personality Psychology), and Psychology at the Faculty of Law and Criminology. She is also a lecturer in Postgraduate Education Programs, such as the Postgraduate 'Forensic Diagnostics & Counseling' at University College Lessius and the inter-university program 'Clinical Psychodiagnostics'. Her research focus is mainly in the domain of personality, especially personality psychopathology and personality assessment. In addition, she also has interest in forensic psychology. She has published her work in well-established journals such 'Journal of Personality Disorders', 'Journal of Personality Assessment', 'Criminal Justice and Behavior', etc. She is reviewer for several journals and consulting editor of 'Journal of Personality Assessment', 'International Journal of Offender Therapy and Comparative Criminology', and associate editor of 'Psychologica Belgica'.

Contents

Preface

Editing this book was a pleasant, but challenging job. I enjoyed reviewing chapters from different domains, bringing up-to-date empirical research studies, excellent literature reviews and controversial issues. This was an instructive experience for me and the authors. We both learned from each other, making different backgrounds a gain-gain situation, by evaluating each chapter critically from different perspectives. We are sure the reader will enjoy the end result: a selection of chapters from different psychology domains.

We start off with two papers on alcoholism. Dr. Dorrian discusses the self-reinforcing feedback loop, pointing out that a holistic, bio-psycho-social approach is necessary to address alcohol use disorders. Mr. Noël underlines the importance of impulsivity in predisposing and developmental factors in alcohol related disorders, bringing an overview of recent inhibition studies. Three papers concern issues relevant to clinical interventions. Dr. Mellsop and Howard introduce diagnoses and the clinical process, and stress the importance of contextualizing the diagnosis with thorough and reflective formulation to optimize the recovery plan. Dr. Kwiatkowski discusses the ongoing controversy on the positive effects of hypnosis and reviews the application in oncology. He concludes that hypnosis does help in psychosocial matters, but not for survival. Dr. Russell and Ms. Fechter-Leggett disentangle the mutual regulation dyad between parents and infants in the context of inconsolable crying. They are convinced of the benefits of dialectical behavior therapy in case of emotion dysregulation. The next chapters specifically focus on the treatment of depression. Dr. Guilloux, Dr. Samuels, Dr. David, Dr. Gardier, and Dr. Guiard show out that current SSRI antidepressant treatments are not sufficient, since the insensitivity of many patients. New methods, like triple reuptake inhibitors should be investigated more thoroughly. Dr. Mutlu, Dr. Ulak, Dr. Celikyurt, Dr. Akar, and Dr. Erden examine new approaches for the treatment of refractory depression. They conclude that nitric oxide synthase inhibitors are a promising approach.

Personality psychology is covered from two approaches. Dr. Mikołajczak-Degrauwe, Dr. Brengman, Dr. Wauters, and Dr. Rossi examine how personality affects compulsive buying. Issues are addressed on how the Big Five Personality model can be applied in this context. Dr. De Weerdt and Dr. Rossi investigate how emotional intelligence and psychopathology relate to each other. They approach emotional intelligence from a perspective integrating personal, emotional, and social competencies in coping successfully with life demands.

Next, the paper of Dr. Biggerstaff introduces qualitative research methods in psychology. She focuses on important concepts, the growing importance of these methods in the field, and strengths and limitations of these methods. This is followed by two practical applications. Dr. Gushin, and Dr. Yusupova analyse communication in space flights. They more specifically address issues of information exchange in long-term space flights. Dr. Lima reveals the connection between topic grounds or lexical worlds and themata from the theory of social presentations by an analysis using the ALCESTE algorithm. Finally, we bring some excellent chapters from social psychology. Ms. Dickel and Dr. Bohner demonstrate how theorizing on automatic associations and persuasion research can be integrated into the research of minority and majority influence on attitudes. Dr. Bocchiaro and Dr. Zamperini bring recent studies on the power of the situation in the context of conformity, obedience and disobedience. Dr. Klose and Dr. Lasser review which social psychological phenomena influence group decision making in an educational context. Dr. Dubois and Dr. Beauvois depart from an evaluative approach. They outline theory and applications related to the social value of persons. As such we have interesting blend of studies from experts from a diverse array of psychology fields. The selected chapters will take the reader on an exciting journey in the domains of psychology. I'm sure the content will appeal to a great audience!

Dr. Gina Rossi
Vrije Universiteit Brussel (VUB)
Belgium

Section 1

Alcoholism

1

Alcoholism: The Self-Reinforcing Feedback Loop

Jillian Dorrian
Senior Lecturer in Psychology, Social Work and Social Policy
University of South Australia
Australia

1. Introduction

Healthcare in the 18th and 19th centuries was primarily focused on infectious illnesses, such as smallpox, influenza, measles and polio. The development of the biomedical model (which specifically acknowledged that diseases could be explained by physical processes connected with injury, imbalance, or infection) represented a major advance in healthcare, facilitating the development improved hygiene practices, vaccines and antibiotics. In contrast to such historical healthcare priorities, in developed countries today, the major reasons for medical treatment and mortality are chronic illness and accidents (Catalbiano, Sarafino, & Byrne, 2008). Indeed, the current health priority areas in Australia are cancer, cardiovascular disease, diabetes, mental health, obesity, injury prevention/control, arthritis/ musculoskeletal conditions and asthma (AIHW, 2011). The risk factors for these contemporary health priorities are not only physical, but include important and complex behavioural and social interactions. Therefore, a biopsychosocial approach (Fig 1) is required in the current healthcare climate, acknowledging the contribution of physical, behavioural and social factors to health (Catalbiano et al., 2008).

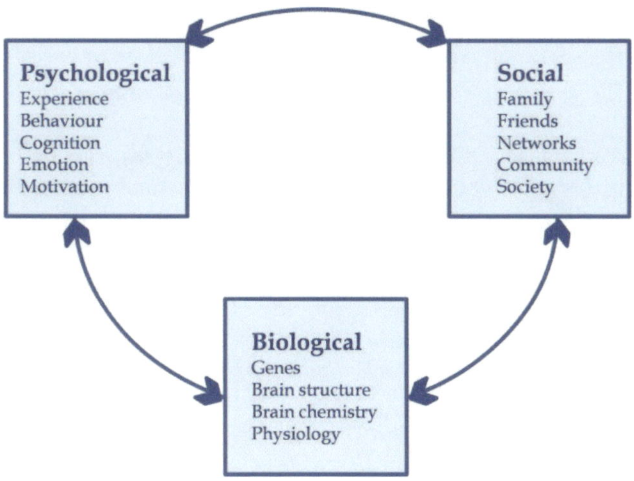

Fig. 1. Biopsychosocial model (adapted from Catalbiano et al., 2008).

Elevated alcohol consumption (along with smoking, lack of exercise and poor diet) represents an key behavioural risk factor for chronic illness and accident and injury, as well as many other costs at the personal and social level (Anderson, Chisholm, & Fuhr, 2009; Carr, 2011; Casswell & Thamarangsi, 2009; Room, Babor, & Rehm, 2005). Alcohol-use disorders are a particularly disabling contributor to the global disease burden (Rehm et al., 2009). Alcohol-use disorders include issues of alcohol *dependency* and *abuse* (Carr, 2011; Rehm et al., 2009), defined in Table 1.

Definitions of Alcohol Abuse and Dependence

Alcohol Abuse

a. *"A maladaptive pattern of substance use leading to clinically significant impairment or distress, as manifested by one (or more) of the following, occurring within a 12-month period:*
   1. *Recurrent [alcohol] use resulting in a failure to fulfil major role obligations at work, school, or home*
   2. *Recurrent [alcohol] use in situations in which it is physically hazardous*
   3. *Recurrent [alcohol]-related legal problems*
   4. *Continued [alcohol] use despite having persistent or recurrent social or interpersonal problems caused or exacerbated by the effects of [alcohol]*

b. *The symptoms have never met the criteria for [Alcohol] Dependence"*

DSM-IV-TR, p199.

Alcohol Dependence

"A maladaptive pattern of substance use leading to clinically significant impairment or distress, as manifested by three (or more) of the following, occurring at any time in the same 12-month period:

1. *Tolerance, as defined by either of the following:*
   a) *A need for markedly increased amounts of [alcohol] to achieve intoxication or desired effect*
   b) *Markedly diminished effect with continued use of the same amount of [alcohol]*
2. *Withdrawal, as manifested by either of the following:*
   a) *The characteristic withdrawal syndrome for [alcohol]*
   b) *The same (or a closely related) substance is taken to relieve or avoid withdrawal symptoms*
3. *[Alcohol] is often taken in larger amounts or over a longer period than was intended*
4. *There is a persistent desire or unsuccessful efforts to cut down or control [alcohol] use*
5. *A great deal of time is spent in activities necessary to obtain [alcohol], use [alcohol], or recover from its effects*
6. *Important social, occupational, or recreational activities are given up or reduced because of [alcohol] use*
7. *The [alcohol] use is continued despite knowledge of having a persistent or recurrent physiological or psychological problem that is likely to have been caused or exacerbated by [alcohol]"*

DSM-IV-TR, p199

Table 1. DSM-IV definitions of Alcohol Abuse and Dependence

The predictors of alcohol-use disorders are varied and complex, including family history (Eve 1989), genetics (Ginter & Simko, 2009; Hansell et al., 2009) and social and familial learning environment (Fergusson, Lynskey et al., 1994; Fergusson & Horwood 1998). The physical and cognitive consequences of alcohol-related problems impact negatively on the ability to engage with treatment (Dorrian, 2010; Williamson, 2009a). Stigma and stereotypes surrounding alcohol-related problems frequently damage crucial support relationships with friends and family (Dorrian, 2010; Schomerus et al., 2011) and healthcare professionals (Crothers & Dorrian, 2011; Durand, 1994). Despite this, research suggests that, at a global level, attempts to address alcohol-related issues are inadequate (Casswell & Thamarangsi, 2009). Problematic alcohol use represents a critical issue in global healthcare.

This chapter will discuss the prevalence and cost of alcohol *abuse* and *dependence*, the effects on brain and body, risk factors for the development of alcohol-use disorders, family and social support, current treatment approaches and the importance of positive, supportive interactions with healthcare professionals. This discussion will feed into the development of a biopsychosocially-grounded self-reinforcing feedback model of alcoholism, where the very nature of the illness serves to perpetuate its development and presents barriers to treatment.

2. Prevalence and cost of alcoholism

Alcohol is an important part of the economy in many countries, giving rise to employment and trade. Alcohol also represents an important part of social and family culture for many people, having associations with celebration, commiseration and relaxation (NAS, 2006). Most of the global population abstain, or drink at levels that do not warrant concern. Approximately 50% of men and two in three women have abstained from alcohol during the last year (WHO 2011). However, alcohol, which has been referred to as "*the oldest drug of abuse*" (Carr, 2011, p9), can lead to serious harm.

Approximately one in ten drinkers engages in *heavy episodic* drinking (consuming >60g of alcohol, approximately 5 standard drinks, on a single occasion). This type of drinking pattern is highly associated with short term risks, including injury. The male:female ratio of heavy episodic drinking is approximately 4:1. Indeed, men substantially outnumber women in all measures of alcohol consumption (WHO, 2011), including rates of alcohol-use disorders. The global estimate of prevalence of alcohol-use disorders among 15 to 64 year-olds in 2004 was 6.3% for men, 0.9% for women and 3.6% overall (Rehm et al., 2009). In the US, it has been estimated that alcohol-use disorders affect up to 25 million adults (Carr, 2011).

Evaluations in the US suggest that one in three adults consume alcohol at risky levels, and that approximately 15% binge drink, and 5% drink heavily (Carr, 2011). A recent report indicates that in Australia, one in five people drink at risky levels for lifetime harm (>2 standard drinks daily), and nearly one in three drink at risky levels for short-term harm (>4 standard drinks per occasion). More than other drugs, alcohol consumption has been cited as the greatest serious community concern in Australia (AIHW, 2010).

Alcohol is in the top 12 risk factors for global causes of disease burden in both developing and developed countries (NAS, 2006). Globally, nearly 4% of deaths have been attributed to alcohol. Further, 4.6% of Disability Life Years (which take into account years lost through early death as well as years lived with disability) have been ascribed to alcohol consumption (Rehm et al., 2009).

A recent study, which estimated the total economic impact of alcohol across 12 countries (Australia, Canada, France, Germany, Japan, The Netherlands, New Zealand, Portugal, Sweden, South Korea, Thailand, USA), found that it equated to between 0.45 and 5.44% of Gross Domestic Product (Thavorncharoensap, Teerawattananon, Yothasamut, Lertpitakpong, & Chaikledkaew, 2009). For high income countries, productivity loss has been identified as accounting for the largest proportion of alcohol-attributable costs (72%), followed by direct health costs (13%)(Rehm et al., 2009).

The yearly cost of alcohol-related social issues in Australia in 1998-99 was estimated to be $7.6 million, with $5.5 billion tangible costs. The greatest proportion of this (34%) occurred in the workplace, through lost productivity and reduced capacity due to absenteeism. This was followed by road accidents (33%), crime (22%), lost production in the home (7%) and health costs (4%)(NAS, 2006).

Alcohol results in increased risk of accident and injury, not only for the individual, but for those around them. It is also associated causally with more than 60 diseases. Table 2 displays a quote from the most recent World Health Organisation (WHO) report on alcohol and health, which summarises these effects.

World Health Organisation statement, 2011
"The harmful use of alcohol results in approximately 2.5 million deaths each year, with a net loss of life of 2.25 million, taking into account the estimated beneficial impact of low levels of alcohol use on some diseases in some population groups...Alcohol consumption is the world's third largest risk factor for disease and disability; in middle-income countries, it is the greatest risk. Alcohol is a causal factor in 60 types of diseases and injuries and a component cause in 200 others. Almost 4% of all deaths worldwide are attributed to alcohol, greater than deaths caused by HIV/AIDS, violence or tuberculosis. Alcohol is also associated with many serious social issues, including violence, child neglect and abuse, and absenteeism in the workplace."
World Health Organisation (WHO), 2011, p10-11.

Table 2. Quote from the WHO regarding the negative impact of harmful use of alcohol.

3. Brain and body effects

Alcohol stimulates the reward centres of the brain, heavily influencing dopamine, as well as other neurotransmitters. It activates similar pathways to other addictive drugs including benzodiazepines, barbiturates and opiates (Carr, 2011). Alcohol induces relaxation and euphoria, while at the same time impairing motor skills and judgement (NAS, 2006).

3.1 Brain damage

Neuronal damage due to chronic alcohol use is widespread, however, much research attention has focused on the diencephalon, limbic system, and in particular, the frontal lobe

(Carr, 2011). Studies suggest reduced glucose-utilisation in the frontal lobes (Kopelman, 2008; Moselhy, Georgiou, & Kahn, 2001). Autopsies of individuals with chronic drinking patterns reveal frontal volume loss and decreased neuronal counts (Kopelman, 2008). Neuropsychological testing indicates that individuals with alcohol-use disorders display reduced functioning on frontal lobe tasks (Kopelman, 2008).

Table 3 shows a list of some of the characteristics of individuals who experience frontal lobe dysfunction. Such difficulties are common among individuals with alcohol-use disorders. As can be seen from this list, these types of impairments can have a direct negative impact on risk-taking behaviours (e.g. impulsivity, disinhibition, reduced attention), and relationships with friends and family (e.g. abnormalities of emotion, apathy, shallowness), as well as the capacity to decide to reduce or cease drinking, and engagement with healthcare professionals and treatment programs (e.g. decrease in will and energy, problems with planning and problem solving, poor motivation and decision making).

Characteristics of frontal lobe dysfunction	
• Disorders of categorising	• Decrease in will and energy
• Decrease in voluntary motor behaviour	• Tendency to engage in perseverative behaviour
• Difficulty shifting response set	• Problems with short-term memory
• Abnormalities in emotion	• Problems with problem-solving
• Apathy	• Impulsivity
• Indifference	• Disinhibition
• Shallowness	• Poor motivation
• Difficulty in creative thinking	• Problems with decision-making
• Reduced capacity to plan future actions	• Poor language and motor control
• Reduced artistic expression	• Reduced ability to sustain attention
• Poor spatial working memory	
	Reviewed in Moselhy et al., 2001

Table 3. Summary of characteristic indicators of impairment in individuals with frontal lobe deficits.

Further, alcohol effects the formation of new long-term memories and can induce black-outs (Lee, Roh, & Kim, 2009; White, 2003). It has been suggested that black-outs may contribute to the likelihood of developing alcohol-use disorders, as perception of the effects of alcohol may be limited to the positive effects, and negative impact may be forgotten during black-out periods (Lee et al., 2009).

3.2 Illness, disease and injury

Continuing alcohol issues are associated with a 200-300% increase in the likelihood of early death. Among the most frequent causes of death are cirrhosis of the liver, heart disease, cancer, stroke and accidents and injuries, which include burns, falls and drowning (Carr, 2011; Schuckit, 2009). It has been estimated that alcohol-use disorders may be causally related to approximately 50% of liver disease-related deaths. Alcohol-use disorders have been implicated in head and neck cancer. It has also been estimated that people with alcohol-use disorders have twice the risk of oesophagus, rectum and breast cancers (Schuckit, 2009). While low to moderate alcohol consumption has been shown to have a protective effect on the cardiovascular system, higher levels of consumption are related to stroke and heart failure (reviewed in Room et al., 2005; Carr, 2011).

Alcohol has also been associated with impaired endocrine function, resulting in problems with libido and reproductive capability, and increased risk of spontaneous abortion (Carr, 2011). Excessive alcohol consumption also interferes with vitamin and mineral absorption, often resulting in thiamine deficiency, which can lead to Wernicke's encephalopathy, characterised by problems with balance, gait, confusion and memory loss. Severe thiamine deficiency can also lead to Korsakoff 's syndrome, which is characterised primarily by severe anterograde amnesia. When the two sets of symptoms are present together, this is typically referred to as Wernicke-Korsakoff Syndrome (Carr, 2011; Schuckit, 2009).

Withdrawal from alcohol and the detoxification process are also associated with a spectrum of health issues. Symptoms may include anxiety, sleep problems, vivid dreams, headache, nausea, dangerously increased heart rate, elevated blood pressure, sweating, tremors, impaired heat regulation, seizures and delirium tremens (delirium and shaking). These symptoms may be fatal in up to 5% of cases (Carr, 2011). Further, repeated detoxification may result in reduced brain plasticity and longer healing times for frontal/executive processes (Loeber et al., 2010).

Failure to diagnose and address an alcohol-use disorder can result in complications with other illnesses, including psychiatric problems (Schuckit, 2009). Even when alcohol-use disorders have been identified, managing concomitant alcohol-related chronic illness can be very difficult. Patients with alcohol-use disorders are more likely to have post-operative complications related to bleeding and infection (Carr, 2011). An individual experiencing one or more of the chronic illnesses mentioned above will be likely to require several medications. Such medications may interact with alcohol, and a patient with alcohol-related memory impairments may have reduced capacity to remember to take correct numbers of medications at the right time of day, in the right dosage (Dorrian, 2010).

The physical, medical, risk, psychological and family/social implications of alcohol-use disorders are summarised, in alignment with the biopychosocial approach, in Table 4.

4. Risk factors for alcoholism

As with many other mental illnesses, family history is an important risk factor for alcohol-abuse disorders, with studies suggesting a heritability rate as high as 60% (Eve, 1989; Ginter & Simko, 2009). This raises classic nature versus nurture questions about whether it is the genes or the family environment that is responsible (Morrison, Bennett, Butow, Mullan, & White, 2008). Certainly, research has identified genetic factors which predispose an individual to developing alcohol-related issues (Ginter & Simko, 2009; Hansell et al., 2009). This is further supported by adoptee studies (Morrison et al., 2008).

The biopsychosocial spectrum of alcoholism-related consequences

bio--psycho------------------------social

Direct physical damage	Associated diseases	Risk	Cognitive/ Psychological	Family/Social
Brain	Cancers	Motor vehicle accident	Frontal lobe dysfunction (see Box 4)	Family deprivation
Gastrointestinal system (in particular, the liver)	Epilepsy	Falls	Unipolar depressive disorders	Unintentional injury
Cardiovascular system	Cardiovascular disorders (heart disease, stroke)	Drowning	Suicidal ideation	Interpersonal violence
Endocrine system	Gastrointestinal disease (cirrhosis of the liver)	Poisoning	Anxiety	Injury/fatality caused through drink-driving
Vitamin and nutrient absorption	Diabetes mellitus	Trauma	Korsakoff's Psychosis	Reduced job performance
Immune system	Wernicke's Encephalopathy	Burns	Confusion	Absenteeism
Dehydration	Infections		Hallucinations	Spread of STD
Blood thinning				Maternal and perinatal disorders
				Judgments from others

Summary from reviews: Anderson et al., 2009; Government of Australia, 2006; Room et al., 2005; Carr, 2011; Rehm et al., 2009; Schuckit, 2009

Table 4. Summary of negative physical consequences, associated disease and illness, risks, cognitive and psychological issues and family and social problems associated with alcohol-use disorders.

On the other hand, family and social learning experience are also predictors of alcohol consumption patterns later in life. Exposure to alcohol before 6 years approximately doubles the likelihood of reporting frequent, heavy or problem drinking during adolescence (Fergusson, Lynskey, & Horwood, 1994). Not only do parental drinking behaviours increase risk of developing problematic alcohol behaviours (Eve 1989), but also violence between parents, particularly violence initiated by the father (Fergusson & Horwood, 1998), and maltreatment and abuse as a child (Gilbert et al., 2009; Magnusson et al., 2011). Taken together, these studies suggest that permissive attitudes to alcohol in the home environment, as well as violence or trauma in the home, may increase the likelihood of later development of problem drinking behaviours (Fergusson, Boden, & Horwood, 2008).

A recent study suggests that early drinking behaviours may be more strongly determined by family environment, whereas, later in life, genetics may be more important (Kendler, Schmitt, Aggen, & Prescott, 2008). Other research suggests an interaction, where early exposure to alcohol may enable expression of genes related to vulnerability (Agrawal et al., 2009). Clearly, both genes and the environment are important.

Psychopathology has also been heavily implicated in alcohol-use disorders. Depression and alcohol-use disorders are frequently comorbid (Fowler, 2006). Indeed, in adolescents comorbidity between depression, suicide and alcohol abuse has been estimated to be as high as 73% (Ganz & Sher, 2009). Alcohol problems are also frequently comorbid with anxiety and post-traumatic stress disorders (Carr, 2011). Mood may provide a motive for drinking (Young-Wolff, Kendler, Sintov, & Prescott, 2009). Indeed, a self-medication hypothesis has been proposed, where individuals may be using alcohol to reduce anxiety, depression, or negative mood more generally (Ganz & Sher, 2009). This is supported by studies of negative mood and behaviour, including evidence for use of alcohol to reduce nervousness (Swendsen et al., 2000), depression in adolescents (Deykin, Levy, & Wells, 1986), psychological distress as a result of sexual assault (Miranda, Meyerson, Long, Marx, & Simpson, 2002), and anxiety in individuals with social phobia (Carrigan & Randall, 2003). However, it is important to note that psychopathologies such as depression and anxiety can be symptoms of alcohol withdrawal or detoxification, and that such disorders may simply tend to have an earlier onset age, and therefore appear to be predisposing factors (Swendsen et al., 2000).

Not only has trauma early in life been identified as a risk factor for alcohol-related problems (Gilbert et al., 2009; Magnusson et al., 2011), alcohol-use disorders with an onset later in life may be triggered by an unpleasant or traumatic event in adulthood (Johnson, 2010; Sacks & Keks, 1998). Alcohol abuse has been associated with disaster, exposure to grotesque death, physical and sexual abuse in adulthood, and combat in military service (reviewed in Stewart, 1996). Increased volume and frequency of alcohol consumption has been linked to loss of a spouse in older men (Byrne, Raphael, & Arnold, 1999). Pilot work has also suggested that females who have recently lost spouses who themselves had alcohol issues, and who also had unresolved marital problems or were socially isolated, may be more likely to experience alcohol issues as a response to grieving (Adele, 1989).

Overall, there are many factors that may, at least partially, explain why individuals develop alcohol-use disorders.

5. Family and social effects

Traditional stereotypes of people with alcohol problems include scruffy, derelict, amoral, weak-willed individuals without friends or family (Carr, 2011; Catalbiano et al., 2008). However, while people in lower socioeconomic groups are at increased risk of alcohol-use disorders, large proportions of individuals with such problems are highly functioning professionals (Catalbiano et al., 2008). Further, British research indicates that higher education level is a risk factor for problem drinking and daily alcohol consumption (Huerta & Borgonovi, 2010). In addition, as discussed in Section 4, there is increasing evidence for multiple predisposing factors that may render individuals particularly vulnerable to alcohol-use disorders, such as genetics (Kendler, Myers, Dick, & Prescott, 2010), early exposure to patterns of drinking in the home (Fergusson et al., 1994; Kendler et al., 2008), and trauma (Sacks & Keks, 1998).

Despite this information, a recent review revealed persistent stigma associated with alcohol dependence. Compared with other mental illnesses that are not linked to substance abuse, individuals with alcohol dependence were more likely to trigger negative emotions and social rejection, and were also less likely to be perceived as having a mental illness. The level of danger attributed was equivalent to that associated with schizophrenia. The authors concluded that alcohol dependence was particularly stigmatised, that individuals were more likely to be blamed for their condition (Schomerus et al., 2011). Given the current context, with understanding of the biopsychosocial determinants of alcohol-use disorders, the question remains, why do stigma and negative stereotyping persist?

One possible explanation may lie in the fact that alcohol-use disorders often involve behaviour which puts others at risk. In a large scale Australian survey completed by more than 26,000 respondents, recent drinkers were asked whether they had done certain potentially harmful activities during the past year while drunk. Thirteen per cent reported that they had driven a vehicle, 6% reported engaging in verbal abuse, 5% reported going to work, 4% reported that they created a disturbance, damaged or stole goods, and 1% reported engaging in physical abuse. Overall, one in five recent drinkers reported engaging in at least one potentially harmful activity while intoxicated (AIHW, 2010). The same study revealed that, within the preceding year, one quarter of participants over the age of 14y had been verbally abused, 8% had been physically abused, and 14% had been put in fear by someone under the influence of alcohol (AIHW, 2010). In addition, there may be specific negative impacts on those caring for an individual with an alcohol-use disorder. A survey of 110 concerned family members and significant others (CSOs) of people with alcohol or other substance abuse reported one or more problems in emotional, family, relationship, financial, health or violence domains (Benishek, Kirby, & Dugosh, 2011).

Another potential reason for the continued negative feeling towards patients with alcohol-use disorders may be alcohol-induced impairment of social cognition. Indeed, in line with the frontal lobe impairment discussed earlier, research indicates that excessive alcohol use may result in difficulties with understanding the stress, rhythm and intonation of speech, problems understanding emotional content of facial expressions, theory of mind impairment and issues with humour processing (Uekermann & Daum, 2008). Further, consistent with other addiction-related disorders, alcohol-use disorders are frequently characterised by deceit, guilt and shame (reviewed in Shaffer et al., 2004). Coupled with emotional abnormalities, indifference, shallowness and apathy (Table 3), this can clearly have a negative impact on interpersonal communication, and ultimately result in damage to crucial support relationships.

6. Alcohol-use disorders, prevention and treatment

At a societal level, there is evidence that alcohol price increases and reductions in alcohol availability and advertising, as well as legally enforced drink-driving penalties may be beneficial in the prevention of alcohol-use disorders (Rehm et al., 2009; Room et al., 2005).

Prevention and treatment approaches at the individual level, and the importance of the relationship between individuals with alcohol-use disorders and healthcare professionals are discussed below.

6.1 Individual-level treatment approaches

Early moral perspectives on alcohol-use disorders considered alcohol-related behaviours to be under the control of the individual, and those with problem behaviour patterns were blamed and punished (Morrison et al., 2008). It is clear that such perspectives are out-dated and counterproductive. A goal in alcohol-use disorder treatment today is to maintain a non-judgemental attitude (Sacks & Keks, 1998), and to acknowledge the importance of the biology, experience and social environment of the individual (Morrison et al., 2008).

Comprehensive care necessitates support and management at intervention, in detoxification and withdrawal, during acute alcohol-related health threats, and throughout on-going follow-up care. This process should include education, individual and possibly group therapy, and special care to address comorbid psychopathologies (Carr, 2011). Family involvement and other sources of psychosocial support are also critical (Carr, 2011; Sacks & Keks, 1998). Medications such as acamprosate and naltrexone, which help to reduce dependence, may be included. However, these should not be employed in isolation. While they are aimed at addressing physical dependence issues, psychological dependence must also be treated (Garbutt, West, Carey, Lohr, & Crews, 1999; Graham, Wodak, & Whelan, 2002).

Central to the success of current treatment approaches is the patient's readiness and willingness to change, and their resulting level of engagement and compliance (Catalbiano et al., 2008; Holmwood, 2002; Sacks & Keks, 1998). Willingness predicts retention in treatment and positive change in substance use (Erickson, Stevens, McKnight, & Figueredo, 1995). Conversely, those who are less willing to change are less motivated and report lower treatment demand (Ekendahl, 2007). It is important to note that, due to the physiological effects of alcohol, especially the frontal lobe impairment (e.g. decrease in will and energy, problems with planning and problem solving, poor motivation and decision making, Table 3), it may be particularly difficult for patients, particularly those with advanced alcohol-use disorders, to make the decision to change, and to comply with treatment. Even indications of readiness to change may not be indicative of future treatment involvement (Yonas et al., 2005). Indeed, "*waiting for the addict to 'be ready' for treatment can be dangerous*" (Clay, 2008, p1).

Many treatments for alcohol-use disorders focus on abstinence. However, there has been a great debate in the literature as to whether individuals with alcohol-use disorders, following a period of abstinence can learn to modify their behaviour and engage in controlled drinking (Catalbiano et al., 2008). This approach has been argued to be most appropriate for young people, with fewer alcohol-related problems (McMurran, 1991), but may not be appropriate for individuals with longer-term chronic alcohol issues (Catalbiano et al., 2008). Nevertheless, it must be recognised that abstinence may not be a realistic goal for all individuals and that relapse is frequent (Graham et al., 2002; Sacks & Keks, 1998). This may be particularly important to acknowledge in situations where individuals have alcohol-related chronic illness, where medications may have reduced efficacy, or even become harmful, with high or fluctuating levels of alcohol in the bloodstream. In such cases, open acknowledgement that abstinence may not be observed, and non-judgemental discussion of alcohol consumption, may lead to safer and more efficacious pharmacological management of the concomitant chronic illness (Dorrian, 2010).

6.2 Interactions with healthcare professionals

Table 5 displays a quote, which summarises many of the current issues related to attitudes and training of healthcare professionals in treatment of individuals with alcohol-use disorders. Research suggests that positive, supportive, non-judgemental interactions with healthcare professionals are critical (Sacks & Keks, 1998). However, healthcare professionals may have negative attitudes to working with patients with alcohol-use disorders (Clay, Allen, & Parran, 2008; Durand, 1994), particularly professionals without specialist training in working with individuals with substance use problems (Albery et al., 1996). Among doctors, including General Practitioners, reported barriers include lack of training, inadequate expertise and time constraints (Durand, 1994; Geirsson, Bendtsen, & Spak, 2005), prejudice against individuals with alcohol-use disorders, and negative perceptions about the potential efficacy of treatment (Carr, 2011). To address some of these negative attitudes, it has been argued that understanding pharmacological as well as cognitive-behavioural treatments should facilitate practitioner optimism in treatment of people with alcohol-abuse issues, specifically, *"an understanding of the biological reality of addiction allows physicians to understand addicts as having a brain disease"* (Clay et al., 2008, p1).

Carr, 2011
"Historically, we have attributed addictive illness, including alcoholism, to wilful misconduct, character flaws, weak will, moral turpitude, or just bad people. Science does not support these outdated stereotypes. In 1956, the American Medical Association declared alcoholism an illness. Hampered by prejudice, misinformation, and an outdated sense of hopelessness at our supposed inability to effect meaningful intervention, the medical community has been slow to respond. Even today, most medical students and residents complete training without benefit of a rudimentary working knowledge of addictive illness; an illness they will see in their office almost daily for the rest of their careers."   *Carr, 2011, p9-10.*

Table 5. Quote from Carr, 2011 summarising issues in the medical community.

Nurses are at the coal-face of healthcare, and also have the potential to make a substantial contribution to alcohol-use disorder prevention, screening and treatment (George, 1988). While overall, recent studies find evidence for neutral or positive attitudes toward the care of patients with alcohol-use disorders, suggestions remain of negative, stereotyped attitudes towards these patients. For example, studies have demonstrated that nurses may be more likely to describe patients labelled as being 'alcoholics' as more unsocial, boring, uncooperative and unpleasant (Wallston et al., 1976). In a recent study of Australian nurses, 14% reported that they did not want to work with drinkers, and 13% did not feel that they would find working with drinkers rewarding. In this study, none of the participants reported receiving drug and alcohol training (Crothers & Dorrian, 2011). In contrast, in a study in a small community hospital with a specialised inpatient drug and alcohol program, nurses reported positive attitudes to working with drinkers (Allen, 1993). Indeed, similar to studies in doctors, nursing studies have consistently indicated gaps and opportunities for training in the identification, treatment and ongoing support of patients with alcohol-related issues (Anderson, Eadie, MacKintosh, & Haw, 2001; Owens, Gilmore, & Pirmohamed, 2000). Studies yield expressions of interest from nursing staff in working more in this area, and requests for more training (Anderson et al., 2001; Owens et al., 2000). This is clearly an important area for development, since education results in more positive attitudes to care (Allen, 1993; Geirsson et al., 2005).

Emergency department staff may also play a particularly critical role. A study of Scottish Accident and Emergency Departments found that one in seven admissions were related to alcohol consumption. However, 40% of departments did not routinely screen for alcohol problems, or keep related records (Anderson et al., 2001). In an Australian study of emergency department staff, including doctors and nurses, only 5% reported routinely screening for alcohol problems, 16% reported routinely directing short interventions, and 27% reported routinely referring for specialist treatment. A primary barrier identified by staff was motivational deficiency on the part of the patients. Again, this study highlighted a requirement for additional training (Indig, Copeland, Conigrave, & Rotenko, 2009). In another Australian study, interns failed to identify 84% of heavy drinkers who attended a casualty department, which was not in alignment with their perceptions of what was required in terms of quality healthcare. This further highlights shortcomings with training (Gordon, Fahey, & Sanson-Fisher, 1988).

Therefore, without further training and support (infrastructure, time, evidence-based techniques) for healthcare professionals, specific treatment of alcohol-use disorders may be inadequate or overlooked. There is evidence that treatment may be so focused on the acute, and potentially life-threatening, related health problems experienced by individuals with alcohol-use disorders, longer-term, consistent follow-up to treat the underlying alcohol-use issues themselves may not occur (Baird, Burge, & Grant, 1989; Dorrian, 2010). This can be conceptualised as a reactive treatment of symptoms as they arise, as opposed to addressing the cause.

A further barrier to working with patients with alcohol-use disorders is that they may not seek treatment. Only 13% of individuals with alcohol dependency will receive specific treatment for their addiction (Carr, 2011). Only one in four people with alcohol-use disorders will pursue treatment, and most will approach their General Practitioner (Schuckit, 2009). Patients may be worried about health care professionals maintaining confidentiality (Gordon, Ettaro, Rodriguez, Mocik, & Clark, 2011), or may be concerned about the treatment approaches (Durand, 1994). However, the difficulties that the patient must contend with relating to stereotyping and stigma from the general community as well as healthcare professionals should not be underrated. *"People living with dependency problems must strive for recovery (often relapsing along the way) within communities and families which often despise them and/or their condition"* (Williamson, 2009, p9). This stigma may represent a significant hurdle for treatment. Further, as discussed earlier, alcohol-related brain damage can harm individual ability to understand risk and to plan, commit and be motivated to change behaviour. This issue of impaired agency and a reduced capacity to "*choose health*" has been largely overlooked in treatment and public policy (Dorrian, 2010; Williamson, 2009a, 2009b).

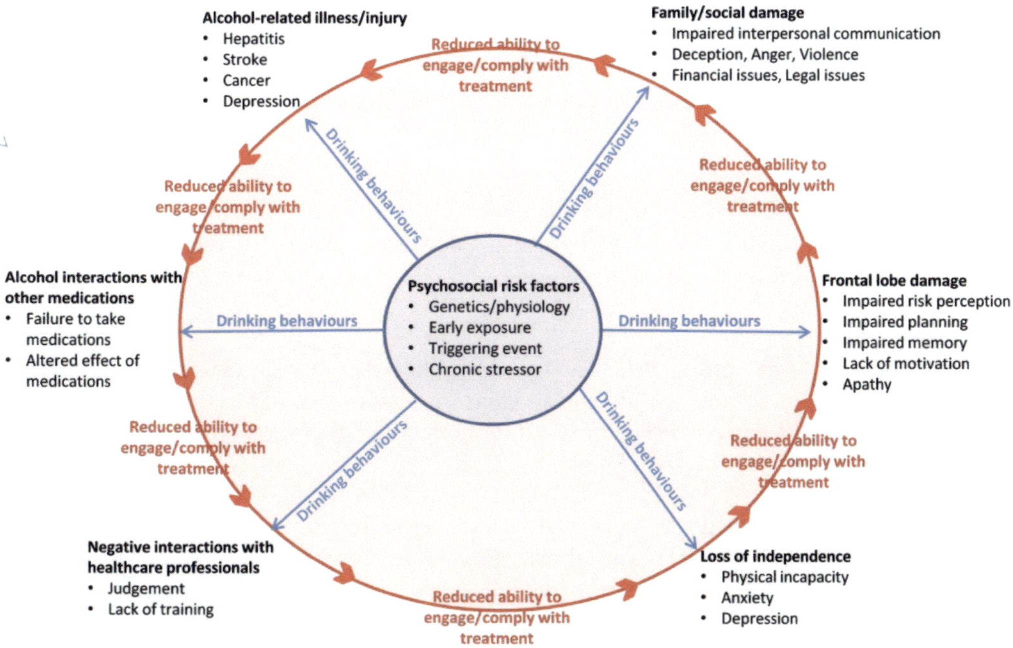

Fig. 2. Alcohol-use disorders as a self-reinforcing (positive) feedback loop.

7. Conclusions

Taken together, alcohol-use disorders can be seen as a self-perpetuating feedback loop, where all aspects of the disease serve to reduce the ability to engage and comply with treatment. This is illustrated in Figure 2, which displays psychosocial risk factors for developing alcohol-use disorders at the centre. Negative outcomes associated with alcohol-use disorders are displayed around the perimeter of the circle. Each outcome— frontal lobe damage, family/social damage, alcohol-related illness, alcohol interactions with other medications, negative interactions with healthcare professionals and loss of independence, all amplify the other effects of the disease, and make it increasingly difficult for the individual to move towards positive behaviour change. It is clear that holistic, biopsychosocial thinking is required to address problems with alcohol-use disorders. In particular, it must be acknowledged that the most seriously ill patients will have progressed further in this loop, and current treatment approaches and public policy which emphasise individual choice will likely be completely inadequate. Final recommendations resulting from the review are displayed in Table 6.

Recommendations
• The importance of support from friends, family and the wider community for those with alcohol-use disorders cannot be overstated. This support is required at times when these relationships are put under particular strain. Stigma and stereotypes of individuals with alcohol-use disorders must be addressed at a community level, and among healthcare professionals, as they are out-dated, unhelpful and present barriers for treatment
• Education for healthcare professionals in evidence-based identification, treatment and follow-up for individuals with alcohol-use disorders is absolutely required and desired by the professionals themselves
• This education must emphasise the importance of positive, supportive, non-judgemental interactions and provide a clear understanding of alcohol addiction as a relapsing brain disease, with recognised biological and social risk factors
• Education will also facilitate increased routine screening for patients particularly those who may be identifiable as 'at-risk' (e.g. older, bereaved individuals, those with frequent hospital admissions for burns, falls or common alcohol-related chronic illness)
• Public level policies and education may be demonstrably effective, as may current treatments with a central focus on readiness to change, but these may have limited influence for those with impaired cognitive capacity who may not be able to "*choose health*"
• We cannot overlook the most ill patients of alcohol-use disorders, and dedicated and innovative research and development of treatments and support systems for those who have reduced agency is crucial

Table 6. Summary recommendations

8. References

Adele, B. (1989). Grief, alcohol dependence and women. *Drug Alcohol Depend, 24*(1), 45-49.

Agrawal, A., Sartor, C. E., Lynskey, M. T., Grant, J. D., Pergadia, M. L., Grucza, R.,Bucholz, K. K., Nelson, E. C., Madden, P. A., Martin, N. G., & Heath, A. C.. (2009). Evidence for an interaction between age at first drink and genetic influences on DSM-IV alcohol dependence symptoms. *Alcohol Clin Exp Res, 33*(12), 2047-2056.

Australian Institute of Health and Welfare (AIHW). (2010). *2010 National Drug Strategy Household Survey report* (Cat. no. PHE 145). Canberra, Australia: Australian Institute of Health and Welfare.

Australian Institute of Health and Welfare (AIHW). (2011, 2011). *National Health Priority Areas*. Canberra, Australia: Australian Institute of Health and Welfare. Retrieved September 17, 2011, from http://www.aihw.gov.au/health-priority-areas/

Albery, I. P., Heuston, J., Durand, M. A., Groves, P., Gossop, M., & Strang, J. (1996). Training primary health care workers about drugs: a national survey of UK trainers' perceptions towards training. *Drug Alcohol Rev, 15*(4), 343-355.

Allen, K. (1993). Attitudes of registered nurses toward alcoholic patients in a general hospital population. *Int J Addict, 28*(9), 923-930.

Anderson, P., Chisholm, D., & Fuhr, D. C. (2009). Effectiveness and cost-effectiveness of policies and programmes to reduce the harm caused by alcohol. *Lancet, 373*(9682), 2234-2246.

Anderson, S., Eadie, D. R., MacKintosh, A. M., & Haw, S. (2001). Management of alcohol misuse in Scotland: the role of A&E nurses. *Accid Emerg Nurs, 9*(2), 92-100.

Baird, M. A., Burge, S. K., & Grant, W. D. (1989). A Scheme for Determining the Prevalence of Alcoholism in Hospitalized Patients. *Alcohol Clin Exp Res*, 13(6), 782-785.

Benishek, L. A., Kirby, K. C., & Dugosh, K. L. (2011). Prevalence and frequency of problems of concerned family members with a substance-using loved one. *Am J Drug Alcohol Abuse, 37*(2), 82-88.

Byrne, G. J. A., Raphael, B., & Arnold, E. (1999). Alcohol consumption and psychological distress in recently widowed older men *Aust NZ J Psychiat, 33*, 740-747.

Carr, G. D. (2011). Alcoholism: a modern look at an ancient illness. *Prim Care, 38*(1), 9-21.

Carrigan, M. H., & Randall, C. L. (2003). Self-medication in social phobia: A review of the alcohol literature. *Addict Behav, 28*(2), 269-284.

Casswell, S., & Thamarangsi, T. (2009). Reducing harm from alcohol: call to action. *Lancet, 373*(9682), 2247-2257.

Catalbiano, M. L., Sarafino, E. P., & Byrne, D. G. (2008). *Health Psychology: Biopsychosocial Interactions* (Second Australasian Edition ed.). Australia: John Wiley and Sons.

Clay, S. W., Allen, J., & Parran, T. (2008). A review of addiction. *Postgrad Med, 120*(2), E01-07.

Crothers, C., & Dorrian, J. (2011). Determinants Of Nurses' Attitudes Toward The Care Of Patients With Alcohol Problems. *International Scholarly Research Network (ISRN) Nursing, Article ID 821514*, 11 pages.

Deykin, E. Y., Levy, J. C., & Wells, V. (1986). Adolescent Depression, Alcohol and Drug Abuse. *Am J Public Health 76*, 178-182.

Dorrian, J. (2010). Alcoholism: disease or symptom? The challenges of managing advanced alcoholism and chronic illness. *Med J Aust, 192*(11), 661-662.

Durand, M. A. (1994). General practice involvement in the management of alcohol misuse: dynamics and resistances. *Drug Alcohol Depend, 35*(3), 181-189.

Ekendahl, M. (2007). Will and skill - an exploratory study of substance abusers' attitudes towards lifestyle change. *Eur Addict Res, 13*(3), 148-155.

Erickson, J. R., Stevens, S., McKnight, P., & Figueredo, A. J. (1995). Willingness for treatment as a predictor of retention and outcomes. *J Addict Dis, 14*(4), 135-150.

Eve, S. I. (1989). A psychotherapeutic approach to treatment of a population at high risk for alcoholism: adult children of alcoholics. *Med Law, 8*(4), 357-363.
Fergusson, D. M., Boden, J. M., & Horwood, L. J. (2008). The developmental antecedents of illicit drug use: evidence from a 25-year longitudinal study. *Drug Alcohol Depend, 96*(1-2), 165-177.
Fergusson, D. M., & Horwood, L. J. (1998). Exposure to interparental violence in childhood and psychosocial adjustment in young adulthood. *Child Abuse Negl, 22*(5), 339-357.
Fergusson, D. M., Lynskey, M. T., & Horwood, L. J. (1994). Childhood exposure to alcohol and adolescent drinking patterns. *Addiction, 89*(8), 1007-1016.
Fowler, T. L. (2006). Alcohol dependence and depression: advance practice nurse interventions. *J Am Acad Nurse Pract, 18*(7), 303-308.
Ganz, D., & Sher, L. (2009). Suicidal behavior in adolescents with comorbid depression and alcohol abuse. *Minerva Pediatr, 61*(3), 333-347.
Garbutt, J. C., West, S. L., Carey, T. S., Lohr, K. N., & Crews, F. T. (1999). Pharmacological Treatment of Alcohol Dependence. *JAMA - J Am Med Assoc, 281*(14), 1318-1325.
Geirsson, M., Bendtsen, P., & Spak, F. (2005). Attitudes of Swedish general practitioners and nurses to working with lifestyle change, with special reference to alcohol consumption. *Alcohol Alcohol, 40*(5), 388-393.
George, V. D. (1988). Nurses' attitude toward alcohol abuse and alcoholism. *J Natl Black Nurses Assoc, 3*(1), 12-22.
Gilbert, R., Widom, C. S., Browne, K., Fergusson, D., Webb, E., & Janson, S. (2009). Burden and consequences of child maltreatment in high-income countries. *Lancet, 373*(9657), 68-81.
Ginter, E., & Simko, V. (2009). Alcoholism: recent advances in epidemiology, biochemistry and genetics. *Bratisl Lek Listy, 110*(5), 307-311.
Gordon, A. J., Ettaro, L., Rodriguez, K. L., Mocik, J., & Clark, D. B. (2011). Provider, patient, and family perspectives of adolescent alcohol use and treatment in rural settings. *J Rural Health, 27*(1), 81-90.
Gordon, J. J., Fahey, P., & Sanson-Fisher, R. W. (1988). Interns' identification of patients' health risks in a casualty department. *Med J Aust, 148*(12), 615-619.
Graham, R., Wodak, A. D., & Whelan, G. (2002). New pharmacotherapies for alcohol dependence. *Med J Aust, 177*(2), 103-107.
Hansell, N. K., Agrawal, A., Whitfield, J. B., Morley, K. I., Gordon, S. D., Lind, P. A., Pergadia, M. L., Montgomery, G. W., Madden, P. A., Todd, R. D., Heath, A. C., & Martin, N. G. (2009). Can we identify genes for alcohol consumption in samples ascertained for heterogeneous purposes? *Alcohol Clin Exp Res, 33*(4), 729-739.
Holmwood, C. (2002). Alcohol-related problems in Australia: is there a role for general practice? *Med J Aust, 177*(2), 102-103.
Huerta, M. C., & Borgonovi, F. (2010). Education, alcohol use and abuse among young adults in Britain. *Soc Sci Med, 71*(1), 143-151.
Indig, D., Copeland, J., Conigrave, K. M., & Rotenko, I. (2009). Attitudes and beliefs of emergency department staff regarding alcohol-related presentations. *Int Emerg Nurs, 17*(1), 23-30.
Johnson, B. A. (2010). Medication treatment of different types of alcoholism. *Am J Psychiatry, 167*(6), 630-639.

Kendler, K. S., Myers, J., Dick, D., & Prescott, C. A. (2010). The relationship between genetic influences on alcohol dependence and on patterns of alcohol consumption. *Alcohol Clin Exp Res, 34*(6), 1058-1065.

Kendler, K. S., Schmitt, E., Aggen, S. H., & Prescott, C. A. (2008). Genetic and environmental influences on alcohol, caffeine, cannabis, and nicotine use from early adolescence to middle adulthood. *Arch Gen Psychiatry, 65*(6), 674-682.

Kopelman, M. D. (2008). Alcohol and frontal lobe impairment: fascinating findings. *Addiction, 103*(5), 736-737.

Lee, H., Roh, S., & Kim, D. J. (2009). Alcohol-induced blackout. *Int J Environ Res Public Health, 6*(11), 2783-2792.

Loeber, S., Duka, T., Welzel Marquez, H., Nakovics, H., Heinz, A., Mann, K., et al. (2010). Effects of repeated withdrawal from alcohol on recovery of cognitive impairment under abstinence and rate of relapse. *Alcohol Alcohol, 45*(6), 541-547.

Magnusson, A., Lundholm, C., Goransson, M., Copeland, W., Heilig, M., & Pedersen, N. L. (2011). Familial influence and childhood trauma in female alcoholism. *Psychol Med,* 1-9.

McMurran, M. (1991). Young offenders and alcohol-related crime: what interventions will address the issues? *J Adolesc, 14*(3), 245-253.

Miranda, R., Meyerson, L., Long, P., Marx, B., & Simpson, S. (2002). Sexual Assault and Alcohol Use: Exploring the Self-Medication Hypothesis. *Violence Victims, 17*(2), 205-217.

Morrison, V., Bennett, P., Butow, P., Mullan, B., & White, K. (2008). *Introduction to Health Psychology in Australia.* NSW, Australia: Pearson Education.

Moselhy, H. F., Georgiou, G., & Kahn, A. (2001). Frontal lobe changes in alcoholism: a review of the literature. *Alcohol Alcohol, 36*(5), 357-368.

National Alcohol Strategy (NAS). (2006). *National alcohol strategy 2006-2009.* Ministerial Council on Drug Strategy, Commonwealth of Australia.

Owens, L., Gilmore, I. T., & Pirmohamed, M. (2000). General practice nurses' knowledge of alcohol use and misuse: a questionnaire survey. *Alcohol Alcohol, 35*(3), 259-262.

Rehm, J., Mathers, C., Popova, S., Thavorncharoensap, M., Teerawattananon, Y., & Patra, J. (2009). Global burden of disease and injury and economic cost attributable to alcohol use and alcohol-use disorders. *Lancet, 373*(9682), 2223-2233.

Room, R., Babor, T., & Rehm, J. (2005). Alcohol and public health. *Lancet 365*, 519-530.

Sacks, T. L., & Keks, N. A. (1998). Alcohol and drug dependence: diagnosis and management. *Med J Aust, 168*(7), 355-360.

Schomerus, G., Lucht, M., Holzinger, A., Matschinger, H., Carta, M. G., & Angermeyer, M. C. (2011). The Stigma of Alcohol Dependence Compared with Other Mental Disorders: A Review of Population Studies. *Alcohol Alcohol, Vol. 46*(2), 105-112.

Schuckit, M. A. (2009). Alcohol-use disorders. *Lancet, 373*(9662), 492-501.

Shaffer, H. J., LaPlante, D. A., LaBrie, R. A., Kidman, R. C., Donato, A. N., & Stanton, M. V. (2004). Toward a Syndrome Model of Addiction: Multiple Expressions, Common Etiology. *Harv Rev Psychiatry 12*, 367–374.

Stewart, S. H. (1996). Alcohol Abuse in Individuals Exposed to Trauma: A Critical Review. *Psychol Bull 120*(1), 83-112.

Swendsen, J. D., Tennen, T., Carney, M. A., Affleck, G., Willard, A., & Hromi, A. (2000). Mood and Alcohol Consumption: An Experience Sampling Test of the Self-Medication Hypothesis. *J Abnorm Psychol, 109*(2), 198-204.

Thavorncharoensap, M., Teerawattananon, Y., Yothasamut, J., Lertpitakpong, C., & Chaikledkaew, U. (2009). The economic impact of alcohol consumption: a systematic review. *Subst Abuse Treat Prev Policy, 4*, 20-31.

Uekermann, J., & Daum, I. (2008). Social cognition in alcoholism: a link to prefrontal cortex dysfunction? *Addiction, 103*(5), 726-735.

White, A. M. (2003). What happened? Alcohol, memory blackouts, and the brain. *Alcohol Res Health, 27*(2), 186-196.

World Health Organisation (WHO). (2011). *Global Status Report on Alcohol and Health 2011* (ISBN 978 92 4 156415 1). Geneva, Switzerland.

Williamson, L. (2009a). Alcohol dependence in public policy: towards its (re)inclusion. *Clin Ethics* 4, 74-78.

Williamson, L. (2009b). Public policy on alcohol in the United Kingdom: Towards a safety net for the alcohol-dependent. *J Law Med, 17*(3), 386-399.

Yonas, M., Baker, D., Cornwell, E. E., 3rd, Chang, D., Phillips, J., Paradise, J., Sutton, E., & Elihu, A. (2005). Readiness to change and the role of inpatient counseling for alcohol/substance abusing youth with major trauma. *J Trauma, 59*(2), 466-469.

Young-Wolff, K. C., Kendler, K. S., Sintov, N. D., & Prescott, C. A. (2009). Mood-related drinking motives mediate the familial association between major depression and alcohol dependence. *Alcohol Clin Exp Res, 33*(8), 1476-1486.

2

Alcoholism: An Impulsive/Disinhibition Disorder?

Xavier Noël
Belgium Fund for Scientific Research (F.R.S./FNRS)
Psychological Medicine Laboratory
Université Libre de Bruxelles
Belgium

1. Introduction

In a broad sense, response inhibition represents as a useful concept to investigate impulsivity, a term referring to "behavior that is performed with little or inadequate forethought" (Evenden, 1999). Impulsivity has been studied for many decades as a trait variable of human personality that is stable within an individual and varies normatively across the healthy population (Barratt, 1995). Following the development of neuropsychology and cognitive neuroscience, impulsivity is often replaced with "disinhibition", a term referring to the idea that top-down control mechanisms ordinarily suppress automatic or reward-driven responses that are not appropriate to the current demands (Aron, 2007).

Such a definition gives weight to the idea that alcoholism and other addictive behaviors might be the consequence of increased impulsivity, that is to say, when top-down mechanisms necessary to suppress actions, emotions and thoughts related to alcohol use are disrupted (e.g., Verdejo-Garcia et al., 2008; de Wit, 2008; Jentsch & Taylor, 1999). Throughout the present chapter, I discuss the relevance of impulsivity/disinhibition concept in order to investigate both risk factors to become alcoholics (as a trait) and acquired component of the development of alcoholism (as a state). Numerous reasons may lead to use alcohol recreationally including peer influence, personality characteristics, alcohol availability, which together tell something about how much of alcohol will be consumed. But once dependent, alcoholics persist in alcohol-taking despite awareness that their alcohol use is directly harmful to their health, their finances and their interpersonal relationships (American Psychiatric Association, 2000). Frequent unsuccessful attempts to quit drinking are a classic and this relapse phenomenon could also have something to do with deficient inhibitory control over a response that provides immediate positive consequences.

From the information-processing perspective, cognitive factors are seen as mediators involved in the development of alcoholism (e.g., Finn, 2002; Tiffany, 1990) as well as relapse (e.g., Noël et al., 2002; Bowden-Jones et al., 2005). An emerging view considers impairment of response inhibition as contributing significantly to the development of alcoholism (e.g., Lyvers, 2000) and to a variety of cognitive impairments (e.g., planning, mental flexibility) (e.g., Noël et al., 2001). The concept of response inhibition refers to the ability to suppress responses (i.e. action, thoughts, emotions) that are inappropriate, unsafe, or no longer required, which supports flexible and goal-directed behavior in ever-changing environments (e.g., Miyake et al., 2000; Stuphorn & Schall, 2006). In everyday life, there are many examples of the importance of response inhibition, such as stopping yourself from crossing a street when a car comes around the corner without noticing you. This idea has been documented by poor performance on a variety of cognitive tasks assessing dominant response inhibition in abstinent alcoholics (e.g., Noël et al., 2001) and in children of alcoholics (e.g., Habeych et al., 2006) as well as by abnormal brain electrophysiology (e.g., Kamarajan et al., 2006) and brain metabolism (e.g., Scheinsburg et al., 2004) while performing response inhibition tasks. In addition, poor response inhibition has been demonstrated to be a predictor of problem drinking in adolescents at risk for alcoholism (e.g., Nigg et al., 2006) and maintenance of abstinence after alcohol detoxification treatment (Noël et al., 2002).

Inhibition plays a central role in theorizing about human cognition and is often regarded as a key component of executive control (e.g., Miyake et al., 2000; Nigg, 2000;Baddeley, 1996). However, inhibition may represent a family of functions rather than a single, unitary construct (Friedman & Miyake, 2004; Nigg, 2000). Indeed, according to Friedman & Miyake (2004), a distinction should be made between the inhibition of a prepotent response that implies to deliberately suppress dominant/automatic responses and the resistance to proactive interference defined as the capacity to resist to memory intrusion of information no longer relevant. In the same vein, Nigg (2000) has suggested that response inhibition may range between intentional/effortful and unintentional/automatic response inhibition. In other terms, intentional/effortful inhibition would occur on mental representations loaded in working memory whereas unintentional/automatic would prevent the intrusion of mental representations irrelevant with the current situation. In addition, within effortful inhibition, a distinction has been made between the suppression of prepotent/automatic response and the suppression of no longer relevant information loaded in working memory. In addition, choice impulsivity, as reflected by rapid temporal discounting may represent a separate impulsivity component (e.g., Verdejo-Garcia et al., 2008; de Wit, 2008).

A very important question raised by research on impulsivity/disinhibition concerns the source of these deficiencies observed in these individuals in trouble with their alcohol use. One possibility is that the repeated use of alcohol may cause a gradual attrition of behavioral self-control, plausibly mediated by structural changes in the prefrontal cortex (e.g., Bechara 2003; Goldstein & Volkow, 2002). An alternative explanation is that deficient inhibitory control may be present prior to alcohol initiation, thus acting as a predisposing factor. This vulnerability pathway has been increasingly recognized by neuroscientific models. Indeed, adolescents' brain is relatively immature on these systems responsible for reward processing, motivation and regulation of these responses (e.g., inhibition). The reasons of these individual differences in term of brain maturation are beyond the scope of this paper, but the developmental pathway of brain maturation and its failures are fascinating topics. For instance, by using a cocaine self-administration procedure, Belin and colleagues (2008) found that, in rodents, high impulsivity predicts the switch to compulsive cocaine-taking. It is likely that vulnerability and attrition ways are not mutually exclusive; poor inhibitory control prior to the onset alcohol use may lead to increase the risk to become an addict, the excessive use of alcohol (e.g., repeated binge drinking episodes) may in turn accentuate this premorbid inhibition weakness. It is also possible that deleterious effects of alcohol are more pronounced in these individuals with poor inhibitory control.

2. Alcoholism: An impulsive/disinhibition disorder?

2.1 Impulsivity measured by self-report questionnaires

Cognitive-motivational theory of personality vulnerability to alcoholism describes impulsivity/novelty seeking and sensation/excitement seeking as fundamental personality dimensions that are distinguished in terms of the motivation, emotional, and cognitive processes that mediate or moderate vulnerability to alcohol use disorders (for a review, see Finn, 2002). For instance, a substantial body of research emphasised that exaggerated levels of novelty-seeking, which is highly correlated with impulsivity and aggressivity (e.g., Finn et al., 2002) and of excitement-seeking mediate alcohol use disorders (for reviews, see Mulder, 2002; Finn, 2002). In young alcoholics, high levels of disinhibited and appetitive personality traits, such as impulsivity, boredom susceptibility, thrill and adventure seeking, excitement-seeking (Finn et al., 2002; von Knorring et al., 1985); novelty-seeking (Finn et al., 2002); and aggressiveness (Babor et al., 1992; von Knorring et al., 1987) were reported. High impulsivity sub-scale of novelty seeking, which reflects poor control of appetitive and aggressive impulses, difficulties delaying gratification, acting without thinking and increased activity and assessed at 3 years of age predict the development of alcohol abuse in early adulthood (Kirisci et al., 2007).

Sensation seeking, as defined as a strong need for varied, novel, and stimulation experiences, and willingness to take risks for the sake of such experiences (Zuckerman, 1979), is another of the personality traits associated with high levels of alcohol and drug use (Andrucci et al., 1989).

Although useful, the questionnaire-based methodology introduces a number of caveats in the context of alcoholic population. The most meaningful may be that impulsivity itself could directly interfere with the completion of the questionnaires themselves, such that an impulsive subject may give less consideration to responses than a non-impulsive subject, the former having possibly less insight capacities than the latter. In addition, self-report questionnaires are susceptible to be highly dependent to social desirability that may naturally differ between alcoholic inpatients and healthy participants.

For all these reasons, direct measurement of inhibitory control processes using laboratory tasks has considerably developed over the past decade.

2.2 Impulsivity measured by laboratory tasks

2.2.1 Chronic effects of alcohol on response inhibition

One of first elements of impulsivity is acting without thinking, which may be operationalized as poor behavior inhibition in a variety of rapid stimulus-discrimination tasks. In this category of tasks, participants are required to respond to target stimuli and not to non-target ones. For instance, on a tasks consisting to click a button when presented whit a five-digit number he or she thought was identical to the preceding number, alcohol-dependent patients made more commission errors, thus indicating that these participants are more impulsive than controls (Bjork et al., 2004). In line with this idea, patients also had faster response times to target, which were inversely correlated with error rates across all subjects, which seemed to point to a 'fast-guess' mechanism of impulsive response. On a go/no-go task for which participants had to respond to a target by pressing a button as quickly as possible (go trials) and withholding their response when a non-target displayed (no-go trials), authors found that (1) the statistical difference between the No-Go and Go conditions was more robust in controls than in alcoholics; (2) relatively less anteriorization of current source density polarity in alcoholics during No-go processing indicating an impaired/decreased frontal lobe contribution. Interestingly, in comparison with patients with late onset of problem drinking and no problem-drinking parent, those alcoholics with earlier age of problem drinking and who reported a problem-drinking father (type 2-like alcohol dependence according to Cloningers' typology) demonstrated faster response latencies and more responses to non-target stimuli in the prepotent motor-response task. Regarding the relationship between these impulsivity measures and clinical indices of alcoholism, the age of onset of alcohol use/heavy drinking and measures of alcohol severity (for a review of the question, see Verdejo-Garia et al., 2008).

A deficit of inhibitory control has been identified consistently as a feature of dependence to alcohol. For instance, in a previous study (Noël et al., 2001), the re-examination of the 'frontal lobe vulnerability' hypothesis of alcoholism with tasks designed to assess separately non-executive and specific executive operations (which proved to be sensitive to frontal dysfunction) highlighted impaired intentional inhibition in recently detoxified alcoholics. The theoretical framework on which this study was based is the control to action model developed by Norman and Shallice (2000) in which two control to action mechanisms are distinguished. The first, contention scheduling, is involved in routine situations in which actions are triggered automatically. The second, the Supervisory Attentional System, (SAS) is needed in situations where the routine selection of action is unsatisfactory, and they conceived it as carrying out a variety of processes allowing the genesis of plans and willed actions. Reflecting this two control to action processes model, the Hayling task assesses the capacity to both activate a habitual response and to suppress (inhibit) this response (Burgess & Shallice, 1996). The test consisted of two sections (A and B) of 15 sentences each read aloud by the experimenter, in which the last word was missing. In section A (initiation/automatic) subjects were asked to give the word that made sense, which contrasts to the section B (inhibition), in which participants were asked to give a word that made no sense at all in the context of the sentence. On this task, non-amnesic alcoholics were as fast and accurate as their controls to produce the expected words but slower and less accurate when the expected word was to be suppressed. As suggested by a PET study (Collette et al., 2001), bilateral median frontal activation occurs during section B of the Hayling test, thus suggesting that alcoholics' inhibition deficits might be due to frontal lobe abnormalities.

Other results of this study were consistent with the existence of an inhibition deficit. In the Trail-Making test, alcoholics were slower than controls on the section B but not on the section A. Similarly, they showed poor performance in the alternate fluency task. Finally, patients spent more time to complete the flexibility condition of the Stroop test. The trail B requires inhibiting current realization strategy (1, 2, 3...) to switch between numbers and letters (1A, 2B, 3C...). Performance in the alternate fluency task requires, notably, that subjects inhibit one search strategy to switch to another. In the Stroop test, the flexibility condition requires the subject to switch between two rules alternatively, that is to inhibit the current rule.

On go/no-go paradigms, alcoholics made more commission errors, thus indicating that they are less efficient suppressing the most common motor action to press key in presence of a target (Bjork et al., 2004; Kamarajan et al., 2005). On the stop signal task, Goudriaan and colleagues (2006) found increased stop signal reaction time in alcoholic patients, which indicates weaker inhibition efficiency.

In contrast to the inhibition of prepotent response for which responses to be inhibited are strongly automatic, the suppression of no longer relevant mental contents (cognitive inhibition) is appropriately assessed by the directed-forgetting procedure. In this procedure (Andrés et al., 2004), memory performance of letter trigrams in three conditions is compared: presented alone (*single-item* condition); followed by a second trigram to be recalled (*double-item* condition); followed by a second trigram to be forgotten (*directed-forgetting* condition). In addition, participants are instructed to perform a distracter task, thus requiring simultaneous maintenance and processing of information. Therefore, low performance in directed-forgetting would reflect impaired ability to inhibit a mental content held in working memory. In alcoholism, this type of inhibition could be of great importance; difficulty suppressing repetitive thoughts about drinking and drinking expectations might represent the core of a craving episode for alcohol (May et al., 2004). In a recent article (Noël et al., 2009), we examined 3-4 weeks abstinent alcoholic's ability to inhibit irrelevant information in working memory by the mean of a directed-forgetting procedure. Results showed that despite similar performances between groups in the *double-item* (interference) condition of the task, alcoholic participants did not improved their performance in the *directed-forgetting* condition relatively to the *double-item* condition, whereas control participants did. In addition, we also highlighted that alcoholics were more sensitive to intrusion errors in the *directed-forgetting* condition. Finally, we found that the inhibition score (measured by the difference in recall performance between the single-trigram and directed-forgetting conditions) was positively correlated with the duration of alcoholism.

These findings are interesting because they complete previous works showing prepotent response inhibition (e.g., Noël et al., 2001; Gaudriaan et al., 2005). Indeed, abstinent alcoholics exhibited poor performance on a variety of dominant response inhibition tasks (e.g., Stop Signal task, Goudriaan et al., 2006; Hayling task, Noël et al., 2001). As shown by Friedman and Miyake (2004) in the first study attempting to empirically evaluate proposed taxonomy of inhibition-related functions, inhibition of dominant response and inhibition of proactive interference may be considered as distinct processes. Therefore, alcoholism would be associated with deficit on those two types of inhibition. However, each of inhibition deficits could be involved in separate aspects of the development and the maintenance of alcoholism. For instance, in Obsessive Compulsive Disorder (OCD), compulsions symptoms may be related with failures in behavioral inhibitory processes leading to repetitive stereotyped behaviours (*e.g.*, ritualistic checking behaviour) whereas obsessions may be related with failures in cognitive inhibitory processes resulting in frequent intrusive thoughts and ideas entering into consciousness (*e.g.*, mental rituals) (Chamberlain et al., 2005). In the same vein, we hypothesized that prepotent response inhibition could prevent alcoholics in resisting to automatically triggered alcohol-related behaviours (i.e., to take a drink) (e.g., Goldstein & Volkow, 2002; Whiteside & Lynam, 2003) whereas inhibition of proactive interference deficit observed on the directed-forgetting procedure in our experiment may lead to enhance occurrence of irrelevant and/or intrusive alcohol-related thoughts. In turn, when alcohol-related representation break through into awareness (being loaded into working memory) and experienced as a craving episode for alcohol (e.g., May et al., 2004), alcoholics would also be in trouble to suppress them and resist drinking because of an impairment to inhibit dominant response. It is obvious that this model remains largely speculative and that further investigations are needed to investigate the relationship between clinical phenomena characterizing alcoholism and different types of cognitive inhibition.

In a recent research (Noël et al., unpublished data), we aimed to reexamine the disinhibitory hypothesis of alcoholism in light of the model proposed by Friedman and Miyake (2004) and this in using several response inhibition tasks tapping into both the automatic suppression of proactive interference and the intentional inhibition of dominant response. One proactive interference inhibition task was Brown-Peterson variant in which participants had to learn four lists of eight words each. The first three lists were taken from the same semantic category, thus generating proactive interference to-be-inhibited for better performance. As an example of intentional prepotent response inhibition task, the antisaccade task (adapter from Roberts et al., 1994) assesses the capacity to minimize the reflexive response (proactive saccade) of looking at the initial cue. Our main finding was that, compared to non-alcoholics, patients had poor performance on cognitive tasks requiring the inhibition of prepotent response. In contrast, alcoholics performed normally on tasks exploring the resistance (inhibition) to proactive interference. The second major finding was that we found a relationship between inhibition of dominant response and alcoholics' greater tendency to act impulsively in particular when facing with their negative feelings.

An intriguing and important question remaining to be clarified if the relationship between enhanced attention for alcohol cues (cognitive bias) and impaired prepotent response inhibition (cognitive deficit). Studies having used the alcohol Stroop task did not report difference between light and heavy drinkers (Sharma et al., 2001) and between alcoholics and healthy participants (Lusher et al., 2004) in terms of the number of errors made when words are related to alcohol. One reason for the absence of cognitive disinhibition in the alcohol Stroop task is that both problematic users of alcohol and healthy participants made very few errors, thus reflecting a ceiling effect. Another limitation of the Stroop task is the questionable nature of inhibitory; whereas the Stroop task has generally been considered as examining resistance to interference (Nigg, 2000), it might also be viewed as taxing mechanisms of inhibitory control, i.e., the suppression of pre-potent responses (i.e., to read the alcohol related words rather than the color). In order to overcome these limitations, we designed an alcohol version of a go/no-go paradigm (the Alcohol Shifting task), which examines distinctly motor response inhibition, shifting of attention and the influence of alcohol-related stimuli's processing on these functions (Noël et al., 2005). We hypothesized that alcoholic subjects exhibit impairments in tasks requiring inhibitory control, as well as shifting. The aim was to test the ability of alcoholics to discriminate between alcohol-related and neutral words. Sometimes, the alcohol-related words were the targets for the "go" response, with neutral words as distracters, sometimes the reverse. Several shifts in the type of the target occurred during the task. More precisely, in our go/ no-go task, words are briefly displayed, one by one, in the center of the screen. Half of the words are targets and half are distracters. Subjects are instructed to respond to targets by pressing the space bar as quickly as possible, but not respond to distracters. Words are presented for 500ms, with an inter-stimulus interval of 900 ms. A 500 ms/450 Hz tone sounds for each false alarm (i.e., a response to a distracter), but not for omissions (i.e., failures to respond to a target). The task comprises two practice blocks followed by eight test blocks of 18 stimuli each composed of nine 'neutral' (N) and nine 'alcohol related' words (A). In each block, either neutral or alcohol related words are specified as targets, with targets for the 10 blocks presented either in the order NNAANNAANN or AANNAANNAA. Due to this arrangement, four test blocks are 'non-shift' blocks, where subjects must continue responding to stimuli in the same way. Four test blocks, however, are 'shift' blocks, where subjects must begin responding to stimuli, which had been distracters, and cease responding to stimuli, which had been targets. These results demonstrate that alcoholics exhibit a basic prepotent response inhibition deficit accentuated when the response to be suppressed is related to alcohol (Noël et al., 2007). Increased impulsivity by alcohol cues observed at the end of a detoxification treatment in ALC might have some clinical implications. Indeed, alcohol-drinking practice in individuals suffering from alcoholism can be viewed as encompassing stimulus-driven automatic behaviors (e.g., Tiffany, 1990). Besides, the intensity of the alcohol-related response may be stronger because of the behavioral sensitization phenomenon described by Robinson and Berridge (2003). In these circumstances, moderating or stopping alcohol drinking might require the inhibition of a prepotent response. The present findings show that the response inhibition deficit seen in ALC is more pronounced when a response associated with alcohol-related stimuli is to be suppressed. Thus, psychopharmacological and psychological strategies consisting to improve the prepotent response inhibition capacities would be fruitful for attenuating the severity of alcoholism and to prevent alcohol relapse.

2.2.2 Sensitivity to delay discounting

On a delay discounting task, subjects are given choices between a small, sooner reward and a larger, delay reward. Traditionally, the outcomes of a series of such choices are used to estimate the present subjective value of a delayed reward as a function of delay time, yielding hyperbolic temporal discount curves (Mazur, 1987; Rachlin, 2000). On this task, the temporal discounting functions are significantly different between groups with alcoholics demonstrating steeper discounting curves (Mitchell et al., 2005). This tendency to discount delayed rewards was positively correlated with subjective reports of both alcohol addiction severity and impulsivity (as assessed by the Barratt Impulsivity Scale). Interestingly, in the same study, alcoholic patients did not differ on motor impulsivity, which means that their inabilities to delay gratification and to inhibit a prepotent response are dissociated. In a study comparing early-onset alcoholics (EOAs) and late-onset alcoholics (LOAs) on sensitivity to delay discounting task (Dom et al., 2006), EOAs had higher discount rates than both the non-substance-abusing subjects and the LOAs, with these two groups performing similarly. This differentiation between EOAs and LOAs in terms of impulsive decision making emphasized the heterogeneity of individuals with alcoholism on the one hand and the existence of distinct pathways leading to alcoholism on the other. Both research and treatment programs should take into account the existence and differences observed in the two alcoholism subtypes.

2.3 Acute effect of alcohol on cognitive inhibitory processes

It is now widely accepted that variable doses of alcohol can affect reaction times (RTs) (Holloway, 1995). Indeed, 80% of the 23 RT studies observed impaired (slowed) RT at different blood alcohol concentrations (BACs). Actually, results may depend considerably on the complexity level of the tasks used, which raises the question as to whether specific cognitive mechanisms are impaired by moderate doses of alcohol. There is a huge difference in terms of the interference of small doses of alcohol on RT between such very simple tasks as pressing a key as quickly as possible when a cross displays on the centre of a computer screen and more complex tasks, such as pressing the same key only when a target symbol appears among distractors, which requires the participants to withhold the response (Holloway, 1995). When compared according to task complexity, RTs on complex tasks are impaired at lower BACs than RTs on simple tasks (Mitchell, 1985). Since the motor execution is similar for both tasks, pre-motor RTs (i.e., cognitive processes) are likely to be more affected by acute affects of alcohol than are the motor functions. Recent findings have in fact supported this idea. Indeed, one study examined directly the possibility that moderate BACs may impair cognitive processes before disturbing motor functions (Hernandez et al., 2006). To do so, RT to the presentation of a stimulus or to the omission of a regularly occurring visual, auditory, or tactile stimulus was fractionated into independent premotor (cognitive) and motor (movement) components. The main finding was that rising BACs slowed premotor RT and had no detectable effect on motor reaction time, thus indicating that moderate doses of alcohol affect cognitive processing more than motor execution (Hernandez et al., 2006).

Alcohol is known for its acute "disinhibiting" effects on behaviour, which may be the consequence of impaired basic cognitive inhibitory mechanisms that normally serve to suppress inappropriate behaviour (Fillmore, 2003). It has been shown to induce perseveration in an attentional set-shifting task, namely the Wisconsin Card Sorting task, and to disrupt inhibition of prepotent behaviour in "Stop-Signal" tasks (Mulvihill et al., 1997). For instance, the cued Go/No-Go reaction time task models behavioural control as the ability to activate a response to a Go-signal quickly and suddenly inhibits a response when a stop-signal occurs (Logan & Cowan, 1984; *Logan, 1994*). On these types of tasks, alcohol produces dose-dependent impairment on both execution (Go response) and motor inhibition (No-Go response) (Marczinski, Abroms, Van Selst, & Fillmore, 2005). Accordingly, the "No-Go P3" event-related potential (ERP) has been identified as one of the markers for response inhibition (Smith et al., 2006). In alcoholic subjects, a decreased amplitude and a delayed latency of this P3 component to task-relevant target (Go) stimuli has been widely observed, particularly over parietal regions (e.g., Begleiter et al., 1984). Other studies (e.g., Kamarajan et al., 2005) have documented not only low amplitude P3b components to target stimuli, but also reduced frontally distributed P3 amplitudes to No-Go stimuli. These deficits observed in both Go and No-Go conditions suggest that both response activation and response inhibition are dysfunctional in alcoholic individuals. Furthermore, while normal controls manifest their largest P3b amplitudes in response to targets over parietal regions of the scalp, and their largest P3a amplitudes in response to rare non-targets over frontal regions, alcoholics manifest poor differentiation (i.e. similar low-amplitude P3s) between task conditions (Kamarajan et al., 2005). Assessing the amplitude and topographic features of ERPs and Current Source Density (CSD) in a Go/No-Go task, Kamarajan et al. (2005) also found less anteriorization of CSD polarity in alcoholics during the No-Go processing. The reduced No-Go P3 along with the less anteriorized CSD topography during the No-Go condition suggests poor inhibitory control in alcoholics, perhaps reflecting underlying central nervous system hyperexcitability (Begleiter & Porjesz, 1999).

Indeed, the inhibitory aspects of behavioural control are more vulnerable to the acute effects of alcohol than the activational aspects (e.g., Abroms, Fillmore, & Marczinski, 2003).

Research in cognition has shown that learned information can be retained and guides behaviour consciously or unconsciously (e.g., Norman & Shallice, 1986). Research investigating the respective influence of alcohol on controlled processes and automatic processes has shown that intentional processes are impaired by alcohol, whereas automatic processes are essentially unchanged (Holloway, 1995; Fillmore, 2007). The same distinction between intentional and automatic processes has been made for cognitive response inhibition (Friedman & Miyake, 2004). Intentional response inhibition is under the control of the individual, and operates at the level of awareness (e.g., trying not to press the spacebar in the presence of a distractor on a Go/No-Go task). By contrast, automatic response inhibition occurs below the consciousness threshold in a reflexive manner evoked for instance by the presence of previously learned but no longer relevant information (e.g., negative priming tasks).

Several studies have shown that cognitive response inhibition that depends on control/intention is more vulnerable to the impairing effects of alcohol than response inhibition dependent upon automatic processes (Fillmore & Vogel-Sprott, 2006; Fillmore, 2007; Abroms, Gottlob & Fillmore, 2006). For instance, Abroms et al., (2006) used a delayed ocular response task and a saccadic interference task, which are similar in their response requirements (the ability to execute a saccade to a target location) but different in the nature of the inhibitory mechanism implicated (intentional vs. automatic). Indeed, on the delayed ocular response task (Ross, Hommer, Breiger, Varley, & Radant, 1994), people were required to inhibit intentionally their tendency to make a reflexive saccade toward the sudden appearance of a visual stimulus on a computer screen. Indeed, while participants attended to the fixation point, a bright target stimulus was presented in the periphery, which normally causes a reflexive saccade, which the participant needs to inhibit while maintaining their gaze on the fixation point until it disappears. Automatic inhibition was assessed by the saccadic interference task (Reingold & Stampe, 2002), which measures the ability of a subject to execute a saccade in the presence of an irrelevant, interfering stimulus. The rationale for this task is that it takes longer to execute a saccade to targets on trials with a distractor compared with trials with no distractor, because the distractor interferes with the generation of the saccade by compromising its programming in the superior colliculus. Also, automatic inhibitory processes located in this region are reflexively executed to suppress this interference. Results indicated that moderate doses of alcohol (i.e., 0.45 g/kg of body mass, that is, around 3 regular beers for a participant weighing 70 kg) impaired the intentional but not the automatic inhibition (Abroms et al., 2006). Moreover, this impairment was quite pronounced; the number of controlled/intentional inhibition errors under the highest dose (0.65 g/kg) was nearly three times greater than in response to placebo.

The deleterious power of moderate doses of alcohol on response inhibition and increased impulsivity could be responsible for other cognitive impairments (Weissenborn & Duka, 2003). For instance, on a planning task, the Tower of London (Shallice, 1982), subjects are presented with two sets of three coloured 'balls', one in the top half of the screen and one in the bottom. They are instructed to move the balls in the bottom array so that they match the pattern in the top array, which requires making and executing plans. On this task, alcohol decreased the thinking time prior to initiating a solution, which may reflect greater impulsivity (Weissenborn & Duka, 2003). But alcohol also impacted planning not only by decreasing the number of correct trials to solve the Tower of London task, but also by increasing the time spent thinking about moves once a solution had been initiated. It is reasonable to assume that, in the absence of alcohol-impaired spatial working memory, acute doses of alcohol dramatically disrupt planning capacities notably by decreasing intentional/controlled response inhibition.

The relationship between acute effects of alcohol and disinhibition is likely to be moderated by numerous cognitive and affective factors (Finn et al., 1999; Ernst et al., 2006; Dom et al., 2006; Hittner & Swickert, 2006). For instance, executive functions other than inhibition-related ones could impact the relationship between acute effects of alcohol and response inhibition. Indeed, only subjects with low capacity to manipulate information stored in working memory (as assessed by counting digits backwards) showed alcohol-induced motor inhibitory control as attested by a greater number of false alarms in a Go/No-Go task after they ingested moderate doses of alcohol (Finn et al., 1999).

Another main moderator of the relationship between acute effects of alcohol and response inhibition would be some personality characteristics (Fillmore et al., 2008; Ray et al., 2006). This line of research has been justified by growing evidence that impulsivity might play an important causal role in problem drinking (Lacono et al., 1999). For instance, longitudinal studies of children and adolescents have shown that impulsivity predicts early onset drinking age and development of heavy drinking and alcohol dependence in young adults (Ernst et al., 2006). In particular, sensation-seeking, considered as a neurobiologically based tendency to seek novel, complex, intense sensations was positively correlated with increased alcohol use and alcohol-related problems (Dom et al., 2006; Hittner & Swickert, 2006). This greater risk to experience alcohol and other substance abuse may be that these individuals are more responsive to the rewarding effects of alcohol as expressed by its more subjective stimulant-like effects (Ray et al., 2006). Interestingly, a study also found that those non-alcoholic students high on sensation-seeking demonstrated increased sensitivity to the subjective rewarding effects of alcohol and also less motor inhibition than those low on sensation-seeking (Fillmore et al., 2008).

3. Conclusion

The present article emphasized the relevance of impulsivity/disinhibition for investigating both predisposing and developmental factors leading to alcohol-related disorders. The association between response inhibition weaknesses prior to the onset of alcohol use with the disinhibitory acute effects of alcohol and its deleterious chronic effects may dramatically improve the likelihood to loss control over alcohol use.

However, one main problem with the use of one or two cognitive tasks is that the construct validities of most commonly used inhibition tasks are not well established. For instance, go/no-go and stop-signal paradigms are generally considered as investigating a same construct, namely intentional prepotent motor response inhibition. However, an important contribution was that these tasks can both rely on both bottom-up control and top-down control (Verbruggen & Logan, 2008). Automatic and controlled inhibition can work together to guide goal-directed behavior. Indeed, Indeed, when a no-go stimulus (in the go/no-go paradigm) or a stimulus that was previously accompanied by a stop signal (in the stop-signal paradigm) is repeated, the stop goal is activated through the retrieval of stimulus-stop associations, and it suppresses automatically the go response. In other terms, a stopping action might be reflecting either the need for top-down executive control processes or the need for bottom-up automatic processes. One way to overcome the fact that an entire task does not tap into one single psychological construct may be to perform analyses within a single task to extract the relative contribution of automatic versus intentional inhibition to the interruption of an action. Then, it will be easy to perform between group comparisons with dependent variables assessing either automatic or intentional response inhibition.

Another way to draw more robust conclusions about the failure of alcoholics to inhibit response could be based on the methodology proposed by Friedmann and Miyake (2004). Indeed, a latent variable analysis makes it possible to "extract" what is common among the tasks selected to tap a putative executive function and use that "purer" latent variable to examine how different executive functions relate to one another. By doing this, these authors showed that prepotent response inhibition and resistance to distractor interference were closely related, but both were unrelated to resistance to proactive interference (Friedman & Miyake, 2004). By using inhibition tasks selected from this theoretical framework, we found that recently detoxified alcoholics exhibit a massive prepotent response inhibition disruption despite preserved bottom up/automatic inhibition (Noël et al., unpublished data).

Another promising avenue of research refers to the notion of "inhibition biases" that reflects performance decreasing while information to-be-inhibited is associated with alcoholism. It is the case when the action suppression associated with alcohol-related words results in the increasing of the number of commission errors in alcoholics compared to non-alcoholics (e.g., Noël et al., 2007). Thus, the investigation of "inhibition deficits" (i.e., disruption of inhibition regardless the kind of information processes) could be advantageously complement with research focused on "inhibition biases".

Finally, it has been more and more obvious that alcoholism is a heterogeneous disease. As a striking example, we reviewed in this chapter that individuals with early onset of alcoholism (EOAs) are generally more impulsive that those with late onset of alcoholism (LOAs). Dom's studies have robustly showed that EOAs had higher discount rates than both the non-substance-abusing subjects and the LOAs, with these two groups performing similarly. This differentiation between EOAs and LOAs in terms of impulsive decision making emphasized the heterogeneity of individuals with alcoholism on the one hand and the existence of distinct pathways leading to alcoholism on the other.

Taken together, it is highly recommendable that research on impulsive decision and behavior should be intensified within more robust theoretical frameworks and updated methodologies. Further understanding of psychological and neurobiological underpinnings of inhibitory control offer obvious promise for improving pharmacological and psychological treatment for individuals with alcoholism.

4. References

Abroms, B. D., Fillmore, M. T., & Marczinski, C. A. (2003). Alcohol-induced impairment of behavioral control: effects on the alteration and suppression of prepotent responses. *Journal of Studies on Alcohol, 64*(5), 687-695.

Abroms, B. D., Gottlob, L. R., & Fillmore, M. T. (2006). Alcohol effects on inhibitory control of attention: distinguishing between intentional and automatic mechanisms. *Psychopharmacology, 188*(3), 324-334. doi:10.1007/s00213-006-0524-y

Andrés, P., Van der Linden, M., & Parmentier, F. B. R. (2004). Directed forgetting in working memory: age-related differences. *Memory, 12*(2), 248-256. doi:10.1080/09658210244000612

Andrucci, G. L., Archer, R. P., Pancoast, D. L., & Gordon, R. A. (1989). The relationship of MMPI and Sensation Seeking Scales to adolescent drug use. *Journal of Personality Assessment, 53*(2), 253-266. doi:10.1207/s15327752jpa5302_4

Aron, A. R. (2007). The neural basis of inhibition in cognitive control. *The Neuroscientist: A Review Journal Bringing Neurobiology, Neurology and Psychiatry, 13*(3), 214-228. doi:10.1177/1073858407299288

Babor, T. F., Hofmann, M., DelBoca, F. K., Hesselbrock, V., Meyer, R. E., Dolinsky, Z. S., & Rounsaville, B. (1992). Types of alcoholics, I. Evidence for an empirically derived typology based on indicators of vulnerability and severity. *Archives of General Psychiatry, 49*(8), 599-608.

Bechara, A. (2003). Risky business: emotion, decision-making, and addiction. *Journal of Gambling Studies, 19*(1), 23-51.

Begleiter, H, & Porjesz, B. (1999). What is inherited in the predisposition toward alcoholism? A proposed model. *Alcoholism, Clinical and Experimental Research, 23*(7), 1125-1135.

Belin, D., Mar, A. C., Dalley, J. W., Robbins, T. W., & Everitt, B. J. (2008). High impulsivity predicts the switch to compulsive cocaine-taking. *Science, 320*(5881), 1352-1355. doi:10.1126/science.1158136

Bjork, J. M., Hommer, D. W., Grant, S. J., & Danube, C. (2004). Impulsivity in abstinent alcohol-dependent patients: relation to control subjects and type 1-/type 2-like traits. *Alcohol, 34*(2-3), 133-150.

Bowden-Jones, H., McPhillips, M., Rogers, R., Hutton, S., & Joyce, E. (2005). Risk-taking on tests sensitive to ventromedial prefrontal cortex dysfunction predicts early relapse in alcohol dependency: a pilot study. *The Journal of Neuropsychiatry and Clinical Neurosciences, 17*(3), 417-420. doi:10.1176/appi.neuropsych.17.3.417

Burgess, P. W., & Shallice, T. (1996). Response suppression, initiation and strategy use following frontal lobe lesions. *Neuropsychologia, 34*(4), 263-272.

Chamberlain, S. R., Blackwell, A. D., Fineberg, N. A., Robbins, T. W., & Sahakian, B. J. (2005). The neuropsychology of obsessive compulsive disorder: the importance of failures in cognitive and behavioural inhibition as candidate endophenotypic markers. *Neuroscience and Biobehavioral Reviews, 29*(3), 399-419. doi:10.1016/j.neubiorev.2004.11.006

Collette, F., Van der Linden, M., Delfiore, G., Degueldre, C., Luxen, A., & Salmon, E. (2001). The functional anatomy of inhibition processes investigated with the Hayling task. *NeuroImage, 14*(2), 258-267. doi:10.1006/nimg.2001.0846

de Wit, H. (2009). Impulsivity as a determinant and consequence of drug use: a review of underlying processes. *Addiction Biology, 14*(1), 22-31. doi:10.1111/j.1369-1600.2008.00129.x

Dom, G., D'haene, P., Hulstijn, W., & Sabbe, B. (2006). Impulsivity in abstinent early- and late-onset alcoholics: differences in self-report measures and a discounting task. *Addiction, 101*(1), 50-59. doi:10.1111/j.1360-0443.2005.01270.x

Ernst, M., Luckenbaugh, D. A., Moolchan, E. T., Leff, M. K., Allen, R., Eshel, N., London, E. D., et al. (2006). Behavioral predictors of substance-use initiation in adolescents with and without attention-deficit/hyperactivity disorder. *Pediatrics, 117*(6), 2030-2039. doi:10.1542/peds.2005-0704

Evenden, J. L. (1999). Varieties of impulsivity. *Psychopharmacology, 146*(4), 348-361.

Fillmore, M. T. (2003). Drug abuse as a problem of impaired control: current approaches and findings. *Behavioral and Cognitive Neuroscience Reviews, 2*(3), 179-197. doi:10.1177/1534582303257007

Fillmore, M. T. (2007). Acute alcohol-induced impairment of cognitive functions: past and present findings. *International Journal on Disability and Human Development, 6*, 115-125.

Fillmore, M. T., Ostling, E. W., Martin, C. A., & Kelly, T. H. (2009). Acute effects of alcohol on inhibitory control and information processing in high and low sensation-seekers. *Drug and Alcohol Dependence, 100*(1-2), 91-99. doi:10.1016/j.drugalcdep.2008.09.007

Finn, P R, Justus, A., Mazas, C., & Steinmetz, J. E. (1999). Working memory, executive processes and the effects of alcohol on Go/No-Go learning: testing a model of behavioral regulation and impulsivity. *Psychopharmacology, 146*(4), 465-472.

Finn, Peter R. (2002). Motivation, working memory, and decision making: a cognitive-motivational theory of personality vulnerability to alcoholism. *Behavioral and Cognitive Neuroscience Reviews, 1*(3), 183-205.

Friedman, Naomi P, & Miyake, A. (2004). The relations among inhibition and interference control functions: a latent-variable analysis. *Journal of Experimental Psychology. General, 133*(1), 101-135. doi:10.1037/0096-3445.133.1.101

Gazzaniga, M. (2000). *Cognitive neuroscience : a reader*. Malden Mass.: Blackwell.

Goldstein, R. Z., & Volkow, N. D. (2002). Drug addiction and its underlying neurobiological basis: neuroimaging evidence for the involvement of the frontal cortex. *The American Journal of Psychiatry, 159*(10), 1642-1652.

Goudriaan, A. E., Oosterlaan, J., de Beurs, E., & van den Brink, W. (2005). Decision making in pathological gambling: a comparison between pathological gamblers, alcohol dependents, persons with Tourette syndrome, and normal controls. *Brain Research. Cognitive Brain Research, 23*(1), 137-151. doi:10.1016/j.cogbrainres.2005.01.017

Goudriaan, A. E., Oosterlaan, J., de Beurs, E., & van den Brink, W. (2006). Neurocognitive functions in pathological gambling: a comparison with alcohol dependence, Tourette syndrome and normal controls. *Addiction, 101*(4), 534-547. doi:10.1111/j.1360-0443.2006.01380.x

Habeych, M. E., Folan, M. M., Luna, B., & Tarter, R. E. (2006). Impaired oculomotor response inhibition in children of alcoholics: The role of attention deficit hyperactivity disorder. *Drug and Alcohol Dependence, 82*(1), 11-17. doi:10.1016/ j.drugalcdep.2005.07.012

Hernández, O. H., Vogel-Sprott, M., Huchín-Ramirez, T. C., & Aké-Estrada, F. (2006). Acute dose of alcohol affects cognitive components of reaction time to an omitted stimulus: differences among sensory systems. *Psychopharmacology, 184*(1), 75-81. doi:10.1007/s00213-005-0237-7

Hittner, J. B., & Swickert, R. (2006). Sensation seeking and alcohol use: a meta-analytic review. *Addictive Behaviors, 31*(8), 1383-1401. doi:10.1016/j.addbeh.2005.11.004

Holloway, F. (s. d.). Low-dose alcohol effects on human behavior and performance. *Alcohol, Drugs and Driving, 11*(1), 39-56.

Iacono, W. G., Carlson, S. R., Taylor, J., Elkins, I. J., & McGue, M. (1999). Behavioral disinhibition and the development of substance-use disorders: findings from the Minnesota Twin Family Study. *Development and Psychopathology, 11*(4), 869-900.

Jentsch, J. D., & Taylor, J. R. (1999). Impulsivity resulting from frontostriatal dysfunction in drug abuse: implications for the control of behavior by reward-related stimuli. *Psychopharmacology, 146*(4), 373-390.

Kamarajan, C., Porjesz, B., Jones, K., Chorlian, D., Padmanabhapillai, A., Rangaswamy, M., Stimus, A., et al. (2006). Event-related oscillations in offspring of alcoholics: neurocognitive disinhibition as a risk for alcoholism. *Biological Psychiatry, 59*(7), 625-634. doi:10.1016/j.biopsych.2005.08.017

Kirisci, L., Tarter, R. E., Reynolds, M., & Vanyukov, M. (2006). Individual differences in childhood neurobehavior disinhibition predict decision to desist substance use during adolescence and substance use disorder in young adulthood: a prospective study. *Addictive Behaviors, 31*(4), 686-696. doi:10.1016/j.addbeh.2005.05.049

Logan, G D, Cowan, W. B., & Davis, K. A. (1984). On the ability to inhibit simple and choice reaction time responses: a model and a method. *Journal of Experimental Psychology. Human Perception and Performance, 10*(2), 276-291.

Logan, Gordon D. (1994). On the ability to inhibit thought and action: A user's guide to stop signal paradigm. *Inhibitory processes in attention, memory and language* (Academic Press., p. 189-239). San Diego, CA: D. Dagenbach, T.H. Carr.

Lusher, J., Chandler, C., & Ball, D. (2004). Alcohol dependence and the alcohol Stroop paradigm: evidence and issues. *Drug and Alcohol Dependence, 75*(3), 225-231. doi:10.1016/j.drugalcdep.2004.03.004

Lyvers, M. (2000). « Loss of control » in alcoholism and drug addiction: a neuroscientific interpretation. *Experimental and Clinical Psychopharmacology, 8*(2), 225-249.

Marczinski, C. A., Abroms, B. D., Van Selst, M., & Fillmore, M. T. (2005). Alcohol-induced impairment of behavioral control: differential effects on engaging vs. disengaging responses. *Psychopharmacology, 182*(3), 452-459. doi:10.1007/s00213-005-0116-2

May, J., Andrade, J., Panabokke, N., & Kavanagh, D. (2004). Images of desire: cognitive models of craving. *Memory, 12*(4), 447-461. doi:10.1080/09658210444000061

Mazur, J. (1987). An adjusting procedure for studying delayed reinforcement. The effect of delay and of intervening events on reinforcement value, In: *The effect of delay and of intervening events on reinforcement value, Quantitative analyses of behavior,* M.L.

Commons, J.E. Mazur, J.A. Nevin, H. Rachlin (Ed.), 55-73, Lawrence Erlbaum Associates, Hillsdale, NJ, England.

Mitchell, J. M., Fields, H. L., D'Esposito, M., & Boettiger, C. A. (2005). Impulsive responding in alcoholics. *Alcoholism, Clinical and Experimental Research, 29*(12), 2158-2169.

Miyake, A, Friedman, N. P., Emerson, M. J., Witzki, A. H., Howerter, A., & Wager, T. D. (2000). The unity and diversity of executive functions and their contributions to complex « Frontal Lobe » tasks: a latent variable analysis. *Cognitive Psychology, 41*(1), 49-100. doi:10.1006/cogp.1999.0734

Mulder, R. T. (2002). Alcoholism and personality. *The Australian and New Zealand Journal of Psychiatry, 36*(1), 44-52.

Mulvihill, L. E., Skilling, T. A., & Vogel-Sprott, M. (1997). Alcohol and the ability to inhibit behavior in men and women. *Journal of Studies on Alcohol, 58*(6), 600-605.

Nigg, J T. (2000). On inhibition/disinhibition in developmental psychopathology: views from cognitive and personality psychology and a working inhibition taxonomy. *Psychological Bulletin, 126*(2), 220-246.

Nigg, J. T., Wong, M. M., Martel, M. M., Jester, J. M., Puttler, L. I., Glass, J. M., Adams, K. M., et al. (2006). Poor response inhibition as a predictor of problem drinking and illicit drug use in adolescents at risk for alcoholism and other substance use disorders. *Journal of the American Academy of Child and Adolescent Psychiatry, 45*(4), 468-475. doi:10.1097/01.chi.0000199028.76452.a9

Noël, X., Van der Linden, M., Schmidt, N., Sferrazza, R., Hanak, C., Le Bon, O., De Mol, J., et al. (2001). Supervisory attentional system in nonamnesic alcoholic men. *Archives of General Psychiatry, 58*(12), 1152-1158.

Noël, X., Billieux, J., Van der Linden, M., Dan, B., Hanak, C., de Bournonville, S., Baurain, C., & Verbanck, P. (2009). Impaired inhibition of proactive interference in abstinent individuals with alcoholism. *Journal of Clinical and Experimental Neuropsychology, 31*(1), 57-64. doi:10.1080/13803390801982726

Noël, X., Sferrazza, R., Van Der Linden, M., Paternot, J., Verhas, M., Hanak, C., Pelc, I., et al. (2002). Contribution of frontal cerebral blood flow measured by (99m)Tc-Bicisate spect and executive function deficits to predicting treatment outcome in alcohol-dependent patients. *Alcohol and Alcoholism, 37*(4), 347-354.

Noël, X., Van der Linden, M., d' Acremont, M., Bechara, A., Dan, B., Hanak, C., & Verbanck, P. (2007). Alcohol cues increase cognitive impulsivity in individuals with alcoholism. *Psychopharmacology, 192*(2), 291-298. doi:10.1007/s00213-006-0695-6

Noël, X., Van der Linden, M., d' Acremont, M., Colmant, M., Hanak, C., Pelc, I., Verbanck, P., et al. (2005). Cognitive biases toward alcohol-related words and executive deficits in polysubstance abusers with alcoholism. *Addiction, 100*(9), 1302-1309. doi:10.1111/j.1360-0443.2005.01125.x

Norman, D. A., & Shallice, T. (1986). Attention to action: Willed and automatic control of behaviour, In: *Consciousness and Self-Regulation: Advances in Research and Theory,* R.J. Davidson, G.E. Schwartz, D. Shapiro (Ed.), 1-18, Plenum Press, New York.

Patton, J. H., Stanford, M. S., & Barratt, E. S. (1995). Factor structure of the barratt impulsiveness scale. *Journal of Clinical Psychology, 51,* 768-774. doi:10.1002/1097-4679(199511)51:6<768::AID-JCLP2270510607>3.0.CO;2-1

Ray, L. A., McGeary, J., Marshall, E., & Hutchison, K. E. (2006). Risk factors for alcohol misuse: examining heart rate reactivity to alcohol, alcohol sensitivity, and personality constructs. *Addictive Behaviors, 31*(11), 1959-1973. doi:10.1016/j.addbeh.2006.01.010

Reingold, E. M., & Stampe, D. M. (2002). Saccadic inhibition in voluntary and reflexive saccades. *Journal of Cognitive Neuroscience, 14*(3), 371-388. doi:10.1162/089892902317361903

Robinson, T. E., & Berridge, K. C. (2003). Addiction. *Annual Review of Psychology, 54*, 25-53. doi:10.1146/annurev.psych.54.101601.145237

Ross, R. G., Hommer, D., Breiger, D., Varley, C., & Radant, A. (1994). Eye movement task related to frontal lobe functioning in children with attention deficit disorder. *Journal of the American Academy of Child and Adolescent Psychiatry, 33*(6), 869-874. doi:10.1097/00004583-199407000-00013

Schweinsburg, A. D., Paulus, M. P., Barlett, V. C., Killeen, L. A., Caldwell, L. C., Pulido, C., Brown, S. A., et al. (2004). An FMRI study of response inhibition in youths with a family history of alcoholism. *Annals of the New York Academy of Sciences, 1021*, 391-394. doi:10.1196/annals.1308.050

Sharma, D., Albery, I. P., & Cook, C. (2001). Selective attentional bias to alcohol related stimuli in problem drinkers and non-problem drinkers. *Addiction, 96*(2), 285-295. doi:10.1080/09652140020021026

Stuphorn, V., & Schall, J. D. (2006). Executive control of countermanding saccades by the supplementary eye field. *Nature Neuroscience, 9*(7), 925-931. doi:10.1038/nn1714

Tiffany, S. T. (1990). A cognitive model of drug urges and drug-use behavior: role of automatic and nonautomatic processes. *Psychological Review, 97*(2), 147-168.

Verbruggen, F., & Logan, G. D. (2008). Automatic and controlled response inhibition: associative learning in the go/no-go and stop-signal paradigms. *Journal of Experimental Psychology. General, 137*(4), 649-672. doi:10.1037/a0013170

Verdejo-García, A., Lawrence, A. J., & Clark, L. (2008). Impulsivity as a vulnerability marker for substance-use disorders: review of findings from high-risk research, problem gamblers and genetic association studies. *Neuroscience and Biobehavioral Reviews, 32*(4), 777-810. doi:10.1016/j.neubiorev.2007.11.003

von Knorring, L., Palm, U., & Andersson, H. E. (1985). Relationship between treatment outcome and subtype of alcoholism in men. *Journal of Studies on Alcohol, 46*(5), 388-391.

von Knorring, L., von Knorring, A. L., Smigan, L., Lindberg, U., & Edholm, M. (1987). Personality traits in subtypes of alcoholics. *Journal of Studies on Alcohol, 48*(6), 523-527.

Weissenborn, R., & Duka, T. (2003). Acute alcohol effects on cognitive function in social drinkers: their relationship to drinking habits. *Psychopharmacology, 165*(3), 306-312. doi:10.1007/s00213-002-1281-1

Whiteside, S. P., & Lynam, D. R. (2003). Understanding the role of impulsivity and externalizing psychopathology in alcohol abuse: application of the UPPS impulsive behavior scale. *Experimental and Clinical Psychopharmacology, 11*(3), 210-217.

Zuckerman, M., & Neeb, M. (1979). Sensation seeking and psychopathology. *Psychiatry Research, 1*(3), 255-264.

Section 2

Clinical Interventions

3

Utilizing Psychiatric Diagnosis and Formulation in the Clinical Process: Meeting the Needs and Expectations of Service Users

Graham Mellsop and Fiona Clapham Howard
Waikato Clinical School, University of Auckland and Canterbury District Health Board, New Zealand

1. Introduction

Service users and those who support them, such as family or friends, have an expectation that a clinical or health diagnosis will offer insight into the cause of their symptoms. Diagnosis is expected to allow both prediction of prognosis and determination of treatment options. However, current widely used psychiatric diagnostic systems do not usually provide links to cause or prognosis. This is explicitly stated in the introductions to the two major current systems, the Diagnostic and Statistical Manual of the American Psychiatric Association (APA, 2000) and the 10th revision of the International Classification of Diseases (WHO, 1992).

Within a complex field such as mental health, the diversity of causal or pathogenetic contributors means that both aetiology and prognosis are likely to be highly individualised. As a result, there is a gap between mental health service users' expectations and what can be realistically provided by diagnosis alone.

However, when paired with a thorough and reflective formulation, diagnosis is placed in a context that facilitates the ineluctable logical development of a comprehensive management or recovery plan. This dynamic combination of diagnosis and formulation results in a collaboratively developed management plan, agreed to by clinician and consumer, that is better placed to meet both the needs and the expectations of those seeking help.

2. The clinical process

People are motivated to go to psychological, counselling or psychiatric services by their discomforts or needs. These needs may relate to various forms of distress or dysphoria and/or to decreases in functionality. Such clients or service users are seeking intervention(s) which will improve the way they feel and/or the way they function. Sometimes it will be family or others who approach services on their behalf.

Together, the trained clinician and the service user will develop a plan of action, perhaps with input from family or supporters, as well as from other clinicians. Indeed, it can be argued that the development of a comprehensive management or recovery plan is the major purpose of the clinician-service user interaction (Mellsop and Banzato, 2006).

In order to develop the plan, an assessment of the individual's difficulties and the context in which they occur is required. The term "assessment" is used to cover a wide variety of ways in which information is obtained. Central to the assessment is the clinical interview. This may be brief or lengthy, but ideally will be comprehensive and supplemented by collateral information such as details from family and other key informants, files written by previous clinicians involved in care or treatment, and sometimes by formal, psychometrically credible, evaluations.

However, sometimes the information available may be very limited. Whatever that information is, a plan of how to proceed will need to be drawn up. Sometimes the central part of that plan may be evidence based therapeutic interventions. By contrast, sometimes the main focus will be on further assessment, data gathering, referral to an alternative service provider, or other intermediate variations or combinations.

A clinician utilizing a recovery approach will expect the service user to be an active participant in this process. Their cognitive, attitudinal and behavioural contribution to the clinician's provisional management plan will be major determinants of the success of the resulting collaboration (Chinman et al., 1999).

Gathering the assessment information is a skill taught, at various depths, to medical students, nurses, psychologists, social workers, occupational therapists, trainee psychiatrists and other clinically active disciplines. It is not usually the ability to collect the information which clearly separates students from practitioners. Rather, the skill lies in making coherent, credible, sense of that assessment information, in formulating it, and in making an accurate diagnosis of the condition with which the individual presents.

The role that diagnosis plays in the process of clinical decision making is sometimes pivotal, but its singular significance can be overemphasised. There are in fact two reasoned conclusions to be drawn from the available assessment information: the diagnosis (or diagnoses), and the formulation. These are distinct and quite different from each other; both, however, are essential to the clinical process. Their contributions to the logic which psychologists and psychiatrists apply need to be clearly understood.

The diagnosis is generally a categorical classification of the disorder the person is presenting with, based on evidence collected from the assessment, determined by utilizing the clinician's judgement. It is the disorder which is receiving the label, not the person.

Classification is categorical in the sense that each diagnostic label is expected to apply to a distinct condition, separable from other conditions, and that the boundaries between disorders can be defined and relied upon. The diagnosis is usually drawn from within an accepted, standardized and reliable classification framework such as the International Classification of Diseases (WHO, 1992) or the Diagnostic and Statistical Manual (DSM) of the American Psychiatric Association (APA, 2000).

In contrast, the formulation is more subjective, extensive and idiographic. It can encompass a diagnosis, but it also provides a broader narrative, thereby giving an explanatory context to the presenting problem and foreshadowing the management or recovery plan. It is likely to take account of predisposing, precipitating and perpetuating factors as they relate to the person's presenting symptoms and level of functioning. It will include reference to the person's capacities and strengths, attitudes, values, illness behavior, culture and societal context.

Therefore, it can be argued that formulation is more meaningful and more useful than diagnosis on its own, not just to the clinician, but also to the non-clinical stakeholders in the process, namely the service user and their family or community of support.

The process of the clinical logic of the clinician/service user interaction is displayed diagrammatically below. The link between the assessment information and the management plan is provided by both the diagnosis and the formulation.

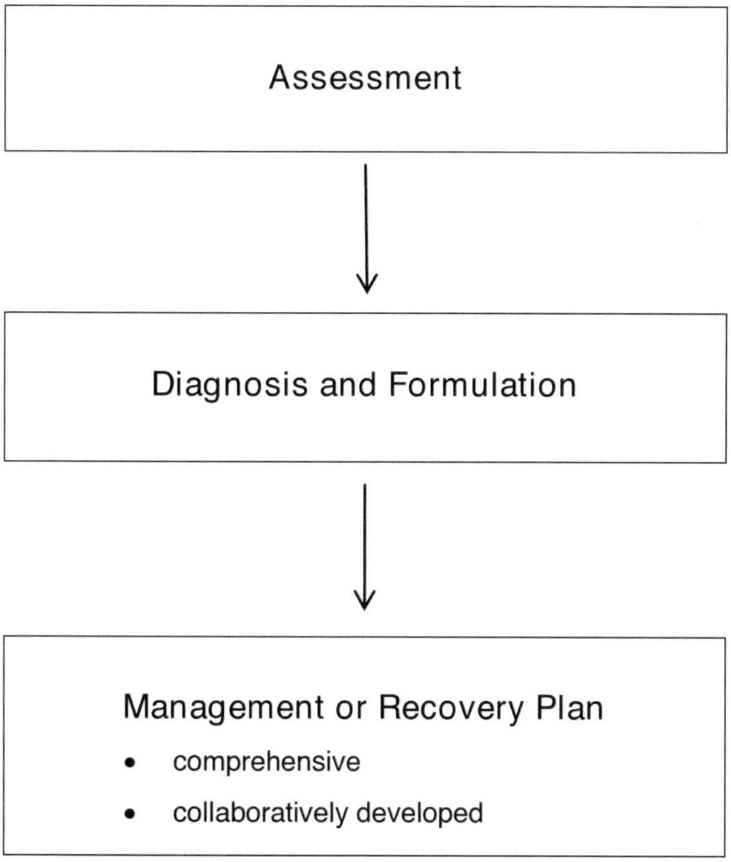

Fig. 1. Diagrammatic display of the essential steps in the clinical process

2.1 Diagnosis and the diagnostic system

Assigning a diagnosis to the symptoms or presentation of psychiatric service users is essential to work in mental health and addictions and important also in counseling services. A diagnosis is not purely clinical in its function. It underpins much of the structure of mental health and addictions work. For example, it can serve a statistical purpose, be taken into account in a public health perspective and is often required for funding, including the funding of research (IAG, 2011; Carey & Pilgrim, 2010).

Because they are determined mainly by the symptoms or phenomenology and ignore much of a person's developmental and contextual information, diagnoses tend to be reductionist in nature. This has the potential for being at odds with therapeutic intentions: diagnosis produces descriptive, generalised labels and can invoke stigma that can be argued is therefore, at least partly, iatrogenic (Carey & Pilgrim, 2010; Hanzawa et al., 2009).

Distinct in its role from diagnosis in other branches of health, a psychiatric diagnosis does not usually have a link to aetiology or to prognosis (Maj 2005; APA, 2000; Mellsop et al, 2007; IAG, 2011).

Classification usually requires a process of creating, defining, and confirming boundaries between concepts. In psychiatry for almost half a century, there have been five widely publicised criteria for judging the validity of the diagnostic categories which make up the classificatory systems. As first suggested by Robins and Guze (1970), these are:

- description of clear and consistent clinical features
- the exclusion of other possible disorders
- a uniform clinical course (including prognosis)
- an increased prevalence in close relatives
- an investigatory marker of the disorder (e.g., laboratory test).

However, it has become clear that for many diagnostic labels the current categorical classificatory systems fail to fulfil most of these criteria (Mellsop et al.,2007; Jorm, 2006; IAG 2011, Hyman, 2010). Recognition of this underpins the planned research programme of the (US) National Institute of Mental Health (Insel et al., 2010).

Three psychometric properties are required of a diagnostic system. In addition to reliability and validity, if the system is going to be used and survive, utility is required. Central to utility in clinical psychiatry is the expectation that knowing the diagnosis allows the selection of the most effective treatment (Nice, 2003; APA 2006; Mellsop et al 2007; Frese and Myrick, 2010).

Psychiatric diagnosis on its own, however, is generally of limited use in the choice of optimal treatment for individual service users. In most cases, multiple characteristics of both the service user and the context will influence a clinician's management plans and treatment choices (Mellsop, & Banzato, 2006; Byrne, 2007; Nice, 2003).

Modern pharmacotherapies are often combined and are remarkably non-specific. For example, 'antidepressants', 'antipsychotics' and 'mood stabilisers' are all used in a range of conceptually and categorically distinct disorders. Most of the different classes of treatment appear to have a place in the treatment guidelines issued by bodies such as the American Psychiatric Association for a variety of different disorders (APA, 2006). Moreover, inter-individual variation in response to these same pharmacotherapies can be striking and usually remains unexplained.

While diagnosis tends to be regarded by the medically trained psychiatrists as fundamental to clinical psychiatry, this is not necessarily the case for other mental health clinicians who embrace the broader field of mental health and its disorders. For example, in psychology practice, diagnosis tends to be underemphasised in favour of formulation (Carey & Pilgrim, 2010).

2.1.1 Significance of diagnosis to the service user and their community

While it may be tempting for all involved to regard diagnosis as a discrete event in the clinical process, for service users and their family or other community it is just one more step (albeit a significant one) on a much longer journey. The service user, along with those whose lives intersect closely with him or her - their family members, friends, those they live or work with - are often highly invested in the outcome of the diagnostic process.

Service users, for example, report the clinical process and its resulting diagnosis as impacting on their self esteem, their sense of self and identity, and influencing their hopefulness for their future (Frese and Myrick, 2010; Crumlish and Kelly, 2009; Barnett and Lapsley, 2006).

These comments offer an insight into the high expectations these "ultimate stakeholders" can bring to the clinical process. For example, many people think it reasonable to believe that following the assessment they will be given an explanation for what they are experiencing. But more importantly, they are likely to hope that there will be a cure, help will be provided, the problem will be fixed and health will be restored (Moeke-Maxwell et al., 2008; Laird et al. 2010).

Service users and others closely affected report both positive and negative consequences stemming from the process of receiving a diagnosis. Some will experience initially favourable outcomes that are not sustained over time, leading to a more sober, sometimes cynical, appreciation of the process.

In terms of positive consequences, service users talk of a diagnosis providing them with a sense of validation: that their experiences, often frightening or confusing to them and those around them, are normalized by receiving a clinical explanation (Moeke-Maxwell et al., 2008). Family members likewise report a sense of relief, and express hope that the burden of care they experience will now be reduced (Laird et al., 2010; Hanzawa et al., 2009).

This concept of clinical validation may at times also lead to a reduction in stigma, both internal and external, and judgements about a person's behaviour or the reasons for it. For example, some family members report having more tolerance for behaviour they might have judged negatively before knowing the diagnosis. The service user's distress may now be explained in terms that are more socially acceptable. As well, having a clinical explanation can mean that others in the wider community are seen as less likely to judge the family as a whole e.g. behaviour is now attributed to a medical condition rather than to "bad parenting" (Laird et al., 2010; Barnett and Lapsley, 2006; Carey and Pilgrim, 2010).

There is often a welcome sense for service users and the others affected of positive action occurring, with the expectation that a diagnosis will go hand-in-hand with some form of treatment, particularly medication (Barnett and Lapsley, 2006; Moeke-Maxwell et al., 2008; Laird et al., 2010).

The diagnosis is also acknowledged as potentially opening doors to specialist (secondary or tertiary) services, as well as to other supports (Carey and Pilgrim, 2010). This has particular significance for family members who often have a "paraprofessional" role in supporting a relative or loved one through illness, and can experience considerable burdens, both objective and subjective, as a result (Laird et al., 2010).

Following a diagnosis family members and supporters report increased understanding of what the service user is experiencing. Many feel more alert to the service users' symptoms, better able to respond and empathize (Laird et al., 2010). Service users can also experience an increased sense of personal competence from working with a new understanding of their experience based on the diagnostic/symptomatic framework.

Some may only experience a downside if treatment turns out to be harder than expected, or not as effective as hoped, or when a relapse or crisis changes their initially favourable perception of the clinical process. For others, however, the negative response to a particular diagnosis is immediate.

The negative stigma associated with mental illness and addiction, and with some diagnoses in particular, is a common theme in service user and family/carer literature (Frese and Myrick, 2010). In particular, psychotic spectrum disorders, such as schizophrenia or some bipolar disorders, as well as personality disorders, tend to come with more unfavourable associations (Hartnell and Lapsley, 2006; Laird et al., 2010).

Families and service users may find themselves struggling with perceptions of "dangerousness" and instability, which can make it difficult for the service user to access meaningful occupation such as employment or study. In some countries such heavily stigmatized associations have been seen as sufficiently important as to require a disorder being renamed, by national fiat (Sato, 2006).

Those affected also have to contend with the limited expectations that can come hand-in-hand with some diagnoses, based on the symptomatic prognosis. Gillian, a young woman diagnosed with an Axis II disorder, sums it up like this:

> *"[Being diagnosed with] personality disorder, it's horrible to get because it's just kind of stuck with you and it suggests that there's something intrinsically wrong with you and it's not something you can change."* (Barnett and Lapsley, 2006)

Keith, a forensic service user, comments on the behavioural consequences of diagnosis:

> *"I think the labelling that goes on is really limiting. Once you get a person to accept a label you also get them to accept the behaviour which is attached to that label. To be called a schizophrenic or a bipolar...turns you into just that."* (O'Hagan, 2000)

It is not uncommon for the service user to disagree with the diagnosis they are given. Both family members and service users report at times that the diagnosis did not match their interpretation of their experience, and came with too many negative associations to be accepted (Frese and Myrick, 2010; Moeke-Maxwell et al., 2008; Laird et al., 2010). Some felt that clinicians did not communicate with them in a way that allowed hope for the prospect of future health.

It can be seen that psychiatric diagnosis cannot stand on its own in terms of pointing to useful interventions for the service user, or in offering a meaningful explanation for the difficulties with which they present. The subsequent steps or consequences that arise from a diagnosis tend to take on much more importance, particularly over time, than the diagnosis itself.

Formulation therefore, along with diagnosis, forms an essential link between the assessment process and the ongoing management or recovery plan (Carey & Pilgrim, 2010).

2.2 Formulation

The process of formulating the assessment information is a fundamental skill required of all trained mental health clinicians. The underlying concept is not particularly contentious. However, there is considerable variation both in creating formulations and in describing the techniques involved (Belz, 1967; Varghese and Mellsop, 1983; Nurcombe and Fitzhenry-Coor, 1987; Mellsop and Banzato, 2006). Alternative frameworks abound, and these can be at odds with each other (Mace and Binyon, 2005). There is further confusion about the definition of a formulation. Is it a summary of the descriptive information obtained via the assessment; or an integrated bio-psycho-social synthesis of the assessment information; or purely psychodynamic?

In essence, formulation consists of bringing together those parts of the information derived from the assessment which are most central to understanding why this person has presented in this fashion at this time.

In order to support this objective, the formulation will include reference to relevant information about the person's socio-cultural context including illness behaviour, family of origin, their health beliefs, personality style, significant relationships, life event exposure, likely treatment participation and adherence. The resulting "understanding" or narrative is therefore a highly individualistic, explanatory summary of the assessment information.

A useful formulation will do more than summarize or re-arrange assessment information, however. Ideally it will draw inferences from that information and offer a range of hypotheses. It will inform treatment, by extracting from the assessment information everything that will make a difference to the recovery plan (Mellsop and Banzato, 2006).

Because the process requires judgements by the clinician, formulations are less standardized, reliable or consistent than diagnoses. However, those aspects which influence the recovery plan are generally agreed; for example, social supports, intellectual ability and style, previous medication adherence, medication tolerance, family support, daily living skills, work and accommodation. The person's susceptibilities and resources are likely to be included. In particular, their personal attributes and strengths which can be drawn upon in the therapeutic alliance and clinical management plan will be delineated.

In practice, most aspects of the plan will be informed by details from the formulation. Much of a service user's contextual information needs to be taken into account by them and the clinician, if they want to produce a successful recovery plan. For example, information about a person's living situation, attitudes, habits and health beliefs is important to include because this will be relevant to the individual's ability and willingness to adhere to the plan.

One of the ways an effective formulation can inform the plan is by predicting the individual's response to treatment, by drawing on the understanding of how the individual perceives and responds to being ill, and their theory of change (Duncan et al, 2010). It can also play a vital role in ongoing evaluation of the effectiveness of treatment and can suggest priorities to address or re-consider, should the initial focus prove ineffective (Mace and Binyon, 2005; Eells et al, 1998).

A thorough formulation will also place importance on the clinician's self-reflection, noting any possible counter-transference issues and utilizing de-biasing strategies to counteract cognitive errors and biases (Crumlish and Kelly, 2009).

Providing as it does a context and narrative for what the service user is experiencing, the formulation offers a more meaningful conclusion to the assessment for the non-clinical stakeholders than does diagnosis alone. It can better encompass factors of significance to the service user and their family or community of support, such as the role trauma may have played.

Read et al. (2005) reviewed the available literature and noted the significance of trauma, including childhood physical and/or sexual abuse, to current presentation. Trauma may not be explicitly reflected in the diagnosis alone, although it is expected that the 11th revision of the International Classification of Diseases will have a full section devoted to trauma-consequential disorders.

Relationships between stressors and trauma on one hand, and psychiatric diagnoses on the other, have been debated for 100 years, and still remain contentious (Bebbington, 2011; Sato, 2006). Stressors or trauma can be predisposing, precipitating or perpetuating factors in psychiatric presentations. As such they need to be acknowledged by the clinician, discussed between the clinician and the service user, and above all, be taken into account in the comprehensive recovery plan, the method by which the service user and their supporters will manage their experience day by day.

Culture can also be highly significant to the service user's experience. Much debate about culture has centred on diagnostic issues, for example culture bound syndromes and the pathoplastic effect of culture on disorders (eg Strakowski et al 1993; WHO, 2000; Udomratn, 2009; Mellsop & Smith, 2007). Other literature emphasizes the importance of cultural consistency or safety across the spectrum of psychiatric or psychological clinical activities (McClintock et al., 2011a & 2011b).

However, of more universal relevance is the effect of culture on illness behaviour and on attitudes towards mental health services. These factors cannot be addressed within the, necessarily limited, scope of a diagnostic label; their incorporation into the formulation is essential. Without this context, the chances of developing a recovery plan that will be useful and effective to the service user are much diminished (Sato, 2006; Lim et al, 2011; Elder, 2008; Mellsop et al, 2007; Bhui, 2010).

2.2.1 Significance of formulation to the service user and their community

The major emphasis for the non-clinical diagnostic stakeholders - service users, their families and broader community of support - is on fixing the "problems" posed by symptoms and illness. Those who live with a mental illness and/or addiction experience their "problem" as developing over time, and being contributed to by many psychosocial factors (Barnett and Lapsley, 2006). Therefore clinical assessments tend, for stakeholders, to be too short and not take the psycho-social factors sufficiently into account (Laird et al., 2010; O'Hagan, 2000).

For some the diagnosis is a source of confusion, subject to significant change over time. The conspicuous lack of a definitive "silver bullet" is highlighted by service users and their supporters who comment on the frequency with which a new clinician is assigned to their case. Many experience this as being the cue for an automatic re-assessment of the service user and often a change to their current diagnosis, which flows on to the management plan.

> *"… the new psychiatrist wants to prove that he is a better psychiatrist than the last one… Every time [there's] a new doctor, every time a new diagnosis, and therefore different drugs. … then you are going to have new withdrawal symptoms."* (Moeke-Maxwell et al., 2008)

The mother of a service user comments:

> *"They put labels like 'schizophrenic' on to him, but it seemed superficial, they didn't get down to the depth of what it was… I can't put it into words but I just know that they looked at the mental problem, instead of seeing a whole person with a mental problem."* (O'Hagan, 2000)

Frese & Myrick (2010) undertook what they describe as a "quasi-qualititative" survey of United States and some international service users, that yielded some common themes pointing to the significance of formulation to service users.

In general, service users reported that a psychiatric diagnosis could be useful, but its utility to them was limited when the focus of the clinician-service user interaction was mainly on the diagnostic label/s. They expressed a desire to have a wide range of other factors taken into consideration, for example acute medical conditions, physical disorders, psychosocial, environmental and traumatic factors. The primary diagnosis as a stand-alone focus, was described as "not capturing the full picture" and "ignoring the whole person and the world in which we live".

Formulation can offer a particularly useful bridge to the recovery plan, when the diagnosis is highly stigmatized and/or not accepted. In the article cited above, one of the authors documents a personal account of how she worked with clinicians to reframe an unwelcome diagnosis into a construct that was of more use to her.

Keris J. Myrick, who has an MS in Organizational Psychology, received a first diagnosis of depression as a college student while studying in a master's program. She writes of an initial response of relief.

> *"…the diagnosis provided me with information about what was going on in my life that I had attributed to defects in my character. Further, the diagnosis consisted of a word used in everyday language – depression."* (Frese and Myrick, 2010)

However, over time Myrick found that more diagnoses were added, and some were changed. As the "labels" shifted towards words that tend to be used derogatorily in the popular media, and were prefaced by descriptors such as "persistent", "life-long" and "devastating", her first response could not be maintained.

> *"Stereotypes and stigma impacted my belief that anything in the schizophrenia spectrum was beyond depression, and the change in diagnosis was like a seismic shift moving me into the range of 'crazy'."* (Frese and Myrick, 2010)

The relief and acceptance she had felt on her initial diagnosis were replaced by fear and shame. She describes her rejection of a schizophrenia diagnosis as, "the refusal to be labelled as 'crazy'".

However, unfortunately but perhaps inevitably, her refusal to accept the diagnosis was then viewed as further evidence of symptoms that supported the diagnosis. The resulting "lack of insight" impasse is not untypical, but its effects can be serious. It can lead to a lack of engagement with treatment options on the part of the service user; and/or a lack of willingness to continue the effort of hopeful engagement on the part of the service provider (Chinman et al, 1999).

This need not be the case. Myrick writes that, from her perspective, "accepting my diagnosis was not related to my recovery, to engaging in treatment, and/or to taking (or not taking) medications". A clinical partnership between her psychologist and a psychiatrist allowed a broader view to emerge.

> *"...the focus [moved] from acceptance and diagnosis to 'call it whatever you want' and 'what would you like to do with your life, how would you like to accomplish your goals/dreams, what is getting in the way of achieving those goals and dreams, and how can we partner together to assist [you] in achieving those goals/dreams?'*

> *"Thus, the diagnosis took on less importance and relevance. I used the information about the range of symptoms as a construct (man-made)... that can help me to understand the range of possible treatments that I can choose to help me move forward with my life."*(Frese and Myrick, 2010)

Myrick's experience illustrates the importance of a comprehensive consideration of the service user's contextual factors in applying a recovery approach to clinical work. In order to engage with treatment options and move towards recovery, Myrick needed an approach that considered her as a whole person - one that captured the "full picture", including the fear and shame that caused her to reject a particular diagnosis. She needed, in essence, to "recover" the personhood and hope for the future that the diagnostic label of schizophrenia - with all its associated stigma and negative stereotypes - denied her.

2.3 The comprehensive recovery plan

The ultimate outcome of the clinical process must be a comprehensive plan for managing and addressing the symptoms causing distress and/or functional difficulties for the service user. The plan should emerge as an ineluctable result of the summarizing of the assessment information into a formulation, along with any diagnostic conclusions that can be drawn.

More than just a management plan, however, the result will ideally be better described as a recovery plan. This approach to treatment should allow for the person to "recover" not just from the distress caused by their symptoms, but also to "recover" or regain lost ground in terms of social inclusion, autonomy and self-efficacy.

Therefore, the plan needs to be oriented around the overarching goal of the individual being able to live a life that has meaning to them; a life worth living (Barnett and Lapsley, 2006; Moeke-Maxwell et al., 2008; Mental Health Commission, 1998). Ideally, it will support the service user in maximizing their ability to live as they wish, and to also enjoy the concomitant responsibilities inherent in the concept of autonomy.

The plan needs to be comprehensive in the sense that it includes all the actions which need to be taken by both the person seeking help and by the clinician.

Technological changes over the last 30 years, such as advances in neuro-imaging and genetics, have influenced the conceptualisation of mental illness. In that period, society's expectations of mental health care have shifted also, from a focus on biological or medical treatments, to more encompassing and holistic approaches that take into account the broader contextual and psychosocial factors (Frese and Myrick, 2010).

Parallel with these advances has been the increasing availability of what are essentially psychological treatments or clinical management approaches, that are more and more evidence based. Many of these are founded on empirical research, in contrast to the available psychologically based treatments of the first half of the 20th century.

The developments in what is available to be included, and the breadth of service users' expectations, means that a truly comprehensive recovery plan may encompass much more than what is usually thought of under the narrower heading of therapies. For example, it may include referral to other social, personal or health agencies; it may require actions by other individuals within the service users' community of support; it may require further assessments; it may involve immediate actions, and/or a course of action undertaken over a prolonged period of time.

While diagnosis and symptom stabilization may be factors to be addressed, they will seldom be the only aspects of the clinical process that are addressed by the plan, or even its primary focus.

The impact of various diagnostic labels on the ability of the individual to be socially included needs to be carefully considered. Implications can be serious, for the service user and for those who support and care for them (Crumlish and Kelly, 2009; Frese and Myrick, 2010), and need to be taken into account within the plan.

Service users have recommended that clinicians explicitly convey to them the multiple purposes of the diagnostic system used, and encourage them to see beyond any perceived limitations of a diagnosis to how they can work together to help the service user achieve their goals in life. It has been suggested that this could be achieved by ensuring all of the current five DSM axes are considered in treatment and treatment planning (Frese and Myrick, 2010).

At the time of writing, it is not yet clear what axes will operate in the next edition of the American Diagnostic and Statistical Manual (DSM-V). It is clear, however, that the 11th revision of the International Classification of Diseases, currently being developed by the World Health Organisation, will retain the separate classificatory systems (their version of axes) in separate publications. The diagnostic labels will remain in a separate publication from that which deals with level of functioning and/or disability. In that sense, it will differ significantly from the American Diagnostic Statistical Manuals, where impairment of functioning is usually a requirement for any individual diagnosis to be allocated (APA, 2000).

One approach that has been endorsed by service users for how to engage diagnostic classifications in ways that are useful to them, is the ADDRESSING framework proposed by Pamela Hays (2006; cited in Frese and Myrick, 2010). This approach would add value to whichever diagnostic system the clinician uses, by including consideration of the individual's age, developmental and acquired disabilities, religion, ethnicity, socioeconomic status, sexual orientation, indigenous heritage, national origin, and gender.

Finally, in order to be both comprehensive and recovery-oriented, the plan must be developed and endorsed collaboratively. This may not be a straightforward part of the process, however.

Service providers and service users have been found to differ greatly in their perceptions of service user interest in collaborative treatment planning. In one study, 60% of service providers believed their clients' lack of interest was a barrier to working collaboratively on treatment planning, whereas only 15% of service users thought this was the case.

As perceived by service users, the principal barriers to working effectively together were a lack of time available within the process, lack of knowledge of how to work collaboratively, and uncertainty that setting treatment goals would help (Chinman et al., 1999).

While a collaborative approach may then require time and effort to achieve, this can be seen as a highly worthwhile investment at the front-end of the process that is likely to ensure better engagement and, ultimately, better outcomes for the service user. It is an essential component of the "recovery" philosophy.

3. Conclusion

Diagnosis is an inescapable factor in the clinical process. It carries significance for service users and those who support them, but as a logical conclusion to the clinical assessment it is insufficient, and it cannot stand alone.

The formulation is a summary of the information gathered via the assessment process(es). It provides an extensive, individualistic and idiographic context to aid understanding of what is occurring for this person at this time, and why this may be so. As such, it provides a wealth of information that is not just useful to developing the recovery plan, but essential to it.

Thus, while the diagnosis may suggest a particular course of action, this will be as part of a comprehensive recovery plan underpinned by the narrative provided by the formulation.

By taking care to contextualize the diagnosis with a thorough and reflective formulation, clinicians can better address the gap between what service users expect from a health diagnosis and the limitations of the diagnostic classification system in psychiatry. This process can also ameliorate the effects of stigma and negative media stereotyping that accompany certain diagnoses.

The collaboratively agreed recovery plan that results from this dynamic combination of diagnosis and formulation will then be better placed to effectively meet the service user's needs.

4. References

APA (2000). Diagnostic and Statistical Manual of Mental Disorders (4th edn, text revision). American Psychiatric Association, ISBN 0-89042-024-6, Washington, DC

APA (2006). Practice Guidelines for the Treatment of Psychiatric Disorders: Compendium. American Psychiatric Association, ISBN 978-0-89042-3837, Arlington, Virginia

Barnett, H., & Lapsley, H. (2006). Journeys of Despair, Journeys of Hope. Mental Health Commission, ISBN 0-478-29211-2, Wellington

Bebbington, P., Jonas, S., Kuipers, E., King, M., Cooper, C., Brugha, T., Meltzer, H., McManus, S., Jenkins, R. (2011) Childhood Sexual abuse and Psychosis: data from a cross-sectional national psychiatric survey in England. Brit J Psychiat, 199, 29-36.

Beltz. (1967). A Triad of Conceptual Models for Formulating and Teaching Psychodynamics. American J Psychiatry, 123:1087-1093. ISSN 0002-953X

Bhui, K. (2010) Culture & Complex Interventions: lessons for evidence based policy & practice. Brit J Psychiat, 197, 172-3.

Byrne, P. (2007). Managing the Acute Psychotic Episode. Brit Med J, 334:686-692. ISSN 0959-8146

Carey, T. A., & Pilgrim, D. (2010). Diagnosis and Formulation: What Should We Tell the Students? Clinical Psychology and Psychotherapy, 17, 447-454.

Chinman ,M . J., Allende, M., Weingarten, R., Steiner, J., Tworkowski, S., Davidson, L. (1999). On the Road to Collaborative Treatment Planning: Consumer and Provider Perspectives. *Journal of Behavioral Health Services & Research.* Vol.26, No. 2, May 1999, pp.211-218, ISSN

Crumlish, N., & Kelly, B. D. (2009). How psychiatrists think. Advances in Psychiatric Treatment, 15, 72-79

Duncan, B.L., Miller, S.D., Wampold, B.E., Hubble, M.A. (2010). The Heart and Soul of change: Delivering what works in therapy. Pub Amer Psychol Assoc, Washington

Eells, T. D., Kendjelic, E. M., Lucas, C. P. (1998). What's in a Case Formulation? Development and Use of a Content Coding Manual. The Journal of Psychotherapy Practice and Research, 7, 144-453.

Elder, H, (2008). Ko wai ahau? (Who am I?) How cultural identity issues are experienced by Maori psychiatrists and registrars working with children and adolescents. Australasian Psychiatry 16:200-203

Frese, F. J. and Myrick, K. J. (2010). On consumer advocacy and the diagnosis of mental disorders. Professional Psychology:Research and Practice 41:495-501

Hanzawa, S., Bae, J-K., Tanak, H., Tanaka, G., Bae, Y. J., Goto, M., Inadomi, H., Ohta, Y., Nakane, H., Nakane, Y.,(2009) Family stigma and care burden of schizophrenia patients: Comparison between Japan and Korea, Asia-Pacific Psychiatry, 1:120-129, ISSN 1758-5864

Hyman, S.E. (2010). The diagnosis of mental disorders: The problem of reification. Annual Review of Clinical Psychology, 6,155-79. ISSN 1584-5951

Insel, T., Cuthbert, B., Garvey, M., Heinsein, R., Pine, D.S., Quinn, K., Sanislow, C., & Wang, P. (2010). Research Domain Criteria (RDoC): Toward a new classification framework for research on Mental Disorders. American Journal of Psychiatry, 167, 748-751. ISSN 0002953X

IAG (2011). International Advisory Group for the Revision of ICD-10 Mental and Behavioural Disorders. A conceptual framework for the revision of the ICD-10 classification of mental and behavioural disorders. World Psychiatry,10:86-92

Laird, B., Smith, B., Dutu, G., Mellsop, G. (2010). Views and Experiences of Family/Whanau Carers of Psychiatric Service Users on Diagnosis and Classification. International Journal of Social Psychiatry 56:270-279 0:0020764008101637

Lim, L.L., Chang, W., Yu, X., Chiu, H., Chong, M-Y., Kua, E.H. (2010). Depression in Chinese elderly populations. Asia-Pacific Psychiatry 3:46-53.

Mace, C., & Binyon, S. (2005). Teaching psychodynamic formulation to psychiatric trainees: Part 1: Basics of formulation. Advances in Psychiatric Treatment, 11, 416-423

McClintock, K. K., Mellsop, G. W., Merry, S., Moeke-Maxwell, T. Powhiri process in mental health research (2011a) International Journal of Social Psychiatry. DOI: 10.1177/0020764010387067

McClintock, K. K., Mellsop, G. W., Kingi, Te K. (2011b) Development of a culturally attuned outcome measure for an indigenous population. International Journal of Culture and Mental Health, 1-16. ISSN 1754-2871

Maj, M. (2005). Psychiatric comorbidity: An artefact of current diagnostic systems? British Journal of Psychiatry, 186,182-184. ISSN 0007-1250

Mellsop, G.W., & Banzato, C. (2006). A concise conceptualisation of formulation. Academic Psychiatry, 30, 424-425 ISSN 1545-7236

Mellsop, G.W., Banzato, C.E.M., Shinfuku, N., Nagamine, M., Pereira, N.E.C. & Dutu, G. (2008). An international study of the views of psychiatrists on present and preferred characteristics of classifications of psychiatric disorders. International Journal of Mental Health, 36, 17-25. ISSN 0020-7411

Mellsop, G.W., Menkes, D. & El-Badri, S. (2007). Releasing psychiatry from the constraints of categorical diagnosis. Australasian Psychiatry, 15, 3-5. ISSN 1039-8562

Mellsop, G.W., Smith, B., (2007). Reflections on masculinity, culture and the diagnosis of depression. Australian and New Zealand Journal of Psychiatry, 41:850-853

Mental Health Commission. (1998). Blueprint for Mental Health Services in New Zealand: How Things Need to Be. Wellington, Mental Health Commission.

Moeke-Maxwell, T., Wells, D., Mellsop, G. (2008). Tangata Whaiora/Consumers' Perspectives on Current Psychiatric Classification Systems. International Journal of Mental Health Systems, 2:7. ISSN 1752-4458

NICE (2003). Full National Clinical Guidelines on Core Interventions in Primary and Secondary Care. National Collaborating Centre for Mental Health. Gaskell, ISBN 190467125X, London

Nurcombe, B., Fitzhenry-Coor, I. (1987). Diagnostic Reasoning and Treatment Planning; I. Diagnosis. Australian & NZ Journal of Psychiatry; 21:477-483. ISSN 00048674

O'Hagan, M. (Ed.). (2000). Three forensic service users and their families talk about recovery, Mental Health Commission, ISBN 0-478-11372-2, Wellington

Read, J., van Os, J., Morrison, A. P., Ross, C. A. (2005). Childhood trauma, psychosis and schizophrenia: a literature review with theoretical and clinical implications. Acta Psychiatrica Scandinavia, 112, pp. 330-350, ISSN 001-690X

Robins, E., & Guze, S.B. (1970). Establishment of Diagnostic Validity in Psychiatric Illness: Its Application to Schizophrenia. American Journal of Psychiatry 126, 983-986. ISSN 0002-953X

Sato, M. (2006). Renaming schizophrenia: a Japanese perspective. World Psychiatry 5:1 53-55

Strakowski, S., Shelton, R.C., Kolbrener, M.L. (1993). The effects of race and comorbidity on clinical diagnosis in patients with psychosis. J Clin Psychiatry 54:3, 96-102

Udomratn, P. (2009). How Thailand has modified the section on mental disorders in the International Statistical Classification of Diseases and Related Health Problems 10th Revision (ICD-10).Asia-Pacific Psychiatry 1:88-89

Varghese, F. T., & Mellsop, G. W. (1983). Formulating the Psychiatric Case. Bulletin, R C Psych, March :48:50

WHO (2000). International Consortium of Psychiatric Epidemiology. Cross-national comparisions of the prevalences and correlates of mental disorders: WHO International Consortium in Psychiatric Epidemiology. Bulletin of the World Health Organization 2000; 78:413-426

WHO (1992). Classification of Mental and Behavioural Disorders Clinical Descriptions and Diagnostic Guidelines. World Health Organisation, Geneva.

4

Hypnosis in Cancer Patients: Can We Do Better?

Fabrice Kwiatkowski
University of Psychology, Paris 8,
Centre Jean Perrin, Clermont, Ferrand,
France

1. Introduction

There is an official history of hypnotism: very often it begins with the Scottish surgeon James Braid (1795-1860) who was one of the first physicians to have used this word in 1843. Instead of using the standard magnetic induction popularized by magnetism/mesmerism[1], he proposed his subjects to stare steadily at a shiny object to enter a trance. He tested his method to anesthetize his patients during surgeries (Braid, 1843). The practice of hypnosis, using deliberate techniques to help focus attention, is recent, but trance states have always been part of the human experience. Many kinds of trance phenomena are observed in shamanism, fakirism, witchcraft, and religion but also in psychopathology. After remaining an inglorious stage practice in western countries, hypnosis has begun to gain relevance in

---

[1]There are slight differences between "mesmerism" and "animal magnetism". Here the label "mesmerism" is used as it is more encountered in the USA. In this country as well as in England, a secondary current emerged among "magnetizers" in order to remove all practices that they thought irrelevant or that did not seem to contribute to the cure. However, both derive from the practice first developped by Anton Mesmer (1734-1815) that he himself called "animal magnetism". For our topic, it is refered here to the wide research on "magnetism" that has started later in 1784 with the Marquis de Puységur and lasted for more than one century mostly in France and England. Studies and practices focused on several main points:

- the reproduction of (alleged) results obtained under magnetic trance (cures but also various phenomena such as blind reading, hyperscience, clear-sightedness...)
- the definition of the medium (magnetic fluid, suggestion...) causing both trance and phenomena
- new concepts about the human psyche that these phenomena (if agreed) made necessary.

The controversy that opposed top physicians, scientists and philosophers, ended at the begining of the 20th along with the onset of psychoanalysis. All the very interesting results (although discussed) have suddenly been swept off. The opponents of magnetism argued that alleged phenomena were either caused by gullible practitioners who were abused by their hysterical patients, or originated in manipulations performed by charlatans (Meheust, 1999). Meanwhile, the emerging science of hypnosis has also been put aside as Freud claimed that results obtained by hypnosis did not last as long as those gained in full counsciousness by psychoanalysis... While this field of experimentation was abandonned in Europe, it has regained interest after 1950 both in the USA and USSR with parapsychology, in particular thanks to the financial support of military agencies: for these latter, new means to obtain information or exert an influence were sought. But for scientists, "animal magnetism" is nowadays considered an irrelevant matter of interest, perhaps too rapidly.

medicine as has proven a real efficiency in several domains; thanks to Milton Erickson (1901-1980), it has earned its place as a therapeutic approach in psychology.

Hypnosis is still at the margins of the scientific mainstream. After the eviction of mesmerism and many related phenomena from the list of tolerated experimental fields (Meheust, 1999), some effort is still required to limit the description of emergences under trance to something acceptable and analyzable. Psychology and medicine seem to have satisfied these criteria in their use of hypnosis as sought goals are largely agreed. Although purposes vary widely, their experimental fields overlap because of the very nature of hypnosis. They both use hypnosis for the benefit of patients. They use some of the same scientific methods, including functional imagery and clinical trials or surveys whose design seems sufficient to assure confidence in the conclusions. In relation to psychosomatic troubles, medicine and psychology share a no man's land where medical treatment appears insufficient and where patient support is necessary (for example pain management). The use of hypnosis consists of mild practices that, according to psychologists, are respectful of individuals' will: these range from relaxation techniques coupled with guided imagery and/or suggestions to more complex tailored hypnosis where trance can be deeper. Self hypnosis belongs to this group of techniques, as it is often encountered in educational/behavioral patient management. No discussion will question here the validity of such a grouping of techniques.

Among medical fields, oncology is a particularly good domain for the use of hypnosis, because cancer is typical of the difficult diseases where medicine fails. This chapter reports the different trials and investigations that today build the consensus on which the routine practice of hypnosis thrives. After hoping for a prognostic impact of hypnosis on cancer itself, investigations have changed their target and now focus on alleviating side-effects of the disease and/or its treatment. The issues studied concern immunity and treatment response. Surveys concentrate on patients' well-being as well as more specialized topics such as anxiety, depression, fatigue, and pain. Very specialized issues, such as hot flushes after cancer treatment, are also addressed.

2. The impact of hypnosis on cancer itself

2.1 Survival outcomes

The first trial investigating survival as a main endpoint[2] was reported by Newton (1983). Unfortunately, the design was inappropriate, as patients were not randomized between the treatment conditions (with or without hypnosis). Also, patients who received less than three one-hour weekly hypnosis sessions were compared to those receiving at least three. As expected, life was shorter for the patients dying before they could receive at least 3 sessions. Despite these weaknesses, this investigation launched a long series of prospective research on psychosocial interventions, at a rate of about one per year since 1985 (Kwiatkowski, 2009). Another trial tested hypnosis as the main psychosocial intervention in patients diagnosed with melanoma (Walker, 2000), but it contained the same kind of methodological flaws, and thus the slight difference in favor of hypnosis could not be trusted.

[2]Endpoint is often used in this chapter because its meaning differs slightly from the words goal and purpose. In clinical research, endpoint is the measurable goal (ex. goal = to live longer; endpoint = survival time - goal = to live better; endpoint = score with the quality of life questionnaire)

Four other randomized controlled trials investigated the impact on survival of educational supportive interventions (group therapy) including self-hypnosis to help patients handle pain or anxiety (Spiegel, 1989; Goodwin, 2001; Kissane, 2007; Spiegel, 2007). Intervention consisted of weekly 90 minutes group sessions where women were encouraged to share and confront their problems, strengthen their relationships, discuss strategies for coping with cancer and find enhanced meaning in their lives. But no suggestion was given to let them believe the intervention could increase their odds of survival. Patients were asked to attend sessions during one year in parallel with standard cancer treatments. The first trial that included only 86 patients with metastatic breast carcinoma, was significant, reducing by 24% the risk of death (Spiegel, 1989) while median survival time after randomization was 17 months longer in the intervention group. The three further trials, performed with a similar design to confirm this outcome, included respectively 235, 227 and 122 women. Unfortunately, they did not show any prognostic advantage for the intervention.

2.2 Impact on the response to chemotherapy

The response to chemotherapy is an interesting endpoint because it usually correlates to overall survival: the better the tumor regresses, the longer the patient survives (with or without relapse/metastasis). Walker et al. (1998, 1999) tested a protocol including relaxation training and guided imagery. Before the first course of chemotherapy, patients randomized to the test group were taught a relaxation method that consisted of "progressive muscular and cue-controlled relaxation" (Hutchings, 1980). The patients were given audiotapes with relaxation instructions and asked to look at a portfolio of cartoons to help them imagine their immune cells destroying the cancer. They also kept a diary to record their daily practice duration. Response to treatment and personal practice was evaluated at the end of the chemotherapy. No significant difference in tumor regression was observed between the two treatment conditions, although a weak association was found between the vividness of imagery and clinical tumor response.

2.3 Enhancement of immunity

Immune cells, mainly lymphoid natural killer (NK) cells, play a major role in tumor cell lysis, and provoking an immune response is useful in cancer treatment. Immunity is probably responsible for the spontaneous complete remissions without treatment observed in melanoma, and partial histopathological remissions in breast cancer (Horii, 2005). In addition, metastasis are often discovered but no primitive tumor can be identified: this suggests that the immune system destroyed the initial tumor cells.

Immunity can be thought of as another self, connecting the psychic and physical selves, and capable of learning and memory (i.e. adaptation). For psychologists, a special property of this immune self is that it can be conditioned (Ader, 1993)[3], which makes it a target of choice

[3]Ader's experiment consisted of the combination of an unconditional immune stimulus (the delivery of a dose of Cyclosporin) with a neutral stimulus (ex. a colored light, a bell or some food) and the repetition of their presentation together. Each time after the Cyclosporin infusion, blood was sampled and some immune factors measured: the results showed the expected immune drop. After a certain number of iterations, only the neutral stimulus was given, but surprisingly, there was a similar drop in immune markers without the use of any drug. Immunity can thus be conditioned.

for hypnosis. Hypnosis has already demonstrated a real efficiency against auto-immune disease, including allergy and asthma (Hackman, 2000; Langewitz, 2005) with a significant decrease of symptoms for patients trained for self-hypnosis.

However, the immune system is very complex and many different parameters (white cell count, cytotoxic potential of NK, cytokines, hormones, cell receptors...) need to be taken into account if one wants to discover significant effects. This multiplicity of parameters increases the risk of false positive study outcomes. The immune system is also affected by variations in gene expression, and this expression can itself be altered by hypnosis (Rossi, 2002). Data demonstrate the high level of interaction between biological and psychological functions, and it is noteworthy that influences are bi-directional (Kiecolt-Glaser, 1999; Temoshok, 2002).

Behavior is another lever that can be used to enhance immunity. As immunity is very dependent on circadian rhythms (mainly the activity-sleep cycle) and on the use of psychotropic substances (tobacco, alcohol, hypnotics, drugs...), any behavioral change that aims to reduce addiction or ameliorate circadian rhythms can benefit immunity. Conversely, this probably explains why chronic depression almost doubles cancer risk in the elderly (Penninx, 1998) as it generally disturbs sleep. Many kinds of psychosocial intervention targeting behavior, such as group relaxation training, meditation, are able to influence immunity. Since the immune system appears weak in cancer patients (since mutated cells avoid cellular immunity), psychosocial approaches can be proposed to remedy this deficiency: hypnosis stands in good place among them.

A first trial testing a psychiatric intervention (including relaxation training but without hypnosis) involved patients with malignant melanoma (Fawzy, 1990). Affective changes related to the intervention were correlated to NK levels. Bakke and col. (2002) tested longitudinally relaxation plus guided imagery in stage I-II breast cancer patients. After eight weeks of training, no change in NK cytotoxicity was observed, but the NK lymphocyte fraction increased in parallel to improvements in mood. These results were not sustained after a 3-month follow-up. In 2008, Lengacher et al. performed a pilot study using the same pretest-posttest design in the same kind of population (28 breast cancer patients aged 25 to 75 years). NK cell cytotoxicity was significantly improved four weeks post-surgery. Both trials, although of limited sample size, suggest that hypnosis can positively impact the immune system. Emotions/mood seemed more correlated to immune changes than coping attitudes were: this might be of importance in defining the strategies for suggestions during hypnosis sessions.

3. Hypnosis and patients' well-being

As the trials focusing on overall survival turned out negative, new goals for hypnosis have been proposed. The main issues now addressed include quality of life, mood, depression, anxiety, and of course pain. We review these topics hereafter.

3.1 Quality of life

Quality of life (QOL) is an accurately standardized concept developed over the past 3 or 4 decades. QOL reflects a great variety of parameters among which cancer status, treatments toxicities[4], physical and psychosocial dimensions, sexual functioning and even financial difficulties. Validated self-questionnaires such as QLQ-C30 (Aaronson, 1993) or SF36 (Wade, 1992) enable a good evaluation of patients' QOL in both curative or palliative situations except when the disease becomes too severe and end of life is expected. In the latter, specialized questionnaires are nowadays available (MV-QOLI (Byock, 1998), Qual-E (Steinhauser, 2002)). In palliative situations, QOL is sometimes chosen as surrogate endpoint for survival (Methy, 2010). However, QOL questionnaires find some limitations in childhood (Payot, 2011), especially with the youngest patients who cannot of course fill out questionnaires and with palliative patients who sometimes need the help of a relative or of a nurse to answer the questions or write the answers.

Very interesting research has been performed by Liossi and White (2001) on the impact of tailored hypnosis sessions on QOL among 50 terminally ill cancer patients. Intervention consisted of four 30 minutes weekly personal hypnosis sessions and it was compared to a cognitive-existential support given at the same rhythm. Suggestions were most often made in order to help patient manage his predominant symptoms but ego-strengthening suggestions were also used, either general or specific. Patients were asked to fill out QOL questionnaires (the Rotterdam Symptom Checklist (DeHaes, 1990) and the HADS (Zigmond, 1983)) before and after each session. The protocol duration was four weeks. Hypnosis demonstrated significant superiority over cognitive-existential management, improving QOL scores and reducing depression and anxiety. Other trials included QOL as secondary endpoint (Spiegel, 1989, 2007; Goodwin, 2001), and similar benefits in QOL were reported. Although QOL is a general and easy to use index, too few trials have focused on it. This endpoint should receive more attention in further research.

3.2 Depression and anxiety

Sporadic depression moderately increases (by 20%) cancer risk (Dalton, 2002), while chronic depression seems to have an even greater impact on this risk (Penninx, 1998). Conversely, cancer favors depression, as almost 50% of patients will face this mood disorder during their treatment or in the following years (Derogatis, 1983; Morasso, 2001; Harter, 2001). Depression causes a lot of personal suffering and should be treated for that sole reason. Depression has also been suggested to shorten survival because it reduces treatment compliance, but also because it increases the suicide rate (Reich, 2007). Another reason to manage depression in cancer patients is that this symptom correlates to poor immune response (Lutgendorf, 2008; Steel, 2007) and worse prognosis (Watson, 1999; Hjerl, 2003). This makes depression a major target for psychosocial intervention (Spiegel, 2003).

In the previously cited trials testing the impact on survival of a cognitive-behavioral therapy including self-hypnosis, all authors reported a significant positive impact of this intervention on depression and anxiety among breast cancer patients. In terminally ill cancer patients, Liossi (2001) obtained similar improvements. As cancer survivors may also experience depression, Elkins et al. (2008) performed a trial testing the impact of 5 weekly sessions of hypnosis plus self-hypnosis training, and observed a significant decrease in anxiety and depression scores in the treatment group.

---

[4] Chemotherapy, radiotherapy and even hormonotherapy can induce various side-effects: haematological toxicities (mainly destruction of leucocytes), fatigue, nausea, vomiting, loss of appetite, hot-flushes, hair loss, skin syndrome, paresthesia...

Overall, hypnosis appears to be a good alternative to conventional psychotherapy against depression (Alladin, 2007). Very few other non-pharmacologic approaches reach its efficacy, although meditation plus yoga showed remission rates comparable to those obtained with a combination antidepressants and psychotherapy (Butler, 2008; Kocsis, 2000). This conclusion is not surprising, as meditation is another means to alter consciousness and obtain a trance. These approaches should thus be tested in cancer patients, where the incidence of depression is very high.

3.3 Pain management

Milton Erickson (1959) was the first author to report the efficacy of hypnosis against pain in cancer patients. Pain should not be considered an isolated symptom of the disease or its treatment. Often, pain has a psychosocial dimension in our culture that echoes both social loneliness and personal distress (Zaza, 2000). It therefore requires the intervention of skilled psychologists. Acute pain should be considered separately as it is often a consequence of surgery and may be treated efficiently with analgesic drugs. Two domains are available to hypnosis, as analgesic treatment may expose patients to severe side-effects (for example respiratory complications):

- expected pain during invasive medical procedures
- chronic pain, especially during palliative treatment.

Several trials have demonstrated the utility of hypnosis to counterbalance anticipated aches by children undergoing painful medical procedures such as lumbar puncture or bone marrow aspiration. Hypnotic techniques (guided imagery, direct or indirect suggestions) applied during medical procedures appeared more efficient than behavioral techniques (cognitive-behavioral training, distraction) to reduce fear, anxiety and pain during procedures (Zelter, 1982; Katz, 1987; Smith, 1996; Liossi, 1999). In these studies, patients age ranged from 3 to 15 and sample size of the trials was around 30. In children, the magnitude of the result depends on hypnotizability of these young patients, and switching to self-hypnosis is less efficient than hypnosis induced by a therapist (Hawkins, 1998; Smith, 1996). Butler (2005) tested an interesting hypnosis strategy against pediatric pain when he trained children as well as their parents, observing a significant reduction of pain, procedural time and thus overall costs thanks to hypnosis. In adults, trials addressing this issue are scarce. Montgomery (2002) successfully tested hypnosis to reduce pain and distress in women undergoing breast biopsy. This shows that such an approach should be employed more frequently, instead of assuming that adults are able to manage the transient pain induced by medical procedures, or that short-term pain does not matter.

Chronic pains offer a different context for hypnosis. Cancer pain is usually caused by the tumor invasion or its pressure on nerves. Medical, surgical and radiological treatment of lesions are used to stop the disease and this often controls suffering directly, even if the short-term complementary use of analgesics may be useful. When medical management is not sufficient to durably prevent pain, complementary therapy is necessary, in order to avoid side-effects of long-term analgesic use (Deng, 2005) and frequent depression symptoms associated with both pain and analgesics. Pain complaints also significantly increase the burden for caregivers, whether relatives or professionals.

Self-hypnosis training plus group therapy was found to significantly reduce pain in women with metastatic breast cancer in the previously discribed trial of Spiegel et al. (Spiegel, 1983). A same strategy with breast cancer patients was tested over a four month period (Butler, 2009): it significantly reduced chronic pain intensity over the period but not the frequency of pain episodes or the amount of constant pain. Syrjala (1992) confirmed some of these outcomes in a trial including 94 male or female adult patients diagnosed with leukemia, myelodysplasia or lymphoma, and suffering from persistent oral mucositis pain following bone marrow transplantation. Before hospitalization, training material (information on relaxation, deep breathing and audio-tapes) was presented through one-to-one interaction in two sessions. During hospitalization, patients were seen twice a week, one session including in-vivo relaxation and imagery. Patients were asked to practice daily. Patients of the control group recieved the standard treatment and an other control group was offered therapist support. After 5 weeks, pain was significantly alleviated by hypnosis. This trial tested also, in adjunction to hypnosis, a cognitive-behavioral coping skills training. This training showed no supplementary effect on pain measures.

Controlled trial assessing the impact of hypnosis on chronic pain over the long run are lacking: therapeutic strategies covering longer intervals should be addressed in further studies.

3.4 Treatment side-effects

Typically, to meet treatment goals, antitumor drugs have to be toxic, surgery invasive and radiation aggressive. Targeted treatments such as monoclonal antibodies may not change this situation. Aside from pain, side-effects comprise a large set of symptoms: nausea, vomiting, fatigue, and neuropathy, and psychological disturbances more or less related to these symptoms. They may lower the patient's therapeutic alliance with his physician and/or require dose reductions or delayed schedules, and thus limit the efficacy of treatment. Because these symptoms often appear before the treatment begins, it has been suggested that hypnosis could significantly remedy this problem.

Nausea and vomiting are some of the most frequently encountered side-effects of chemotherapy. A universally effective anti-emetic medication remains elusive (Koeller, 2002), although important advances have been made. Complementary approaches are therefore interesting, especially for anticipatory symptoms. Three trials tested this question using self-hypnosis (Syrjala, 1992; Jacknow, 1994; Hawkins, 1995) that patients were supposed to use before and during treatments, while the other one proposed tailored individual hypnosis (Zelter, 1991) including imaginative fantasy with suggestions (for example, holding or cuddling a pet). All these trials concerned pediatric cancer patients except for Syrjala (1992). Because of the small sample size of the four trials, a meta-analysis was conducted by Richardson (2007) who concluded that hypnotherapy significantly lessened symptoms. Overall, hypnosis was twice more efficient against nausea and/or vomiting symptoms than therapist contact and five times more than cognitive-behavioral management. Trials including pediatric patients contributed the most to the effect size but the other one including adults demonstrated no difference between intervention conditions.

Fatigue is a frequent side-effect of cancer treatments, although the disease itself can concurrently be responsible for it. In one trial of radiotherapy, this symptom was stabilized by cognitive-behavioral therapy plus hypnosis, while the control group showed a linear increase of fatigue scores over the same period (Montgomery, 2009).

Hot-flushes in breast cancer patients are an underestimated symptom that affects almost 80% of the women undergoing chemotherapy and 70% of those treated by hormonotherapy (Carpenter, 2001). It also concerns female patients and survivors of other cancer locations and is often associated with other physical symptoms including headaches, palpitations, or insomnia, and psychological difficulties such as irritation, or a sense of loss of control. Elkins (2008) included 60 females in remission of their breast cancer who suffered from frequent and/or intense hot-flushes. The five weekly sessions of hypnosis defined in the trial protocol consisted of "*mental imagery and suggestions for relaxation; mental imagery for coolness; deepening hypnosis and dissociation from hot flashes; positive suggestions and imagery for the future*". Results showed that hot-flushes frequency could be largely reduced by hypnosis (by 68%) and that this reduction had a significant impact on overall quality of life and sleep.

3.5 Management of digestive symptoms

The digestive system and the treatment of related diseases and symptoms is a particular medical domain where hypnosis and psychosocial intervention can demonstrate their interest and at the same time shed new light on the interactions between mind and body. Thanks to Gershon's findings (1965, 1998) on the importance of what he called "the second brain", we now know that one of the most influential hormones on mood and depression (serotonin) is mainly secreted by enteric neurons, and that these neurons together form a network capable of autonomous responses. The digestive system is known to respond to psychological stress and emotions (Jones, 2006) although gastric troubles as ulcers have recently disappeared from the list of the psychosomatic diseases[5]. In 2008, Charioni et al. reviewed the literature testing the efficacy of hypnosis in the modulation of upper digestive motor and secretory function (more than 20 published reports). This did not take into account previously reported management against nausea and vomiting. Studies investigating the secretory function are not easy. They need nasogastric intubations in order to collect gastric secretion and sampling has to be made before and after the hypnosis intervention. Studies focusing on the gastric motor function needs less invasive procedures: real-time ultrasonography can measure with a good reliability gastric emptying rate using the diameter variation of the gastric antrum in the sagittal plane passing through the aorta. Suggestions must fit targeted funtions: to induce an increase of acid secretions in healthy volonteers, they are asked to visualize and eat the most delicious meal possible, while sensory aspects of the eating process, including food appearance, aroma, texture and taste, are explored and reinforced by hypnotist. On the opposite, the averting-food strategy uses intense imagery to divert one's attention from eating. Imagery may concern lying on a beach, watching a sunset, or meeting a friend in a nice environment. To accelerate gastric motility, water flowing in a river or in a waterfall can be used; suggesting warmth in one hand and placing it over the epigastrium can associate suggestion of improved well being and gastric function mediated by the warmth of the hand.

[5] Most often, peptic ulcers are caused by helicobacter pylori infection of the stomach and/or the use of NSAIDs, but about 20% of cases seem not related to either risk factor, and psychological factors are still suspected for them. Also, it is not impossible that psychological stress may alter gastric metabolism and thus favor the proliferation of the bacteria.

Reported investigations confirmed significant effects of hypnosis. The authors concluded that *"hypnosis delivered in a single session by an expert therapist has been shown capable of modulating gastric secretion and accelerating gastric emptying in healthy volunteers. In addition, hypnosis has improved gastric emptying and epigastric sensations in severe functional dyspepsia. Small bowel transit may also be influenced by hypnosis"* (Charioni, 2008 p.6282) As the delay of resumption of intestinal transit is of major importance in colorectal cancer surgery, hypnosis may be useful to reduce this delay and facilitate recovery. This field of research remains unexplored.

4. Conclusion

Numerous valuable works have been performed to test the use of hypnosis in oncology. Most of the results are encouraging and often durable: despite no definitive effect on the cancer prognosis itself has been objectivized, hypnosis has demonstrated its utility in many aspects of patient's well-being. The methodology used in these cross-sectional studies has largely improved over the past decades (Moyer, 2009), although some authors suggested that hypnotic protocols should be more accurately defined (Wild, 2004). Most published investigations were based on solution-oriented strategies: hypnosis was used to remedy one particular problem (pain, side-effects, hot flushes...). On the other hand, trials with more global goals (depression, quality of life) included hypnosis as a complementary method within a more general cognitive-educational approach. In fact, aside from a study of terminally ill cancer patients (Liossi, 2001), most studies used hypnosis in a very limited scope and/or as one of many psychological tools. Self-hypnosis has been used more often, and is usually taught during group sessions. This is regrettable, as outcomes seem better when sessions are adapted to the patient's needs and desires (Syrjala, 1995) and only individual sessions enable such tailoring. Similarly, relaxation plus guided imagery represents only a small part of the various hypnosis techniques. Other techniques only available with tailored hypnosis enable the management of deeper psychological difficulties, and their resolution could result in a stronger effect on the cancer itself.

Trials performed to test the effect of hypnosis on gastric system were more often done within personal sessions, but for experimental reasons, their goal was limited to localized somatic objectives. Therefore, no study really investigated with a correct methodology the impact of hypnosis on overall survival in cancer patients.

Hypnosis remains an under-exploited therapy that has not revealed its full capacities against cancer. Although medical painful routine procedures and treatments side-effects are valuable targets for short interventions, researchers should be more audacious in the determination of goals. There are large domains that remain unexplored (immunity, genetics) and investigations in these domains could very well help understand how psyche interacts with soma (and vice-versa). Biological research always needs an accurate definition of goals, and parameters that objectivize changes in these goals. This does not imply that associated hypnotic protocols should also be reduced to a single induction type and/or a limited suggestions panel. On the other hand, when a person is taught self-hypnosis within a larger set of tailored hypnosis sessions, it provides him new skills to handle personally his pathology and/or other life problems. In such a strategy, the physical symptom could be considered as the starting point of an evolutive mental process that could benefit the whole personality of the patient. *"For clinician, hypnosis is an opportunity to be inventive, spontaneous and playful and to build a stronger therapeutic relationship with a patient while providing symptom relief*" (Liossi, 2006, p.55).

Hypnotisability, or susceptibility to hypnosis, is often supposed to limit the efficacy of hypnosis (Smith, 1996; Hawkins, 1998; Butler, 2009). Although Erickson claimed that 100% of normal people can be hypnotized and that most unsuccessful protocol failed because a too short time is reserved for the induction (Erickson, 1980; 1982), some studies have questioned if the power of suggestions coud vary with the subject's sensitivity to hypnotic induction. This question seems to have been solved thanks to Raz's experiment with the stroop test[6] where he demonstrated that hightly hypnotisable subjects were more likely to short-circuit neuronal networks managing conflicts than less hypnotisable subjects (Raz, 2005). According to a large meta-analysis of 57 controlled trials testing hypnosis (Flammer, 2003), the hypnotic susceptibility was responsible for about 20% of treatment outcomes. This percentage is not negligible but this means that 80% of hypnosis capacities depend on other parameters: this is a reassuring perspective. To our mind, hypnotisability should be tested if a rather fixed hypnotic protocol is used as sole intervention. With face-to-face tailored inductions, the hypnotist can adapt his suggestions to his subject's characteristics and generally obtain the trance depth or the receptivity he thinks necessary.

As hypnosis requires only a few days training from physicians or nurses that want to use it in specialized contexts, some assume that this technique is rather simple and does not deserve any more effort and learning. Also, because psychological formation of physicians and nurses is rather limited, this can prevent them from engaging a deeper dialog with their patients and incite them to limit their support to what seems sufficient for their medical purpose. In such a situation, well defined and reduced hypnotic procedures may be felt protective: it holds off the threat of crisis that they could not keep under control. The separation between psychology and medicine raises another type of difficulty. For psychologists, symptoms management may represent a minor target compared to patients' psychic well-being and evolution; but they can feel limited if they have to evaluate a physical symptom or make a decision about it. Is seems thus important that research teams include both types of practitioners, the physicians defining the primary endpoint (necessarily restricted if medical) and the psychologists/hypnotists the hypnotic strategy (as large as they wish, that is adaptable to patient's personality and needs) and possible secondary endpoints.

Performed by skilled practitioners, hypnosis has a great potential mostly unexplored in oncology, especially as cancer represents for patients a major threat for life and since many patients are left without efficient medical solution. The consequences of this disease are so extensive that it exhausts psychological resources of individuals, and very often drives them to depression. Hypnosis has proven to be one of the most efficient psychological tools. It can contribute more rapidly than other psychosocial managements to biological changes. It does not expose patients to toxicities or side-effects. It can be delivered at very low expense to patients of almost any age. Hence, the limiting factor for research today is not means but ideas and priorities. When oncologists' priority was the short-term survival, there was no

[6]The Stroop test presents the words red, blue, green and yellow in colored capital letters. The subject has to press a button identifying the real color of the letters. The difficulty is that sometimes the word RED is colored blue. Or the word YELLOW is colored green.

time left for psychological considerations. Nowadays, cancer often becomes a chronic disease (palliative treatments may last years). In curative situations, invasive surgeries have non negligible consequences (body image...) while complete remissions never totally discard the threat of a relapse: both situations considerably impact survivors' psyche. There is therefore, facing cancer, a large place for psychosocial interventions and thus for hypnosis.

As psychological risk factors of cancer are still under debate (depression, life events, coping styles...), research concerning hypnosis in cancer patients could very well bring new evidence about them too. Conversely, because it is easier to demonstrate changes at a biological level than at a psychological one, such research could help discriminate the best psychotherapeutic approaches from the others and give arguments to psychologists for a better integration into medicine and overall health management.

5. References

Aaronson NK, Ahmedzai S, Bergman B, Bullinger M, Cull A, Duez NJ, Filiberti A, Flechtner H, Fleishman SB, de Haes JC et al. (1993) The European Organization for Research and Treatment of Cancer QLQ-C30: a quality-of-life instument for use in international clinical trial in oncology. *J Natl Cancer Inst*; 85(5): 365-76

Ader R, Cohen N (1993) Psychoneuroimmunology : conditioning and stress. *Annu. Rev. Psycho*; 44 : 53-85

Alladin A, Alibhai A (2007) Cognitive hypnotherapy for depression : an empirical investigation. *Int J Clin Exp Hypn*; 55(2): 147-66

Bakke AC, Purtzer MZ, Newton P (2002) The effect of hypnotic-guided imagery on psychological well-being and immune function in patients with prior breast cancer. *J Psychosom Res*; 53(6):1131-7.

Braid J (1843) Neurypnology or the Rationale of nervous lleep considered in relation with animal magnetism. J Churchill; London

Butler LD, Symons BK, Henderson SL, Shortliffe LD, Spiegel D (2005) Hypnosis reduces distress and duration of an invasive medical procedure for children. *Pediatrics*; 115: 77-85

Butler LD, Waelde LC, Hastings TA, Chen XH, Symons B, Marshall J, Kaufman A, Nagy TF, Blasey CM, Seibert EO, Spiegel D (2008) Meditation with yoga, group therapy with hypnosis and psychoeducation for long-term depressed mood: a randomized pilot study. *J Clin Psychol*;64(7): 806-820

Butler LD, Koopman C, Neri E, Giese-Davis J, Palesh O, Thorne-Yocam KA, Dimiceli S, Chen XH, Fobair P, Kraemer HC, Spiegel D. (2009) Effects of supportive-expressive group therapy on pain in women with metastatic breast cancer. *Health Psychol*; 28(5): 579-87.

Byock I, Merriman M (1998) Measuring quality of life for patients with terminal ilness: The Missoula-VITAS Quality Of Life Index. *J Pal Med*; 12:231-244.

Carpenter JS (2001) The hot flash related daily interference scale: a tool for assessing the impact of hot flashes on quality of life following breast cancer. *J Pain Sympt Manag*; 22(6): 979-89

Chiarioni G, Palsson OS, Whitehead WE (2008) Hypnosis and upper digestive function and disease. *World J Gastroenterol*; 14(41): 6276-84

Dalton SO, Boesen EH, Ross L, Schapiro IR, Johansen C (2002) Mind and Cancer: do psychological factors cause cancer ? *Eur J cancer*; 38 : 1313-1323

De Haes JC, Van Knippenberg FC, Neijt JP (1990) Measuring psychological and physical distress in cancer patients: structure and application of the Rotterdam Symptom Checklist. *Br J Cancer*; 62: 1034-8

Deng G, Cassileth BR (2005) Integrative oncology: complementary therapies for pain, anxiety and mood disturbance. *CA Cancer J Clin*; 55: 109-16

Derogatis LR, Morrow GR, Fetting J, Pennam D, Piasetsky S, Schmale AM, Henrichs M, Carnicke CL Jr (1983) The prevalence of psychiatric disorder among cancer patients. *JAMA*; 249(6): 751-7

Elkins G, Marcus J, Stearns V, Perfect M, Rajab MH, Ruud C, Palamara L, Keith T (2008) Randomized trial if a hypnosis intervention against hot flashes among breast cancer survivors. *J Clin Oncol*; 26(31): 5022-6

Erickson MH (1959) Hypnosis in painfull terminal illness. *J Ark Med Soc*; 56(2): 67-71

Erickson MH, Rossi EL (1980) Basis of hypnosis: discussion about hypnosis in:Collected Papers on Hypnosis: Volume 1 - Nature of Hypnosis and Suggestion. Ernest L. Rossi Editor, NY, pp 29-37

Erickson MH (1982) Deep hypnosis and its induction in:Collected Papers on Hypnosis: Volume 3 - Hypnotic Investigation of Psychodynamic Processes. Ernest L. Rossi Editor NY, pp 177-213

Fawzy FI, Kemeny ME, Fawzy NW, Elashoff R, Morton D, Cousins N, Fahey JL (1990) A structured psychiatric intervention for cancer patients. II. Changes over time in immunological measures. *Arch Gen Psychiatry* 47(8) : 729-35

Flammer E, Bongartz W (2003) On the efficacy of hypnosis: a meta-analytic study. *Contemporary Hypnosis*; 20(4): 179-97

Gershon MD, Drakontides AB, Ross LL (1965) Serotonin: synthesis and release from the myenteric plexus of the mouse intestine. *Science*;149:197-9.

Gershon MD (1998) "The Second Brain. The Scientific Basis of Gut Instinct and a Groundbreaking New Understanding of Nervous Disorders of the Stomach and Intestine." Harper Collins Publishers, New York

Goodwin P (2005) Support groups in advanced breast cancer. Living better if not longer. *Cancer*; 104(11): 2596-601

Hackman RM, Stern JS, Gershwin ME (2000) Hypnosis and asthma: a crirical review. *J Asthma*; 37(1) : 1-15

Harter M, Reuter K, Aschenbrenner A, Schretzmann B, Marschner N, Hasenburg A, Weis J (2001) Psychiatric disorders and associated factors in cancer results of an interview study with patients in inpatient, rehabilitation and outpatient treatment. *Eur J Cancer*; 37(11): 1385-93

Hawkins P, Liossi C, Ewart BW, Hatira P, Kosmidis VH (1995) Hypnotherapy for control of anticipatory nausea and vomiting in children with cancer : preliminary findings. *Psycho-Oncology*; 4: 101-6

Hawkins P, Liossi C, Ewart BW, Hatira P, Kosmidis VH (1998) Hypnosis in the alleviation of procedure related pain and distress in paediatric oncology patients. *Contemporary Hypnosis*; 15(4): 199-207

Hjerl K, Andersen EW, Keiding N, Mouridsen HT, Mortensen PB, Jorgensen T (2003) Depression as a prognostic factor for breast cancer mortality. *Psychosomatics*; 44(1): 24-30

Horii R, Akiyama F, Kasumi F, Koike M, Sakamoto G (2005) spontaneous "healing" of breast cancer. *Breast Cancer*; 12(2): 140-4

Hutchings DF, Denney DR, Basgall J, Houston BK (1980) Anxiety management and applied relaxation in reducing general anxiety. *Behav Res Ther*; 18:181-90

Jacknow DS, Tschann JM, Link MP, Boyce WT. Hypnosis in the prevention of chemotherapy-related nausea and vomiting in children: a prospective study. *J Dev Behav Pediatr*; 15(4): 258-64

Jones MP (2006) The role of psychosocial factors in peptic ulcer disease: Beyond Helicobacter pylori and NSAIDs. *Journal of Psychosomatic Research*; 60: 407- 412

Katz ER, Kellerman J, Ellenberg L (1987) Hypnosis in the reduction of acute pain management with pediatric cancer patients undergoing bone marrow aspirations. *J Pediatr Psychol*; 12(3): 379-94

Kiecolt-Glaser JK, Glaser R (1999) Psychoneuroimmunology and Cancers : fact or fiction ? *Eur J Cancer* 35(11) : 1603-7

Kissane DW, Grabsch B, Clarke DM, Smith GC, Love AW, Bloch S, Snyder RD, Li Y (2007) Supportive-expressive group therapy for women with metastatic breast cancer : survival ans psychosocial outcome from a randomize controlled trial. *Psycho-Oncology*; 16: 277-286

Kocsis JH (2000) New strategies for treating chronic depression. *J Clin Psychiatry*; 61(suppl.11) : 42-5

Koeller JM, Aapro MS, Gralla RJ, Grunberg SM, Hesketh PJ, Kris MG, Clark-Snow RA (2002) Antiemetic guidelines: creating a more practical treatment approach. *Support Care Cancer*; 10(7): 519-22

Kwiatkowski F, Uhrhammer N, Bignon YJ., Blanchet, A. (2009). Hypnosis and Cancer: A Dead-End Story? In G. D. Koester & P. R. Delisle (Eds.), *Hypnosis: Theories, Research and Applications*. Nova-Sciences - Hauppauge NY

Langewitz W, Izakovic J, Wyler J, Schindler C, Kiss A, Bircher AJ. (2005) Effect of self-hypnosis on hay fever - a randomised controlled intervention study. *Psychother. Psychosom*; 74(3) : 165-72

Lengacher CA, Bennett MP, Gonzalez L, Glvary D, Cox CE, Cantor A, Jacobsen PB, Yang C, Djeu J (2008) Immune responses to guided imagery during breast cancer treatment. *Biol Res Nurs*; 9(3): 205-14

Liossi C, Hatira P (1999) Clinical hypnosis versus cognitive-behavioral training for pain management with pediatric cancer patients undergoing bone marrow aspiration. *Int J Clin Hypn*; 47,2: 104-16

Liossi C (2001) Efficacy of clinical hypnosis in the enhancement of quality of life of terminally ill cancer patients. *Contemporary hypnosis*; 15(1): 34-8

Liossi C (2006) Hypnosis in cancer care. *Contemporary hypnosis*; 23(1): 47-57

Lutgendorf SK, Lambin DM, DeGeest K, Anderson B, Dao M, McGinn S, Zimmerman B, Maiseri H, Sood AK, Lubaroff DM (2008) Depressed and anxious mood and T-cell cytokine expressing populations in ovarian cancer patients. *Brain Behav Immun*; 22(6): 890-900

Méheust B (1999) Somnambulisme et médiumnité, tome 1, le défit du magnétisme naturel. Coll. *Les empêcheurs de penser en rond*. Edition Institut Synthélabo, Le Plessis-Robinson, France

Methy N, Bedenne L, Bonnetain F (2010) Surrogate endpoints for overall survival in digestive oncology trials: which candidates? A questionnaires survey among clinicians and methodologists. *BMC Cancer*;10:277.

Montgomery GH, Weltz CR, Seltz M, Bovbjerg DH (2002) Brief presurgery hypnosis reduces distress and pain in excisional breast biopsy patients. *Int J Clin Exp Hypn*; 50(1): 17-32

Montgomery GH, Kangas M, David D, Hallquist MN, Green S, Bovbjerq DH, Schnur JB (2009) Fatigue during breast cancer radiotherapy: an initial randomized study of cognitive-behavioral therapy plus hypnosis. *Health Psychol*; 28(3): 317-22

Morasso G, Costantini M, Viterbori P, Bonci F, Del Mastro L, Musso M, Garrone O, Venturini M (2001) Predicting mood disorders in breast cancer patients. *Eur J Cancer*; 37(2): 216-23

Moyer A, Sohl SJ, Knapp-Oliver SK, Schneider S (2009) Characteristics and Methodological Quality of 25 Years of Research Investigating Psychosocial Interventions for Cancer Patients. *Cancer Treat Rev*; 35(5): 475–484

Newton BW(1983) The use of hypnosis in the treatment of cancer patients. *Am J Clin Hypn*; 25: 104-13

Payot A, Barrington KJ (2011) The Quality of Life of Young Children and Infants with Chronic Medical Problems: Review of the Literature. *Curr Probl Pediatr Adolesc Health Care*; 41(4): 91-101

Penninx BW, Guralnik JM, Pahor M, Ferrucci L, Cerhan JR, Wallace RB, Havlik RJ (1998) Chronically depressed mood and cancer in older persons. *J Natl Cancer Inst*; 90(24): 1888-93

Raz A, Fan J, Posner MI (2005). Hypnotic suggestion reduces conflict in the human brain. *Proceedings of the National Academy of Sciences of the United States of America*, 102(28): 9978–9983.

Reich M, Lesur A, Perdrizet-Chevallier C (2007) Depression, quality of life and breast cancer: a review of the literature. *Breast Cancer Res Treat*; 110(1): 9-17

Richardson J, Smith JE, McCall G, Richardson A, Pilkington K, Kirsch I (2007) Hypnosis for nausea and vomiting in cancer chemotherapy: a systematic review of the research evidence.*Eur J Cancer Care* (Engl);16(5):402-12

Rossi EL (2002) Psychobiologie de la guérison. Edition "Le souffle d'or", Barret-sur-Méouge, France. Original edition (1993) WW Norton & Company Inc. New-york

Smith JT, Barabasz A, Barabasz M (1996) Comparison of hypnosis and distraction in severely ill children undergoing painful medical procedures. *J Couns Psychol*; 43:187-95

Spiegel D, Bloom JR, Kraemer HC, Gottheil E (1989) Effect of psychosocial treatment on survival of patients with metastatic breast cancer. *Lancet*; 2 : 211-22

Spiegel D, Butler L, Giese-Davis J, Koopman C, Miller E, DiMiceli S, Classen C, Fobair P, Carlson R, Kraemer H (2007) Effects of supportive-expressive group therapy on survival of patients with metastatic breast cancer. *Cancer*, 11(5) : 1130-8

Spiegel D, Giese-Davis J (2003) Depression and cancer: mechanisms and disease progression. *Biol Psychiatry*; 54: 269-282

Steel J, Geller D, Gamblin TC, Olek MC, Carr B (2007) Depression, immunity and survival in patients with hepatobiliary carcinoma. *J Clin Oncol*;25(17): 2397-404

Steinhauser KE, Bosworth HB, Clipp EC, McNeilly M, Christakis NA, Parker J, Tulsky JA (2002) Initial assessment of a new instrument to measure quality of life at the end of life. *J Palliative Medicine*; 5(6): 829-41

Syrjala KL, Cummings C, Donaldson GW (1992) Hypnosis or cognitive behavioral training for the reduction of pain and nausea during cancer treatment: a controlled clinical trial. *Pain*; 48: 137-46

Syrjala KL, Donaldson GW, Davis MW, Kippes ME, Cart JE (1995) Relaxation and imagery and cognitive-behavioral training reduce pain during cancer treatment: a controlled clinical trial. *Pain*; 63: 189-98

Temoshok LR, Wald RL (2002) Change is complex: rethinking research on psychosocial intervention in cancer. *Integr Cancer Ther*; 1(2): 135-45

Wade JE, Sherbourne CD (1992) The MOS 36-item short-form health survey (SF-36). *Medical Care*; 30: 473-83

Walker L, Ratcliffe M, Dawson A (2000) Relaxation and hypnotherapy: long term effects on the survival of patients with lymhoma. *Psycho-oncolgy*; 9: 39-45

Walker LG, Walker MB, Ogston K, Heys SD, Ah-See AK, Miller ID, Hutcheon AW, Sarkar TK, Eremin O (1998) Psychological, clinical and pathological effects of relaxation training and guided imagery during primary chemotherapy. *British Journal of Cancer*; 80 (1/2): 262-8

Walker LG, Heys SD, Walker MB, Ogston K, Miller ID, Hutcheon AW, Sarkar TK, Ah-See AK, Eremin O (1999) Psychological factors can predict the response to primary chemotherapy in patients with locally advanced breast cancer. *Eur J Cancer*; 35(13): 1783-1788

Watson M, Haviland JS, Greer S, Davidson J, Bliss JM (1999) Influence of psychological response on survival in breast cancer. A population based cohort study. *Lancet*; 354: 1331-6

Wild MR, Espie CA (2004) The efficacy of hypnosis in the reduction of procedural pain and distress in pediatric oncology: a systematic review. *J Dev Behav Pediatr*; 25: 207-13

Zaza C, Baine N (2002) Cancer pain and psychological factors: a critical review of the literature. *Journal of Pains and Symptoms Management* ; 24 : 526-542

Zelter LK, LeBaron S (1982) Hypnosis and nonhypnotic techniques for reduction of pain and anxiety during painful procedures in children and adolescents with cancer. *J Pediatr*: 101(6); 1032-5

Zelter LK, LeBaron S, Zelter M (1984) The effectiveness of behavioural intervention for reduction of nausea and vomiting in children and adolescents receiving chemotherapy. *J Clin Oncol*; 2: 683-90

Zigmond AS, Sanith RP (1983) The Hospital Anxiety and Depression Scale. *Acta Psychiatrica Scandinavia* 67: 367-70

5

Mutual Regulation in the Context of Inconsolable Crying: Promoting Tolerance to Distress

Beth S. Russell[1] and Molly Fechter-Leggett[2]
[1]*University of Connecticut, Department of Human Development & Family Studies, Storrs, CT*
[2]*Stanford Home for Children, Sacramento, CA*
USA

1. Introduction

All parents face a new stressor when an infant joins the family; most have not likely faced the intense and evocative stimuli of an infant in their care crying for prolonged durations. For most parents, their infant's crying takes up a small portion of a day, and as parents learn the cues or signals specific to their infant they become more effective at soothing a cry and preventing situations likely to trigger another bout. Indeed, one might summarize a common conceptualization of crying thusly: Something has triggered the infant's cry, the cry signals a specific need, parents should respond with the appropriate remedy to stop the cry, and parents should learn from these experiences to anticipate and prevent their infant's future distress (Barr, Hopkins, & Green, 2000). Our broader social awareness of crying and our culturally influenced beliefs about parents' role in their infants' cries are communicated explicitly through direct and often verbal means, and through implicit, unspoken exchanges. Parents (perhaps irrationally) fear the demands of the public – *why can't you keep your baby quiet?* – just as they dread the pointed glares shot to them when their infant cries in public. Both types of communication convey a social attitude towards crying: It is the parents' role to meet the needs of their infant to keep crying to a minimum.

As an example of these everyday social pressures, I sat in a waiting area while my car was serviced, checking the grammar in this manuscript on my laptop computer. A father cradled his young infant in his arms nearby and told me his son was 10 weeks old. The infant's limbs were drawn into his body, his eyes clamped tightly shut against the sun pouring through the skylights overhead. In the course of more than 20 minutes, the father maintained a series of soothing behaviors and furtive glances to the 10 or so adults waiting with us. Despite his son's quiet, light sleep and occasional coos, the father shushed and hummed constantly, slightly jiggling his baby while he sat. When the baby grunted or murmured, his father's vocalizations were louder, he rose to his feet and paced, bouncing the baby a bit more vigorously, while glancing up at the rest of us from a lowered gaze. The baby remained in a light sleep, but his father was clearly concerned that his son stay quiet - a goal he achieved - his behaviors were gentle, affectionate, and calming to observe.

For the majority of families, as described in the father-son example above, the social expectations for soothing their infants are readily met; parents are capable of soothing their infants most of the time and are eager to reduce their infants' distress. [A particularly helpful and succinct description of the preoccupation with and fears that arise with the birth of a child concerning parenting, see Stern's (2004) writing on the "motherhood constellation".] In early infancy, this is largely accomplished through the parent's use of soothing techniques, and increasingly over time, "to scaffold an infant's regulatory capacities" by supporting the infant's self-soothing efforts (Tronick, 2007, p.9). But for a portion of families whose infants cry inconsolably, the social expectation that they are responsible for their infant's distress should they fail to soothe a cry is burdensome and unreasonable; for them, the presumption that all cries *can be soothed* if the parent knows what to do is faulty and potentially hurtful, as it places the responsibility for knowing how to soothe a cry - and the guilt for failing to do so - solely on the parent. Papousek and von Hofacker (1998), and Levitzky and Cooper (2000) found that mothers of inconsolably crying infants felt shameful and inadequate in social situations when they could not soothe their infant. By way of definitions, between 16% and 29% of infants experience excessive crying (St. James-Roberts & Halil, 1991) starting as young as 3 weeks of age, peaking in duration at 2 months and decreasing to normal amounts of crying by 3 months of age (Barr, 1990b; Brazelton, 1962). International consensus on the criteria for above-normal or excessive amounts of crying in otherwise healthy infants comes from Wessel and colleagues' (1954) "rule of 3s": crying and fussing for more than 3 hours a day, for more than 3 days a week, for more than 3 weeks. The frequency and duration of crying described by this criterion is extreme, but even parents enduring fewer than 3 weeks of a lot of crying are also at risk for emotional dysregulation – while these clinical criteria are useful for describing infant behavior, there is no consistent characteristic used to predict which parents will be able to cope effectively with the demands of caring for an infant who cries or fusses even average amounts – less than an hour -each day (even when the amount of crying is at its peak during the first 12 weeks of life; Barr, 1990a). The causes for excessive crying remain complicated; there are instances of physiological etiology (i.e., lactose intolerance; Marklund, Ahlstedt, & Nordstrom, 2007), gastrointestinal reflux (Henry, 2004), and prenatal teratogenic exposure (Phillips, Sharma, Premachandra, Vaughn, & Reyes-Lee, 1996), and efforts to establish the contribution of temperament - i.e., irritability or soothability - but this is made complicated by temperament's instability at this young age; and all of this is further confounded by neonates' immature neurobehavioral system, characterized by vast changes in metabolism, thermoregulation, and immunology (Papousek, Schieche, & Wurmser, 2008). Once physiologic causes have been ruled out, infants' excessive cries can be classified as inconsolable – without cause.

Distinct from colic or more general irritability, inconsolable crying is normative for 16% - 29% of the population (St. James-Roberts & Halil, 1991), for simplicity's sake, we can consider this 1 in 5 infants. It occurs without cause, does not signal a specific need or a particularly notable level of physical discomfort, and is considered benign (Miller & Barr, 1991; Stifter & Braungart, 1992). Crying, even at the intense levels associated with inconsolable crying or for prolonged durations, does not put infants at risk – babies can cry vigorously for extended lengths of time without injury - leading to the common prevention slogan in Shaken Baby Syndrome interventions "Crying can't hurt a baby, shaking can". Hence, locating the *problem* of inconsolable crying within the infant is a misinterpretation of the situation. There is nothing wrong with the infant, no problem to be solved, no cure to apply – it is a social convention that needs adjustment. Supporting an inconsolable infant is difficult, stressful, tiring, but normative (St. James-Roberts, 2007) and should not be pathologized because doing so intensifies the pressure parents' feel to perform their role as soothing caregivers who should intuitively know what to do to effectively calm their baby (Barr, 1993; Stern, 2004).

The social convention for interpreting an infant's cry should be expanded to include the possibility that infants' cries are not always indicative of problems to be solved. Instead, the focus should shift to how caregivers with inconsolable infants respond. If caregivers fail to regulate their own reactions to their infant's cry and respond harshly, they risk injury to the infant or establishing dysfunctional patterns of interaction with long-term, deleterious socioemotional consequences for the child (Tronick, 2007). Parents with infants who cry excessively are likely to spend incredible amounts of the day and night cycling through soothing attempts for their crying infant "while at the same time neglecting their own needs to a critical degree" (Papoušek, 2008, p.90). This failure to regulate the self creates a frantic, exhausted, and forlorn parent who is, in turn, less available to meeting their infant's needs in supportive ways.

With regards to parents' self-regulation, objective measures of precisely how many hours the baby cries inconsolably are relatively immaterial; the focus needs to be on how well the parent copes with crying in any perceived long duration. There is evidence (as summarized by Crouch, Skowronski, Milner, & Harris, 2008), that parents who perceive their infant's cries as excessive are more likely to respond abusively, however, since the majority of families with inconsolably crying infants survive these early months safe, healthy, and with secure, responsive parent-infant interactions in place, clearly there is more to consider that the frequency, duration, or intensity of the infant's cry. Parent characteristics that interfere with responsivity in the infant-parent dyad include depression, addiction, and other psychopathology that results in barriers to emotional availability, parent-child intersubjectivity, and parent self-regulation (Beeghly, & Tronick, 1994; Easterbrooks, Biesecker, & Lyons-Ruth, 2000; Kogan & Carter, 1996; Steina et al., 2010; Trevarthen & Aiteken, 2001; Tronick, 2007). Targeting parents who struggle with pathologic obstacles to adaptive dyadic function is a necessary and effective intervention strategy. A focus on secondary prevention approaches based on caregiver demographics or pathology, however, discounts the normative population of parents whose only risk indicator for future failures in dyadic regulation lies within the infant (in the case of normative excessive crying, for example) or within the interaction between infant and parent itself.

As Papoušek (2008) states: "Chronic stress, severe exhaustion, and overstrain may elicit defense mechanisms, including reduced initiative, feelings of powerlessness, burnout, and emptiness, which for a time inhibit the parents' intuitive readiness to respond. Intense negative affects and/or entanglement in insoluble conflicts may so absorb the parents that they no longer perceive their baby's signals" (p.69). There is widespread recognition that an infant inconsolably crying places the parent-infant relationship at risk for dysregulation (as in "persistent mother-infant distress syndrome", Barr, 1998; specific studies presented by Crouch, Skowronski, Milner, & Harris, 2008; Howell, Mora, & Leventhal, 2006; Maxted, et al., 2005; Papousek & von Hofacker, 1998 ; Raiha, Lehtonen, Saleva, & Korvenranta, 2002; more broad literature reviews summarized by Lieberman, 2004; National Research Council

Institute of Medicine, 2000; Tronick, 2007). Accordingly, attention must be paid to the set of skills that we argue are teachable and may serve as protective for the dyad as they mutually regulate one another through an incredibly challenging but normative stretch of time - the peak of infant crying in the first 2-3 months of life (Barr, 1990b, Brazelton, 1962).

1.1 Mutual regulation predicated on self-regulation

Mutual regulation describes dyadic interactions that work towards the goal of reciprocity between parent and infant through affect regulation (Brazelton, Kowslowski, & Main, 1974). This approach acknowledges the contribution of the infant as an actor in the dyad with a differentiated affective system, but also acknowledges that often reciprocity is not achieved. As a result, the focus in mutual regulation research is on how the dyad navigates the negative affect of mis-matched states, and how parent and infant regulate one another to experience the positive affect from reciprocity. In order for the dyad to repair any mis-match, each actor must regulate his or her responses thereby further developing and reinforcing the skills required to communicate with dyadic partners. Over time, the impact of infant-parent mutual regulation on self-regulatory skill has significant impact on the child's socioemotional outcomes.

The most comprehensive considerations of many of the socioemotional difficulties children might manifest acknowledge the power of the affective communication between infant and caregiver (Tronick, 2007). The interactions parents and infants share are bi-directional, giving both actors a sense of who they are and who their partner is, as in Charles Horton Cooley's (1998) "looking glass self", and involve interpersonal/behavioral and intrapsychic/subjective aspects (Stern, 2004). Infants learn intersubjectivity as they build mental representations, or schemas for themselves, objects, and their environment, including the social world. Similarly, parents adapt their existing schemas to accommodate their role as parents. For both members of the dyad, ideas about how relationships work and their impact on the self is an on-going process; in other words, the formation of internal working models begins with interactions in early infancy and continues to shift ever so slightly with an accumulation of interactions over hours, days, weeks, and years (Pietromonaco, & Barrett, 2000). These blueprints for relationships have predictive value across the lifespan and shape expectations and behavior in the interpersonal world (Bowlby, 1982), and while they are fairly consistent over time (Waters, Merrick, Treboux, Crowell, & Albersheim, 2000), they are still flexible and can change with the input of new experiences (Pietromonaco, & Barrett, 2000). Nonetheless, most clinical theories and intervention approaches acknowledge the power of early experiences and the preference to adjust maladaptive relationship patterns early in life to relieve suffering in the present and prevent long-term problems (Sameroff, 2004).

In early infancy, dyadic interactions rely heavily on the skills and resources of the parent - skills and resources that are each heavily taxed by the demands of caring for a new baby. The more available, attentive, and creative a parent can be in meeting their infant's needs, the more likely it is that the dyad will spend time in positive interactions that are synchronistic, mutual, and rewarding. Parents are more likely to have these qualities when they are caring for themselves by self-regulating - they are more likely to observe their infant's cues, interpret them accurately, and attempt multiple responses to bring a distressed, fussy, or disengaged baby back into a more rewarding shared space.

The shared goal that humans strive for from infancy onward is a positive experience in the interpersonal world (Leary, 2004). Infants, with their not-yet-developed self-regulatory capabilities, spend the majority of their time in exchanges that are not inherently rewarding (Tronick, 2007) - states of mis-match between infant signals and caregiver responses that represent the earliest form of miscommunication between individuals. Infants are often inconsistent in their communicative gestures, parents are similarly often poor interpreters of these seemingly random cues, leading them to respond to the infant with behavior that overwhelms, frustrates, or otherwise dysregulates the infant (Tronick, 2007).

Indeed, the research on the coordination of parent-infant interactions illustrates that the majority of dyadic exchanges are not coordinated (see Fogel, 1982; Haley & Stansbury, 2003; Lester, Hoffman, & Brazelton, 1985 as examples). For our purposes, this literature yields a singularly import finding for parent-infant interactions: the reparation of these communicative mis-steps is the telling interpersonal moment (as described by Kogel & Carter, 1996). In other words, the prototypical social exchange between caregiver and infant may be uncoordinated, but any impact this miscommunication may have is dwarfed by the relieving experience of its positive resolution: when an infant fusses to signal she is cold in the night, and her father responds by further exposing the infant to change her soiled diaper, her distress may increase and her father may feel alarmed, confused, or frustrated. But when the father pulls the child to his chest, tucking a blanket around her, she is likely to become warm, comforted, and relaxed - a rewarding snuggle for both members of dyad follows. Tronick's (2007) belief is that this repaired interaction conveys more powerful information to both the daughter and the father about their relationship and themselves than the initial mismatch. He asserts that mutual regulation is predicated on effective self-regulation - particularly of the parent - and that the infant's ability to engage with the inanimate world is predicated on the endogenous, subjective social engagement patterns learned through mutual regulation with a parent (drawing on the work of Mary Ainsworth concerning exploration away from the attachment figure).

1.2 Intervention considerations

Intervention approaches for low-risk families with inconsolably crying babies (those not identified as "at risk" by dint of open cases with Child Protection Services agencies, have no history of mental illness, poverty, or addiction, for example) are rare in the United States as higher risk groups tend to garner more public and fiscal attention. The most common intervention for low-risk families is a brochure lost among the coupons for free diapers and formula passed on to parents upon discharge from the hospital with their newborn (see American Academy of Pediatrics, 2003, for a common example). Although the materials themselves are well designed and provide psychoeducation on infant injuries and crying, they do not target the specific skills sets that all parents will need to develop in response to their infants crying (e.g. self monitoring, emotion regulation, and distress tolerance skills).

After otherwise adaptive and resilient families have identified their struggle with their infant's cry - most often to a pediatrician, as infant mental health struggles during the postnatal period are still largely considered under pediatric purview (Sameroff, 2004) - and physiologic causes for the infant's distress have been ruled out, they are often told there is nothing to do but wait until the 3rd or 4th month after birth, when inconsolable crying typically abates (Barr, 1990a). Inconsolable crying may be a short term struggle, but there is a good deal of risk to the dyad and infant if the parent becomes dysregulated (acutely, in the instance of shaking or otherwise abusing an infant, and chronically in the establishment of dysfunctional relationship patterns - both of which are considered in depth, below). The most readily available advice given to parents in this group is to "take a break" from their infant for a few minutes. The implication is that parents should be taking care of themselves, monitoring their emotions, and practicing their personal coping techniques to remain calm, safe caregivers for their infants - and to do so in 10 minutes or less during a cry bout. Often, these implications are not explicit, nor is guidance given on how to cope with the demands of an inconsolable infant (as found in the otherwise laudable period of PURPLE crying materials; NCSBS, 2004).

1.2.1 Acute risk for the mutually dysregulated dyad

Inconsolable crying has been identified as a risk factor for child abuse of many types, including violent shaking (Levitzky & Cooper, 2000; Reijneveld, van der Wal, Brugman, Hira Sing, & Verloove-Vanhorick, 2004). A significant portion of the infant death rate each year in the United States is accounted for by traumatic head injuries, including infants who die as a result from the injuries sustained from violent shaking (i.e., Shaken Baby Syndrome [SBS]). Shaking an infant younger than 2 years of age results in often-fatal brain injury plus a plethora of secondary injuries caused by gripping the infant during violent shaking (broken ribs, and bruising on the torso and extremities, plus retinal tears and bleeding in the eye; Jentzen, 2001). Research on the perpetration of SBS has identified only one consistent predictor - an infant's inconsolable cry (Lee & Barr, 2007; Barr, Trent, & Cross, 2006).

The case of SBS is extreme, and the consequences of that particular mechanism of injury are particularly lethal, but there are many other missteps parents might take when faced with the fatigue, stress, and other demands of caring for an inconsolably crying infant. As noted by Papoušek and colleagues (2008), infants who cry inconsolably are often paradoxically soothed for short periods of time by stimulating activities (for example, being held while bouncing on a exercise ball, or vigorous rocking in a rocking chair). These caregiving responses to a cry might distract the infant from the intense physiologic rhythm of a cry, but do not provide the organizing qualities the infant needs to settle into either a calm alert state or to down-regulate into the drowsy and deeper sleep states. Thus, strategies effective for halting a cry are not necessarily long-term solutions that support infant self-regulation and can leave the dyad in a frustrating cycle of short periods of calm between periods of fussing or full blown crying bouts (Papoušek et al., 2008).

Parents are at an increased risk for more impulsive, poorly considered responses when their emotion regulation flags, when inattention to or inability to cope with the accumulation of frustration, exhaustion, anger, loneliness, and desperation build in the course of days or weeks of inconsolable crying. When parents are run ragged by their often ineffective attempts to calm a perpetually distressed infant, their responses can become increasingly less nurturing long before their actions become less safe. Even the more seemingly benign response of leaving the child alone for periods of time to rest or emotionally regroup, for example, can set the stage for a pattern of neglectful interaction that can negatively impact how the infant grows to view him or herself and the social world.

1.2.2 Chronic risk for the mutually dysregulated dyad

Infants with generally positive internal working models for themselves and the social world are better prepared to encounter challenging situations later in life and adapt to them successfully, including the ability to work within the challenging context to change the environment itself (Goldhaber, 2000). The qualities that compose these adaptive worldviews are considered in current research programs, but generally build upon a sense of trust in the social world (particularly in caregivers during infancy; i.e., Erikson, 1950). These infants learn that the social world will not be dysregulating, and that intimate relationship partners can be relied upon to respond to distress sensitively and promptly when needed; this gives them a sense of confidence in the environment (Sroufe, 1996) and builds emotional and communicative self-efficacy (as summarized by Goldhaber 2000; Tronick, 2007). Additionally, caregivers who remain emotionally available to their infants by attending to their own needs model these skills for their children, thereby communicating that distress is resolvable and often temporary, that a full range of even intense emotions is a healthy part of social life, and that individuals are capable of manipulating their own affective experiences. In essence, children who observe their parents' adaptive self-regulation learn attitudes and behavior that support their own abilities to engage in a healthy interpersonal life (Leary, 2004). Without experienced others (including parents, siblings and, later, peers and mentors) to model good self-regulatory skill and scaffold infant's own regulatory attempts, and without a sense of trust in their caregivers and the environment as partners in mutual regulation while working towards shard goals, infants lack the confidence to explore their world, to advocate for themselves when they are distressed, or to offer help to peers when they perceive distress in others. These infants are necessarily using their self-regulatory resources on negative affect all the while learning they are ineffective communicators, helpless in interactions with their unavailable and unreliable parents (Tronick, 2007).

2. Strategies to support mutual regulation

There is considerable evidence that social interactions give individuals tremendous amounts of information about themselves across the lifespan. The management of dyadic social interactions is a particularly crucial skill set that supports positive exchanges and repairs to unsuccessful or asynchronous ones. Tronick (2007) includes these skills and the identity implications of both rewarding and unrewarding dyadic interaction between infants and their mothers in his description of a Mutual Regulation Model (MRM). We believe that many of the skills used to regulate parent-infant interactions are teachable, as the early intervention literature on parenting suggests, and that improving parent self regulation is part of the skill set that serves to support dyadic interaction. Cognitive coping mechanisms used to regulate distress when caring for infants are the favored regulatory skill (Russell, Alpert, & Trudeau, 2009). Caregivers of all sorts (babysitters and those in other near-parent roles) describe using coping strategies that predominantly involve mental activity - like counting to ten, and mentally escaping to a "happy place" - and this preference or reliance on cognitive engagement to distract or contain emotional distress is at the root of many therapeutic approaches, including cognitive behavioral therapies (CBT) such as dialectical behavior therapy (DBT). Dialectical Behavior Therapy (DBT) targets emotion regulation as a crucial mechanism for change in behavioral outcomes (Axelrod, Perepletchikova, Holtzman, & Sinha, 2011) and overall psychological well-being.

Emotion regulation is dependent on self monitoring skills because without the ability to take stock of how we feel, both psychologically and physically, we lack information about how to alter our behavior or work to change our environment. In particular, self monitoring skills lead to better distress tolerance and emotion regulation practices which help us adapt to challenging circumstances - and, possibly, even to change those circumstances (Linehan, 1993a; Linehan, 1993b). When a parent is calm and in control of their affect, engaged with their infant, and has the energy/cognitive resources to try new responses to their infant's cues, new patterns of interaction emerge, creating the possibility for less tension, fear, and frustration within the infant-parent dyad. We begin this section with a deeper examination of DBT as an empirically tested tool for supporting parents facing the challenges of their newborn child.

Dialectical Behavior Therapy (DBT), a widely used empirically supported treatment developed by Dr. Marsha Linehan to address the needs of patients with Borderline Personality Disorder (BPD), has been applied to multiple populations to help individuals to develop emotion regulation, self-soothing, mindfulness and crisis management (Linehan, 1993a; Linehan, 1993b). There is a growing body of empirical work demonstrating the effectiveness of DBT for a range of populations (for further information on DBT adaptations for adolescents and children, we suggest Klein, & Miller, 2011 and Perepletchikova, Axelrod, Kaufman, Rounsaville, Douglas-Palumberi, & Miller, 2010, respectively) across a variety of psychiatric needs including ADHD, substance use, suicide risk, PTSD, and eating disorders (Davenport, Bore, & Campbell, 2010; Axelrod, Perepletchikova, Holtzman, & Sinha, 2011; Harned, Chapman, Dexter-Mazza, Murray, Comptois, & Linehan, 2008 or Kotler, Iancu, Efroni, & Amir, 2001; Koons, Robins, Tweed, Lynch, et al., 2001; Safer, Telch, & Agras, 2001 or Telch, Agras, & Linehan, 2001). Although these techniques were first developed to address the symptoms of some of the most difficult to treat client populations, many of the basic tools are useful to *anyone* and appear to target the very vulnerabilities that many new parents face when dealing with an inconsolable infant.

The primary targets of DBT most relevant to parenting infants are: Core Mindfulness, Emotion Regulation, and Distress Tolerance (Linehan, 1993a; Linehan, 1993b). (The fourth target of DBT, Interpersonal Effectiveness, is useful with individuals with chronic emotional dysregulation and crisis, but may not apply to new parents as a whole.) The skill modules in each do not require advanced training in DBT, many of them could be adapted for self-learning if there were additional reinforcers to maintain practice and provide personalized consultation (such as through meetings with a visiting nurse, pediatrician, therapist, or through self-study support groups). DBT combines psychoeducation, specific cognitive techniques, behavioral practice, and mindfulness. The goal of this approach is to help the new parent to feel validated in their experience of distress, and to take a problem-solving stance - not on solving the inconsolable crying, but on solving how it causes parents to get dysregulated. For an identified high-risk group (such as parents with anger management or impulse control problems, or those who have previously engaged in infant abuse), it may make sense to implement DBT closer to its original format with individual, and group clinical support.

2.1 Core mindfulness

The first target in DBT is Core Mindfulness (Linehan, 1993a; Linehan, 1993b). As noted by Lynch, Chapman, Rosenthal, Kuo, and Linehan (2006), this skill set is based on the premise that individuals have to build self-monitoring skills in order to maintain being present in the moment of "crisis" and not reacting impulsively (in the extreme this could be shaking the infant) or shutting down (in the extreme this is depression, withdrawal, neglect). The belief is that all individuals are of two minds- Emotional Mind and Reasonable Mind. The vulnerability lies in being too far in one extreme. When fully in Emotional Mind, we are vulnerable to becoming flooded by our feelings, to act impulsively, and to cause others to feel dysregulated in relationship to us. When fully in Reasonable Mind, we are vulnerable to disregarding our own and other's feelings. DBT teaches the concept of "Wise Mind," a regulated place between Emotional Mind and Reasonable Mind. "Wise Mind" is the area of regulation needed to manage the emotional, cognitive, and physical demands of parenting *any* infant. Identifying triggers and contributing factors to being more in emotional mind (such as high pitched screaming, feeling hopeless, lack of sleep, lack of self-care, being alone), and using cognitive and behavioral strategies to help regulate and return to the balanced state of "Wise Mind" are the goals to coping with an infant's distress.

Core Mindfulness skills combine two sets of skills: "what" skills and "how" skills (Linehan, 1993a; Linehan, 1993b). The "what" skills are learning to observe, describe and participate with awareness. An assumption is that participating without awareness is characteristic of impulsive and mood dependent behavior. Generally, observing, describing, and participating is only necessary when learning a new behavior- such as how a novice piano player learns how to play the piano by paying close attention to their hands and fingers, they may count beats out load or name the keys and chords they are playing. As skills improve, the observing and describing cease to be necessary. But, if a habitual mistake is learned, they may have to revert to the observing/describing to learn a new pattern. Teaching parents to observe/describe/participate in their world helps to build awareness and is a building block for developing self-monitoring skills and self-regulation.

The "how" skills have to do with *how* to attend, describe and participate. Taking a non-judgmental stance helps to eliminate self-blame and negative beliefs such as "I am a bad mother" and offers the opportunity to observe/describe/participate in their experiences without reinforcing negative self-talk. One "how" skill is "Focus on the Moment," it is useful in avoiding the rumination about past negative experiences and ascribing the same outcomes to current ones- such as having had three bad nights of bouts of inconsolable crying and responding in the present to the infant with the thoughts, fears, frustration, and belief that it will happen again. "Focus on the Moment" helps to ground the parent in the current moment and to allow the parent to respond as if the situation was novel- often leading to calmer, more creative, and more patient responses to their infant.

2.2 Emotion regulation: Self-monitoring

Many people attempt to regulate their emotions by telling themselves not to feel what they feel. This oversimplification results in an emotionally invalidating environment that requires people to smile when they are unhappy, be nice when they are angry, and bottle up their feelings until they are so overwhelmed and vulnerable that they are flooded (resulting in depression, rage, and other forms of extreme dysregulation). Emotion regulation, the second target area of DBT, is best taught through the framework of emotional self-validation (Linehan, 1993a; Linehan, 1993b). These skills are taught through a combination of psychoeducation about emotional states and conscious self-practice. In the case of intervening with parents of infants with inconsolable crying, it may make sense to target dominant negative emotional states: hopelessness, fear, anger, and emotional exhaustion. The core tenant of emotion regulation skills is to build self-monitoring. Conscious practice and "homework" assignments increase individual's awareness and monitoring of emotions and, then, inherent in increased awareness and monitoring is increased *action* to regulate.

The Emotion Regulation target in DBT (Linehan, 1993a; Linehan, 1993b) counters emotion dysregulation with 4 skills: 1) Identifying Emotions. Many emotional experiences go unnoticed in the course of day, some of these are fleeting, mild experiences that do not warrant examination or any particular response; but forming the habit of noting and articulating what emotions feel like is an important precursor to having some agency over behavior when feelings are intense and/or unpleasant. 2) Increasing Mindfulness to Current Emotions. This involves practicing experiencing emotions without judging or trying to inhibit, block or distract from those feelings. Judging leads to guilt, anger, anxiety, and impulsivity. If an individual is feeling sad, it is important to make space and time to feel sad. 3) Increasing Positive Emotional Events includes consciously finding ways to increase positive experiences and being mindful of positive moments. This is often accomplished by keeping a daily journal only of the positive experiences of the day. 4) Reducing Vulnerability to Dysregulation, which has two parts. First is to Identify Triggers and Vulnerabilities, for example recognizing that caffeine makes me edgy, or that not feeling supported makes me angry; and second, to Make a Self-care Plan to Reduce Triggering Situations and Personal/Situational vulnerabilities, by avoiding coffee or talking to my partner about alternating care for the baby every half-hour during crying jags.

2.3 Distress tolerance

The third target area taught in DBT is Distress Tolerance (Linehan, 1993a; Linehan, 1993b). These skills address crisis survival when emotion regulation has failed. The mantra for these times is *Make it through the moment without making the situation worse, but hopefully making it better*. Distress Tolerance skills build off of the core mindfulness tenets. Most mental health approaches focus on changing distressing events and circumstances. They often ignore the concepts of acceptance and learning how to *tolerate* distressing emotions. Parents with inconsolable infants cannot always change the events and circumstance of their distress, and thus need skills to manage their emotions effectively. These skills are about accepting current reality both in the situation and in oneself without judging, and taking specific action to reduce the risk of acting impulsively (Davenport, Bore, & Campbell, 2010). Distress tolerance skills focus on several specific strategies. At any given time one may or may not work. Parents are taught to develop a repertoire of skills to try when they have reached the proverbial "end of their rope." There are three main categories of skills that are useful and relevant to parents with infants: 1) Distraction Skills, 2) Improving the Moment, and 3) Self-soothing Skills.

3. Conclusion

Parenting a newborn will involve periods of high-stress that challenge all parents to adapt their self care routines. This component of the transition into the role of "parent" can be supported through two pathways: First, we believe the cultural expectations that *good* parents know how to keep their infant calm and have the skills to do so are harmful to families because all babies cry, and some cry excessively - this is not a reflection on parenting skills but a normative experience (Barr, 1990a). Human service professionals can play an important role is disseminating messages that normalize this experience for parents and encourage communities to be more supportive of families with infants. Second, we believe the growing empirical evidence for the emotion regulation benefits of DBT in clinical populations can lend concrete skills to all parents of infants - even normative, high functioning families may benefit from the lessons learned across 20 years of DBT practice. Although the empirical literature on DBT outcomes is currently centered on clinical populations , future research would be wise to consider the protective distress tolerance and emotion regulation skills gained by normative populations faced with life-expectant stressors (as in the case of the transition to parenthood). Through the use of three target areas of DBT, parents can learn to self-regulate more effectively, co-regulate more effectively, and manage the distressing experience of having a crying infant without becoming dysregulated and risking injury to their child.

4. References

American Academy of Pediatrics (2003). *Prevent Shaken Baby Syndrome* [Brochure]. American Academy of Pediatrics, 141 Northwest Point Blvd., Elk Grove Village, IL, 60007.

Axelrod, S. R., Perepletchikova, F., Holtzman, K., & Sinha, R. (2011). Emotion regulation and substance use frequency in women with substance use and borderline personality disorder receiving dialectical behavior therapy. *American Journal of Drug and Alcohol Abuse, 37,* 37-42.

Barr, R. G. (1990a) The normal crying curve: what do we really know? *Developmental Medicine and Child Neurology, 32,* 356-362.

Barr, R. G. (1990b). The 'colic' enigma: Prolonged episodes of a normal predisposition to cry. *Infant Mental Health Journal, 11,* 340-348.

Barr, R. G. (1993). Normality: A clinically useless concept; the case of infant crying and colic. *Journal of Developmental and Behavioral Pediatrics, 14,* 264–270.

Barr, R. G. (1998). Crying in the first year of life: Good news in the midst of distress. *Child: Care, Health and Development, 24,* 425-439.

Barr, R. G., Hopkins, B., & Green, J. A. (Eds) (2000). *Crying as a Sign, a Symptom, & A Signal.* Mac Keith Press

Barr, R. G., Trent, R. B., & Cross, J. (2006). Age-related incidence curve of hospitalized Shaken Baby Syndrome cases: Convergent evidence for crying as a trigger to shaking. *Child Abuse & Neglect, 30,* 7-16.

Beeghly, M., & Tronick, E. Z. (1994). Effects of prenatal exposure to cocaine in early infancy: Toxic effects of the process of mutual regulation. *Infant Mental Health Journal, 15,* 158-175.

Bowlby, J. (1982). *Attachment and loss: Vol. 1. Attachment* (2nd ed.). New York: Basic Books.

Brazelton, T. B. (1962) Crying in infancy. *Pediatrics, 29,* 579-588.

Brazelton, T. B., Koslowski, B., & Main, M. (1974). The origins of reciprocity: The early mother-infant interaction. In M. Lewis & M. Rosenblum (Eds.), *The effect of the infant on its caretaker: The origins of behavior* (pp. 49-76). New York: Wiley

Cooley, C. H. (1998). *On self and social organization.* Chicago, IL: University of Chicago Press

Crouch, J. L., Skowronski, J. J., Milner, J. S., & Harris, B. (2008). Parental response to infant crying: The influence of child physical abuse risk and hostile priming. *Child Abuse & Neglect, 32,* 702-710.

Davenport, J. Bore, M., & Campbell, J. (2010). Changes in personality in pre- and post-dialectical behavior therapy borderline personality groups: A question of self-control. *Australian Psychologist, 45,* 59-66.

Dimeff, L. A. & Koerner, K. (Eds.) (2007). *Dialectical Behavior Therapy in clinical practice: Applications across disorders and settings.* New York: Guilford Press

Easterbrooks, M. A., Biesecker, G., & Lyons-Ruth, K. (2000). Infancy predictors of emotional availability in middle childhood: The roles of attachment security and maternal depressive symptomology. *Attachment & Human Development, 2,* 170-187.

Erikson, E.H. (1950). *Childhood and society.* New York: Norton.

Fogel, A. (1982). Early adult-infant interaction: Expectable sequences of behavior. *Pediatric Psychology, 7,* 1-22.

Goldhaber, D. E. (2000). *Theories of human development: Integrative perspectives.* Mountain View, CA: Mayfield Publishing Co.

Harned, M., Chapman, A., Dexter-Mazza, E., Murray, A., Comptois, K. A., & Linehan, M. M. (2008). Treating co-occurring axis I disorders in recurrently suicidal women with borderline personality disorder: A 2-year randomized trial of dialectical behavior therapy versus community treatment by experts. *Journal of Consulting and Clinical Psychology, 76,* 1068-1075.

Haley, D. W., & Stansbury, K. (2003). Infant stress and parent responsiveness: Regulation of physiology and behavior during still-face and reunion. *Child Development, 74,* 5134-1546.

Henry, S. (2004). Discerning differences: Gastroesophageal reflux and gastroesophageal reflux disease in infants. *Advances in Neonatal Care, 4,* 235–247.

Hirvikoski, T., Waaler, E., Alfredsson, J., Pihlgren, C., Holmstron, A., Johnson, A., et al., (2011). Reduced ADHD symptoms in adults with ADHD after structures skills training group: Results from a randomized controlled trial. *Behavior Research and Therapy, 49,* 175-185.

Howell, E., Mora, P., & Leventhal, H. (2006). Correlates of early postpartum depressive symptoms. *Maternal and Child Health Journal, 10,* 149–157.

Jentzen, J. M. (2001). Pathological findings in fatal Shaken Impact Syndrome. *Journal of Aggression, Maltreatment, & Trauma, 5,* 199-224.

Klein, D. A., & Miller, A. L. (2011). Dialectical behavior therapy for suicidal adolescents with borderline personality disorder. *Child and Adolescent Psychiatric Clinics of North America, 20,* 205-216.

Kogan, N., & Carter, A. S. (1996). Mother-infant reengagement following the still-face: The role of maternal emotional availability in infant affect regulation. *Infant Behavior and Development, 19,* 359-370.

Koons, C. R., Robins, C. J., Tweed, J. L., Lynch, R. R., et al., (2001). Efficacy of dialectical behavior therapy in women veterans with borderline personality disorder. *Behavior Therapy, 32,* 371-390.

Kotler, M., Iancu, I., Efroni, R., & Amir, M. (2001). Anger, impulsivity, social support, and suicide risk in patients with posttraumatic stress disorder. *Journal of Nervous and Mental Disease, 189,* 162-167.

Leary, M. R. (2004). The sociometer, self-esteem, and the regulation of interpersonal behavior. In R. F. Baumeister & K. D. Vohs (Eds.), *Handbook of self-regulation: Research, theory, and applications* (pp 373-391). New York: Guilford Press.

Lee, C., & Barr, R. G. (2007). Age-related incidence of publicly reported Shaken Baby Syndrome cases: Is crying a trigger for shaking? *Journal of Developmental & Behavioral Pediatrics, 28,* 288-293.

Lester, B., Hoffman, J., & Brazelton, T. B. (1985). The rhythmic structure of mother-infant interaction in term and preterm infants. *Child Development, 56,* 15-27.

Levitzky, S., & Cooper, R. (2000). Infant colic syndrome—Maternal fantasies of aggression and infanticide. *Clinical Pediatrics,* 395–400.

Lieberman, A. F. (2004). Child-parent psychotherapy: A relationship-based approach to the treatment of mental health disorders in infancy and early childhood. In A. J. Sameroff, S. C. McDonough, & K. L. Rosenblum (Eds.), *Treating parent-infant relationship problems: Strategies for intervention* (pp.97-122). New York: Guilford Press.

Linehan, M.M. (1993a). *Cognitive-behavioral treatment of borderline personality disorder.* New York: Guilford Press.

Linehan, M.M. (1993b). *Skills training manual for treating borderline personality disorder.* New York: Guilford Press.

Lynch, T. R., Chapman, A. L., Rosenthal, M. Z., Kuo, J. R., & Linehan, M. M. (2006). Mechanisms of change in dialectical behavior therapy: Theoretical and empirical observations. *Journal of Clinical Psychology, 62,* 459-480.

Marklund, B., Ahlstedt, S., & Nordstrom, G. (2007). Food hypersensitivity and quality of life. *Current Opinion in Allergy and Clinical Immunology, 7,* 279–287.

Maxted, A., Dickstein, S., Miller-Loncar, C., High, P., Spritz, B., Liu, J., & Lester, B. (2005). Infant colic and maternal depression. *Infant Mental Health Journal, 26,* 56–68.

Miller, A. R. & Barr, R. G. (1991). Infantile colic: Is it a gut issue? *Pediatric Clinics of North America, 38,* 1407-1423.

National Center on Shaken Baby Syndrome (2004). *Period of PURPLE crying.* Ogden (UT): National Center on Shaken Baby Syndrome.

National Research Council Institute of Medicine (2000). *From neurons to neighborhoods: The science of early childhood development.* Washington, D.C.: National Academy Press

Papousek, M., & von Hofacker, N. (1998). Persistent crying in early infancy: A non-trivial condition of risk for the developing mother- infant relationship. *Child: Care, Health, and Development, 24,* 395–424.

Papousek, M., Schieche, M., & Wurmser, H. (Eds.). (2008). *Disorders of behavioral and emotional regulation in the first year of life: Early risks and intervention in the developing parent-infant relationship* (K. Kronenberg, Trans.). Washington, D.C.: Zero to Three.

Perepletchikova, F., Axelrod, S. R., Kaufman, J., Rounsaville, B. J., Douglas-Palumberi, H., & Miller, A. L. (2011). Adapting dialectical behavior therapy for children: Towards a new research agenda for pediatric suicidal and non-suicidal self-injurious behaviors. *Child & Adolescent Mental Health, 16,* 116-121.

Phillips, R. B., Sharma, R., Premachandra, B. R., Vaughn, A. J., Reyes-Lee, M. (1996). Intrauterine exposure to cocaine: Effect on neurobehavior of neonates. *Infant Behavior & Development, 19,* 71-81.

Pietromonaco, P. R., & Barrett, L. F. (2000). The internal working models concept: What do we really know about the self in relation to others? *Review of General Psychology, 4,* 155-175.

Raiha, H., Lehtonen, L., Saleva, K., & Korvenranta, H. (2002). Excessively crying infant in the family: Mother-infant, father-infant and mother-father interaction. *Child: Care, Health, and Development, 28,* 419–429.

Reijneveld, S., van der Wal, M., Brugman, E., Hira Sing, R., & Verloove-Vanhorick, P. (2004). Infant crying and abuse. *Lancet, 364,* 1340–1342.

Russell, B. S., Alpert, L., & Trudeau, J. J. (2009). Child abuse prevention during infancy: Intervention implications for caregivers' attitudes towards emotion regulation. *Journal of Human Behavior in the Social Environment, 19*(5), 540-553.

Safer, D., Telch, C. F., & Agras, W. S. (2001). Dialetical behavior therapy for bulimia nervosa. *American Journals of Psychiatry, 158,* 632-634.

Sameroff, A. J. (2004). Ports of entry and the dynamics of mother-infant interventions. In A. J. Sameroff, S. C. McDonough, & K. L. Rosenblum (Eds.), *Treating parent-infant relationship problems: Strategies for intervention* (pp. 3-28). New York: Guilford Press.

Sroufe, L. A. (1996). *Emotional development: The organization of emotional life in the early years.* New York: Cambridge University Press.

Steina, A. Artechea, A. Lehtonena, A., Craskeb, M., Harveyc, A., Counsella,, N., & Murrayd, L. (2010). Interpretation of infant facial expression in the context of maternal postnatal depression. *Infant Behavior & Development, 33,* 273–278.

Stern, D. N. (2004). The motherhood constellation: Therapeutic approaches to early relational problems. In A. J. Sameroff, S. C. McDonough, & K. L. Rosenblum (Eds.), *Treating parent-infant relationship problems: Strategies for intervention* (pp.29-42). New York: Guilford Press.

Stifter, C. A. & Braungart, J. (1992). Infant colic: A transient condition with no apparent effects. *Journal of Applied Developmental Psychology, 13,* 447-462.

St. James-Roberts, I. (2007). Helping parents to manage infant crying and sleeping: A review of the evidence and its implications for services. *Child Abuse Review, 16,* 47–69.

St. James-Roberts, I. & Halil, T, (1991) Infant crying patterns in the first year: normative and clinical findings. *Journal of Child Psychology and Psychiatry, 32,* 951-968.

Telch, C., Agras, W. S., & Linehan, M. M. (2001). Dialetical behavior therapy for binge eating disorder. *Journal of Consulting and Clinical Psychology, 69,* 1061-1065.

Trevarthen, C., & Aitken, K. J. (2001). Infant intersubjectivity: Research, theory, and clinical applications. *Journal of Child Psychology & Psychiatry, 42,* 3-48.

Tronick, E. (2007). *The neurobehavioral and social-emotional development of infants and children.* New York: Springer.

U.S. Department of Health and Human Services, Administration for Children and Families, Administration on Children, Youth and Families, Children's Bureau (2010). *Child Maltreatment 2008.* Available from http://www.acf.hhs.gov/programs/cb/stats_research/index.htm#can

Waters, E., Merrick, S., Treboux, D., Crowell, J., & Albershiem, L. (2000). Attachment security in infancy and early adulthood: A 20-year longitudinal study. *Child Development, 71,* 543-562.

Wessel, M. A., Cobb, J. C., Jackson, E. B., Harris, G. S., & Detwiler, A. C. (1954). Paroxysmal fussing in infants sometimes called "colic." *Pediatrics, 14,* 421-434.

Section 3

Depression

6

Non-Response to Initial Antidepressant Therapy

J.P. Guilloux[1], D.J. David[1], B.A. Samuels[2], I. David[1,2],
A.M. Gardier[1] and B.P. Guiard[1]
[1]*Laboratoire de Neuropharmacologie, Faculté de Pharmacie,
Université Paris Sud XI, Châtenay-Malabry,*
[2]*Department of Psychiatry, Columbia University, New York, NY,*
[1]*France*
[2]*USA*

1. Introduction

Depressive and anxiety disorders are a major burden on society. Mood disorders affect 7% of the world's population, while severe forms of depression impact 2-5% of the US population (Murray and Lopez, 1996; Samuels and Hen, 2011). Furthermore, approximately 32-35 million adults in the US population (16%) experience an episode of major depression in their lifetime (Kessler et al., 2003). While many classes of drugs with antidepressant activity have been developed and approved (Wong et al., 2010), many patients do not respond to treatment (Trivedi et al., 2006). Therefore it is critical for basic research to develop animal models that present behavioral, neurochemical and brain morphological phenotypes reminiscent of depression and anxiety. Given that anxiety and depression have a high comorbidity with co-occurrence rates up to 60% in patients (Leonardo and Hen, 2006), animal models that present signs of both diseases could potentially be the most useful.

When prescribing medication, there is increasing pressure on clinicians to follow decision-tree medical algorithms, such as the Texas Medication Algorithm project (TMAP), in attempts to combat depression in patients that are non-responsive to initial lines of treatment. These involve multiple levels of treatments, each with varying success. Recently, STAR*D, a large study designed to mirror clinical practice, was conducted at 25 different sites. The study enrolled over 4000 patients with a broad range of symptoms and involved 4 possible steps for treatment (Fava and Covino, 2007). If patients failed to achieve remission at any level, they would be randomized for the next step of treatment. As patients moved from levels 2-4 of treatment, remission rates dropped dramatically (from approximately 35% at level 2 to 16% at level 4). Therefore, failure to achieve remission with 2 consecutive treatments is associated with very low remission rates in subsequent treatments. This suggests that the usefulness of current lines of treatment is limited and underscores the need for discovery of new treatments.

The present review defines the notion of non-response/resistance to antidepressants in human and the factors that may influence these clinical aspects. Then it focuses on the preclinical study aimed at developing relevant animal models of resistance including the unpredictable chronic mild stress (UCMS), the social interaction test and the repeated corticosterone exposure. Is it worthwhile to model depression in rodents? Clearly many signs of depression such as guilt, feelings of worthlessness and recurrent thoughts of death are going to be features specific to humans. It is not possible to question animals and give them a score on the Hamilton Rating Scale for Depression (HAM-D) as is often done with humans. However, many other aspects of depressive disorders have been replicated in the laboratory setting. This review also describes the recent findings about the cellular and molecular bases of non-response and resistance to antidepressants. Finally, it synthesizes our current knowledge on the therapeutic activity of a new generation of antidepressant drugs, the triple reuptake inhibitors (TRIs). These pharmacological agents, that simultaneously increase serotonergic, noradrenergic and dopaminergic neurotransmissions, are believed to produce greater antidepressant effects than single- or dual acting-agents such as the selective serotonin reuptake inhibitors (SSRIs) or the serotonin/norepinephrine reuptake inhibitors (SNRIs) (Skolnick et al., 2003; Guiard et al., 2009). Indeed, by treating core and/or residual symptoms of depression, TRIs might provide an interesting alternative to the 50% of depressive individuals that do not respond adequately to conventional antidepressants.

2. Treatment-resistant depression (TRD) – Clinical aspects

SSRIs and SNRIs are the most commonly prescribed drugs for the treatment of major depression (MD). Despite recent advances in the pharmacological treatment of depression, 60% of patients with unipolar major depressive episodes do not respond adequately to SSRIs/SNRIs. Furthermore, as observed in the STAR*D study, treatment resistant depression, i.e. major depressive episodes resistant to antidepressant treatment, as defined by the lack of response to two consecutive and different antidepressant drugs, prescribed at adequate dosages and for adequate durations (Connolly and Thase 2011; Ruhé et al., 2011), occurs in 20% to 30% of MD patients (Gaynes et al., 2008). As compared with major depressive episode responsive to antidepressant drugs, treatment resistant episodes are associated with a 2 to 3-times increase in the use of other psychotropic medications. More importantly, the global medical costs associated with resistance are 6-times higher than those associated with non treatment-resistant depression ($42,344 vs. $6512) and the total depression-related costs of resistance are 19-times higher than those of patients with non-treatment-resistant MD ($28,001 vs. $1455) (Crown et al., 2002; Ivanova et al., 2010).

2.1 From non response to resistance: Definitions

Response to an antidepressant is usually characterized by a decrease of at least 50% from the baseline score in a depression scale at the end of the trial endpoint (Riso et al., 1997). Measurement of depression severity and antidepressant responsiveness is usually performed using scales such as the HAM-D, MADRS (Montgomery-Åsberg Depression Rating Scale), QUIDS (Quick Inventory of Depressive Symptomatology) and CGIs (Clinical Global Impression). However, such a decrease does not qualify a patient as remitted but only as responder, as patients with high scores (>30) at the HAM-D scale would not be consider as remitted (Nierenberg et al., 2001). Oppositely, the threshold for non-response is always hard to set and can exclude various sub-groups such as "non-remitted" responders as well as partial responders. Usually, non-response is considered to be a decrease of less than 25% on depression scale measurements, but in some studies, failure of remission can be set as the threshold to define treatment failure. For instance, one of the largest studies aiming at defining effectiveness of SSRIs and identifying predictors of symptom remission was STAR*D, and its criteria were as following: an exit HAM-D score ≤7 qualified for remission and a reduction of more than 50% in baseline QIDS-SR (Quick Inventory of Depressive Symptomatology-Self Report) at the last assessment was defined as response (Hollon et al., 2005; Trivedi et al., 2006).

The definition of treatment resistance depressed (TRD) patients is still a matter of debate, and numerous definitions have been proposed based either on the duration of the illness, use of augmentation strategies or extent of treatment (Souery et al., 1999; Sackeim, 2001; Fagiolini and Kupfer, 2003), resulting in a possible under-estimation of TRD prevalence (Nemeroff et al., 2007). Furthermore, our knowledge of TRD is also based on naturalistic follow-up studies of the outcome of depressive disorders in general (Souery et al., 1999). The simplest and most widely used definition of resistance is when a current episode of depression has not benefited from at least 2 adequate trials (i.e. appropriate dose, duration and extent) of different classes of antidepressants (Ananth, 1998; Rush et al., 2003; Keller, 2005). Despite limitations (Berlim and Turecki, 2007a), this definition is the most widely accepted. Furthermore, this definition benefits from the strong support brought by the STAR*D study, where response rates after failure to 2 antidepressant strategies dramatically decrease (Ruhé et al., 2006b; Rush et al., 2006).

Staging methods for classifications of TRD have been proposed and reviewed by several authors (Berlim and Turecki, 2007b; Hetrick et al., 2008) and consist of graduating stages of resistance based on response to one or more different therapeutic strategies (Thase and Rush, 1997, see Table 1), but can also include chronic aspects of resistance (European Staging Model: Souery et al., 1999; Antidepressant Treatment History Form (ATHF): Sackeim et al., 1990; Oquendo et al., 2003). More recent models do not implicate an antidepressant hierarchy: for instance, the Massachusetts General Hospital staging method is a more flexible model, based on the number of antidepressant trials performed and their possible adjustments, without taking into consideration the pharmacological class differences of each trial (Fava, 2003). However this does not include duration of the disease. Yet one of the most comprehensive models proposed may be the Maudsley staging method for TRD (MSM). It incorporates the number of failed treatment trials, the chronicity of the disease and also includes measurements of disease severity as an important cofactor (Fekadu et al., 2009a,b). Ruhé et al. (2011) recently compared various staging methods and concluded that overall MSM displays high validity, but its reliability and sensitivity needs to be confirmed in other larger studies.

Stage	Definition
0	Yet no adequate medication trials.
I	Non-response to 1 adequate trial of antidepressant
II	Stage I + non-response to 1 adequate trial of single antidepressant belonging to a distinct pharmacological class from that used in class I
III	Stage II + non-response to an adequate trial of a TCA
IV	Stage III + non-response to an adequate trial of a MAOI
V	Stage IV + non-response to electroconvulsive therapy

Table 1. Staging method, adapted from Thase and Rush, 1997.

2.2 Factors implicated in non-response/resistance

Clinical, biological, and sociodemographic variables have been studied in relation to resistance to antidepressant treatment. However, due to sample size of the studies and methodological variablilities in defining resistance, results are not necessarily consistent and reliable (Berlim and Turecki, 2007a,b; Kornstein et Schneider, 2001).

2.2.1 Sex differences in non-reponse/resistance

Women are twice as likely to experience MD as men (Kornstein et al., 2000) and four times as likely to have recurrent MD (Perugi et al., 1990). Women also have more MD symptoms and greater symptom severity (Angst and Dobler-Mikola, 1984; Frank et al., 1988; Young et al., 1990). Therefore, there is often a preponderance of women in studies, including treatment-resistant depression studies, but there is no evidence that sex is a predictor for resistance (Sotsky et al., 1991; Souery et al., 2007). The only sparse and slight evidence of sex differences might be in response to first antidepressant treatment (Sloan and Korstein, 2003), where women seem to respond slightly less to tricyclics (Hamilton et al., 1996), but respond similarly or slightly better to SSRI treatment (Papakostas et al., 2006; Kornstein et al., 2006). No sex difference to ECT treatment has been reported (Bloch et al., 2004).

2.2.2 Age of onset

There is evidence that age of onset may predispose to a higher risk to develop TRD. Indeed, early onset of depression has been associated with a chronic course of the illness (Akiskal et al., 1981), and often results in higher severity of the disease as well as higher rates of comorbidity (Klein et al., 1999). Furthermore, early onset of first depressive episode has been considered as a risk factor in recent studies including large sample of patients (Dudek et al., 2010; Souery et al., 2007). Onset of depression in patients >60 years has been associated with a greater likelihood of psychotic symptoms and vascular brain changes that may increase the risk to develop to resistance (Kornstein et Schneider, 2001) Similar efficacy rates for antidepressant and psychological therapies have been reported in older adults and those under the age of 60 (Goldberg et al., 1998). TRD is clearly understudied in the elderly, because late-life depression has higher rates of physical and cognitive comorbidity and age-related pharmacodynamic/pharmacokinetic changes add greatly to the complexity of monitoring TRD (Cooper et al., 2011)

2.2.3 Depression subtypes

Despite efforts to elucidate if TRD could be classified as "a unique subtype of depression" (Fagiolini and Kupfer, 2003), no specific endophenotypes or biological markers have been solely associated with TRD. Moreover depressive subtypes such as atypical depression, psychotic depression, and bipolar depression have been associated with poor outcome and a higher degree of resistance to specific types of treatment or to treatment in general, or both. Thus, depression subtypes are important elements as they may influence the rate of TRD, its evaluation and management. For example, patients with bipolar disorder may be misdiagnosed as TRD due to their higher rate of MD compared to manic episodes (Gaynes et al., 2009; Kupfer et al., 2002). Depressed subjects with melancholia have a greater degree of response to TCAs and ECT (Fava, 1996, 2003) whereas atypical depression is known to be more resistant to TCAs but not to MAOIs (Liebowitz et al., 1988; Quitkin et al., 1993; Thase et al., 1991).

2.2.4 Severity of the disease and other comorbid psychiatric disorders

Disease severity has been thoroughly associated with TRD (Souery et al., 2007; Dudek et al., 2010) and patients with greater symptom severity were approximately 3 times less likely to remit than those with mild or moderate depression in the STAR*D study (Rush et al., 2008). Severe depression is usually associated with lower spontaneous remission rate, greater risk of recurrence and higher chronicity of the disease (Thase et al., 2000). Disease chronicity has been also associated with TRD with longer episodes and greater recurrence of episodes (Souery et al., 2007; Dudek et al., 2010).

Comorbid anxiety is one of the most associated symptom coexisting with MD (Clayton et al., 1991) and thus is also one of the highest comorbidity of the disease associated with TRD (Gaynes et al., 1999; Souery et al., 2007; Dudek et al., 2010). Patients with melancholic features also appear more prone to develop TRD (Rush et al., 2008; Mc Grath et al., 2008). Obsessive-compulsive disorders, personality disorders, suicidal risk and substance of abuse (most of all is alcohol) are also among the greatest comorbidity associated with TRD (Souery et al., 2007; Kornstein et Schneider, 2001; Fagiolini et Kupfer, 2003; Sackeim, 2001). Finally, other medical conditions such as weight gain, diabetes, hypertension, hypothyroidism, chronic painful conditions are also considered as risk factors to develop TRD (Gaynes et al., 2009; Kornstein et Schneider, 2001; Berlim and Turecki, 2007a)

3. Animal models of depression and non-response/resistance to monoaminergic antidepressant

Given the problems with current lines of antidepressant treatment in the clinic, it is incumbent upon basic research to yield novel methods of treatment. In order for basic research to provide potential advances, a critical first step is to create useful animal models with relevant phenotypic features to reveal treatment responsiveness. However, some of the original animal models designed to address this problem suffered from a flawed tautological approach in that they were based solely on responsiveness to known antidepressants. Since no genetic variants with high penetrance that cause depression are known, animal models have mainly relied on different means of chronically exposing rodents to stressful experiences, or sensory tract lesions such as in olfactory bulbectomy, to induce behavioral states that present depression-like signs and are responsive to chronic antidepressant treatment.

3.1 Non-response/resistance in the unpredictable chronic mild stress model

The oldest most commonly used paradigm to induce a depression-like state is chronic mild stress (CMS). Initial observations suggested that animals subjected to multiple stressors over a prolonged period of time reduced their intake of saccharine or sucrose, a potential behavioral model of anhedonia (Katz, 1982). Furthermore, this effect was selectively reversed by chronic treatment with the TCA imipramine (Katz, 1982). Further work was able to repeat this result using more mild stressors, such as periods of food and water deprivation, small temperature reductions and changes of cage mates (Willner, 2005; Willner et al., 1987). Following these studies the CMS procedure, and modified versions such as chronic unpredictable stress (CUS or UCMS), became commonly used and much work demonstrated that other depression-like changes were induced in animals, such as decreased sexual and aggressive behavior, decreased self-care, and altered sleep patterns (Willner, 2005). Furthermore these behaviors are all reversible by chronic, but not acute, treatment using multiple classes of antidepressants (Surget et al., 2008). While historically potential pitfalls of the CMS procedure are that it is notoriously labor intensive, and that there has been some difficulty in getting the procedure established and the results replicated across laboratories (Nestler et al., 2002), the modified versions of the CMS have proven more useful.

Recently, there have been some reports using CMS or variants to model treatment resistance in rodents. In one study, CMS significantly decreased sucrose consumption and the proliferation of adult hippocampal neural progenitors (Jayatissa et al., 2006). Following chronic treatment with a SSRI (escitalopram), the subjects were retested for sucrose consumption. A bimodal distribution was found where one group recovered (increased sucrose consumption) while another refracted treatment (no increase in sucrose consumption). Interestingly, there was a correlation between the animals in the group that recovered with a reversal of the decreased proliferation that was absent in the group resistant to treatment (Jayatissa et al., 2006). More recently, follow-up work has taken a proteomic approach in an attempt to find molecular differences in the ventral hippocampus between responders and non-responders (Bisgaard et al., 2007). Another study demonstrated that if animals are on a high fat diet during multiple UCMS procedures they become resistant to treatment with a SSRI (fluoxetine) (Isingrini et al., 2010).

3.2 Non-response/resistance in the social interaction model

A distinct procedure that has gained traction is the usage of a social defeat model. In this paradigm a mouse is forced into the territory of a mouse from a larger, more aggressive strain leading to an interaction resulting in intruder subordination. Repeated defeats over 10 days can result in a long lasting reduced social interaction, sexual dysfunction, sleep dysregulation, anxiety, metabolic deficits and anhedonia (Berton et al., 2006; Tsankova et al., 2006; Krishnan et al., 2007; Krishnan and Nestler, 2008). Interestingly, following the social defeat procedure there remains a large variance in behavior outcomes in spite of using an inbred mouse strain (C57BL/6). Some animals display a resistance to social defeat (resilience) while others are susceptible (determined by interaction with a social target relative to an empty enclosure). If animals are separated based on this measure, susceptible mice demonstrate decreased sucrose intake, a blunted circadian rhythm, and conditioned place preference to cocaine (Krishnan et al., 2007). Furthermore, phenotypes induced by social defeat in susceptible mice can be reversed by antidepressant treatment (Tsankova et al., 2006). Given that molecular mechanisms for resilience to the stressful procedure are now being worked out (Krishnan et al., 2007; Vialou et al., 2010), it would be intriguing to see if similar pathways are necessary for mediating response to antidepressants.

3.3 Non-response/resistance in the corticosterone model

A third procedure for inducing a depression-like state in animals is administration of chronic glucocorticoids in order to mimic the effects of chronic stress. A significant proportion of depressed patients display altered activity of the HPA axis, and stress generally leads to hypersecretion of corticosteroids, which imposes an increased risk for depression (Carroll et al., 1981; Nemeroff et al., 1984; Strohle and Holsboer, 2003; Brown et al., 2004; de Kloet et al., 2005; Antonijevic, 2006; Leonardo and Hen, 2006, 2004). Chronic treatment of rodents with corticosterone effectively induces multiple anxiety- and depression-like changes in behavior, neurochemistry and brain morphology (Ardayfio and Kim, 2006; Gourley et al., 2008; Murray et al., 2008; David et al., 2009). Behaviorally, depression-related changes include suppression of sucrose intake and decreased self-care (Gourley et al., 2008; David et al., 2009), while anxiety-related changes include increased latency to emerge into the light compartment in the light/dark test, decreased time, entries and percent distance in the center of an open field and increased latency to take a bite of food in the novelty suppressed feeding (NSF) test (Ardayfio and Kim, 2006; David et al., 2009). Behaviorally, approximately 85% of C57BL/6 mice demonstrate anxiety and depression-related signs in response to chronic corticosterone, suggesting that, similar to social defeat, there is a small population that is resilient to the manipulation (David et al., 2009; David unpublished data). Interestingly, animal subjects that participate in the Novelty Suppressed Feeding test, a paradigm sensitive to chronic antidepressant, do tend to show a bimodal distribution in response to antidepressant treatment, suggesting a responder and non-responder divide (Samuels et al., 2011). By anthropomorphic analogy, an animal was considered as a responder to fluoxetine when its behavioral response was improved by at least 50%. Similarly to what is observed in humans, it was shown in this model that 30% of the animals did not respond to fluoxetine. These preliminary data argue for the validity of the CORT model in assessing non-response to antidepressants. Furthermore, we propose here a preclinical model for studying non-response/resistance, based on what has been developed in clinic by international consensus statement on major depressive disorder (Nutt et al., 2010) and proposed in therapeutic (Figure 1).

3.4 Current hypotheses on the molecular and cellular bases of non-response/resistance to antidepressants

It is still not clear why some animals are non-responders to antidepressants in these models. However growing evidence suggests that part of the answer lies in the neurogenesis process. At the cellular level, it has been known for several years that antidepressants increase hippocampal neurogenesis (Malberg et al., 2000) and that some of their behavioral effects require adult neurogenesis (Santarelli et al., 2003; Surget et al., 2008; Wang et al., 2008, David et al., 2009). However, in rodents deprived of adult neurogenesis, some behavioral effects of chronic antidepressant treatments remained unaltered suggesting the existence of neurogenesis-dependent and neurogenesis-independent mechanisms (Surget et al., 2008) (Figure 2). The delayed onset of antidepressants response in MD patients led to the hypothesis that their efficacy results from restoration of functional neural networks which are altered in MD patients (Duman et al., 2000). Thousands of new neurons are continuously produced every day in the mammal adult brain, specifically in the dentate gyrus (DG) of the hippocampus and the olfactory bulb (OB) (Lledo et al., 2006). In the DG, stem cells give rise to progenitor cells that migrate to the granular and molecular layers and differentiate into excitatory granule neurons. Neuroblasts fated for the adult OB are produced in the walls of the lateral ventricles (subventricular zone: SVZ). They migrate tangentially toward the core of the OB, forming the rostral migratory stream. Upon reaching the OB, adult born neuroblasts migrate radially within the lamina of the OB to reach their final position and start to differentiate. In several animal models of depression, including the CORT model, chronic antidepressant treatments accelerate the three phases of hippocampal neurogenesis i.e. proliferation, maturation and survival of the newly born neurons (Wang et al., 2008). Interestingly, in some of the neurogenesis readouts (proliferation and maturation), the SSRI fluoxetine is much more effective in corticosterone-treated animals than in normal animals, suggesting that stress may increase the dynamic range in which fluoxetine can exert its effects on specific stages of neurogenesis. In humans, evidence suggests higher levels of neural progenitor cells in the DG of depressed individuals treated with SSRIs compared to untreated patients, who also had 50% fewer dividing cells than controls (Boldrini et al., 2009). Together these data are consistent with the hypothesis that part of antidepressant response is the stimulation of neurogenesis whereas non-response/resistance could potentially be explained by a lower capacity for neurogenesis.

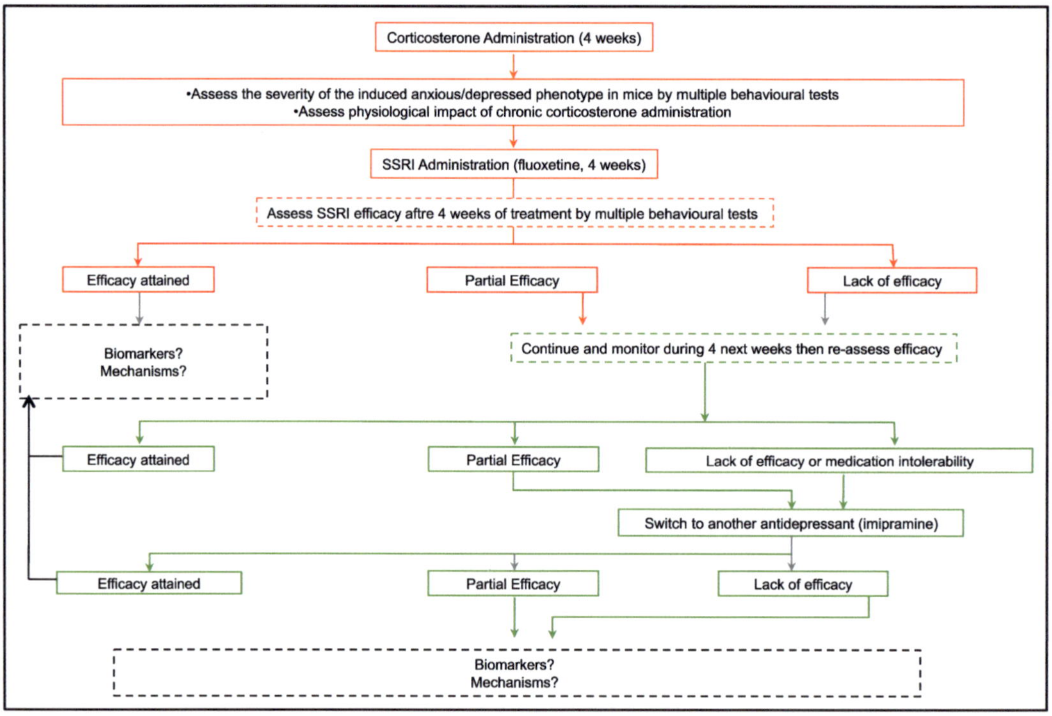

Fig. 1. Algorithm for developing animal model of resistance, based on the CORT model (David et al., 2009)

At the molecular level, Brain-derived neurotrophic factor (BDNF), a member of the neurotrophin family, has been identified as a major candidate involved in the regulation of adult neurogenesis in the DG of the hippocampus and the OB (Duman and Monteggia, 2006; Bath et al., 2011). Indeed, chronic antidepressant treatments produce an increase in hippocampal BDNF levels (Nibuya et al., 1995; Duman & Monteggia, 2006) and a direct infusion of BDNF into the DG exerts antidepressant-like effects (Shirayama et al., 2002; Hoshaw et al., 2005; Kozisek et al., 2008). These observations raised the possibility that BDNF and activation of its high affinity receptor TrkB could be relevant markers of antidepressants response in MD patients, and blunted BDNF neurotransmission a marker of non-response/resistance to these drugs. Among the main signaling pathways implicated in the pathophysiology of MD and antidepressant response, the β-arrestin-signaling cascade has recently gain attention due to the fact that BDNF may indirectly regulate this pathway. To date, four functional members of the arrestin gene family have been cloned, two arrestins (visual arrestin and cone arrestin) are expressed almost exclusively in the retina whereas two β-arrestins, β-arrestin 1 and 2, are ubiquitously expressed proteins with high levels in the brain (Luttrell and Lefkowitz, 2002). β-arrestins display two distinct roles. They constitute important proteins involved in the internalization of various receptors including 5-HT and DA receptors (Li and Jope, 2010). They are also scaffolds for G-protein-coupled receptors (GPCR) to recruit signaling molecules, one of the most fundamental cellular signal transduction processes known. Through this mechanism, β-arrestins activate intracellular kinases such as the protein kinase B (Akt) (involved in cell survival and proliferation), the extracellular-regulated kinase (Erk) (involved in cell proliferation, differentiation and survival) and the Glycogen Synthase Kinase-3β (GSK-3β) (involved in energy metabolism and neuronal cell development) (Lefkowitz and Shenoy, 2005). A substantial body of evidence has accumulated indicating that β-arrestins play a major role in the pathophysiology of mood disorders, as well as in the mechanisms of action of antidepressants. In human, for example, changes in β-arrestins expression are detected in MD patients and in response to stress while various antidepressant drugs reverse these changes (Avissar et al., 2004). Overall, these data suggest that β-arrestins could be major molecular determinants of the effects of fluoxetine, and, more generally, of SSRIs and SNRIs. β-arrestin-1 protein and mRNA levels in mononuclear leukocytes of untreated patients with MD are significantly lower than those of healthy subjects and these levels are significantly correlated with the severity of depressive symptomatology (Avissar et al., 2004; Schreiber et al., 2009). The low β-arrestin-1 protein and mRNA levels were alleviated by antidepressant treatments, whereby normalization of β-arrestin-1 preceded, and thus predicted, clinical improvement. In rodent, SSRIs, SNRIs but also non-selective reuptake inhibitors increase β-arrestin-1 levels. Molecular functions of β-arrestins place them in pathways associated with response to lithium, a drug currently used to treat bipolar disorders (Beaulieu et al., 2008). Caron's group had hinted that β-arrestin KO mice were unable to scaffold a signaling complex. Hence, in these mutants, lithium failed to activate Akt, leading to a loss GSK3 inhibition and to a disruption of antidepressant-like responses. Several sources of evidence suggest that SSRIs promote inhibitory control of GSK3 in several brain regions including the frontal cortex, the hippocampus and the striatum of naïve mice exhibiting a normal, non-depressed phenotype (Emamian et al., 2004; Li et al., 2007; Beaulieu et al., 2008) suggesting that inhibition of this protein play a major role in the antidepressant response. Consistent with this hypothesis, GSK3 inhibitors produce antidepressant-like effects in the mouse FST (Gould et al., 2004). Similar results were observed in GSK3 mutant mice, which display a 50% reduction in the expression of this kinase (Hoeflich et al., 2000). With respect to β-arrestin-2, recent findings show that this protein might be also involved in neurogenesis-dependent and -independent mechanisms (David et al., 2009; Li et al., 2009). Using the "CORT model", it was shown that fluoxetine reversed the neurogenic deficit induced by glucocorticoid elevation and restored expression of β-arrestin-1 and -2 that were blunted by chronic corticosterone (David et al., 2009). These observations further confirm the possibility that β-arrestins are necessary for antidepressant to exert their therapeutic activity. Accordingly, deficient mice for β-arrestin-2 displayed a reduced response to fluoxetine (David et al., 2009). Together, these data led us to postulate that decrease in the expression and/or functional activity of molecular components of β-arrestin-signaling cascades represent biomarkers of non-response and resistance to antidepressant.

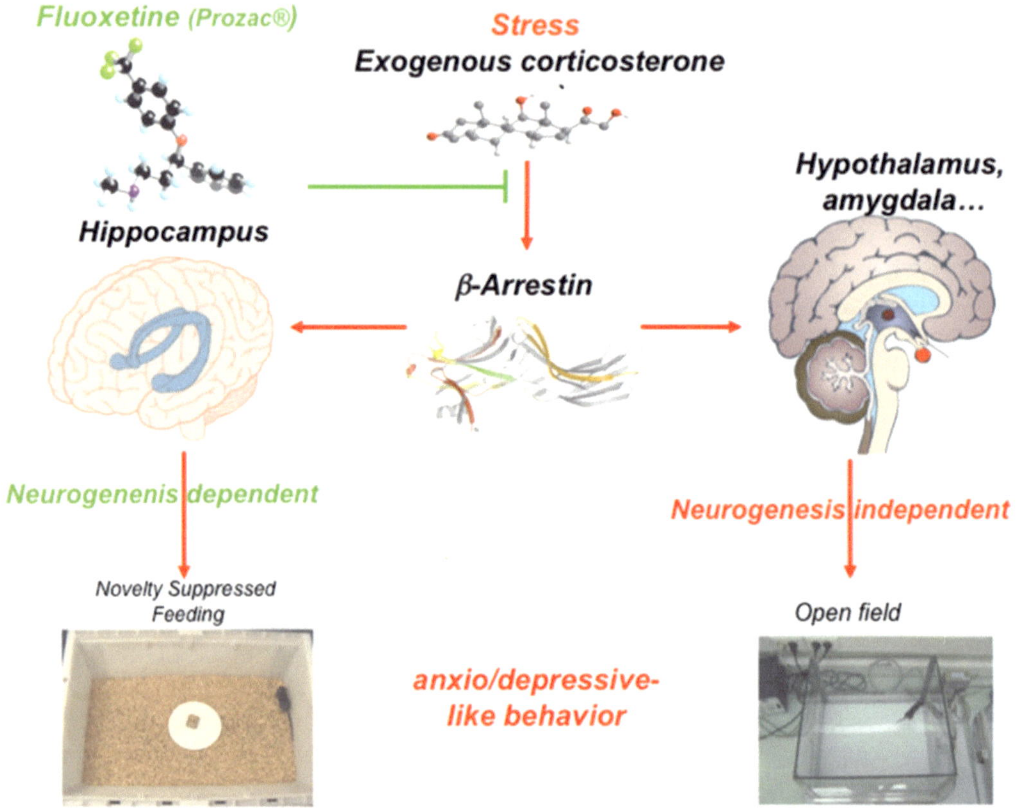

Fig. 2. Chronic fluoxetine reverses the behavioral and neurogenic deficits induced by chronic corticosterone exposure, showing neurogenesis-dependent and neurogenesis-independent effects (Adapted from Rainer et al., 2009).

4. New antidepressant strategy to counteract resistance: The triple reuptake inhibitors (TRIs)

Numerous therapeutic strategies have been proposed to alleviate TRD, including augmentation strategies such as the combination of SSRIs with bupropion or antipsychotics, combination of drugs with ECT or somatic treatments such as repetitive transcranial magnetic stimulation (rTMS), vagus nerve stimulation (VNS), and deep brain stimulation (DBS), or new molecules including the triple reuptake inhibitors (TRIs).

Signs and symptoms of depression can be linked to one or more monoaminergic systems, specifically the 5-HT, the NE and the DA systems. There are considerable reciprocal interactions between these monoaminergic neurons that can produce counterproductive effects (Guiard et al., 2008). When using a SSRI, for example, 5-HT transmission is enhanced, but at the same time there is a dampening of the activity of NE and DA neurons through inhibitory 5-HT2A and 5-HT2C receptors, respectively. This could explain the residual symptoms of fatigue, lack of energy, and anhedonia, often observed after patients present an overall positive response to a SSRI (Blier and Briley, 2011). Using dual-acting agents such as duloxetine, milnacipran or venlafaxine would result in an additional increase in NE activity. However, a risk inherent in increased NE activity is that of provoking anxiety. Hence, the question can be asked as to whether the remaining symptoms observed with SSRI/SNRIs are responsible for a non-response/resistance to these antidepressants or if the lack of significant therapeutic activity results from dysfunction in other neurotransmitters such as a blunted DA neurotransmission? In this context, a new generation of antidepressants named the triple reuptake inhibitors (TRIs) has been developed with the hope of offering a clinically relevant advantage over currently available medications (Guiard et al., 2009). Since TRIs simultaneously enhance extracellular levels of 5-HT, NE and DA neurotransmissions in various brain regions, this class of antidepressants could exert their therapeutic activity by treating more symptoms of MD and/or by attenuating some side effects observed in response to traditional antidepressants. Accordingly, converging lines of evidence indicate that drugs enhancing dopaminergic neurotransmission can diminish anhedonia (Dunlop and Nemeroff, 2007), a symptom that responds poorly to SSRIs (Shelton and Tomarken, 2001). Clinical studies indicate that it is possible to achieve an antidepressant action by enhancing DA. Moreover, the dopamine reuptake inhibitor bupropion has also demonstrated antidepressant activities (Tremblay and Blier, 2006) and its use in combination with SSRIs enhances the antidepressant response in resistant patients (Zisook et al., 2006).

4.1 Preclinical properties of TRIs

A number of compounds with the ability to bind and block all three monoamine transporters have been developed with the hope to produce greater symptomatic relief than single- or dual-acting agents and consequently to reduce non-response and resistance. DOV Pharmaceutical, Inc. is the first company having provided in vitro and in vivo preclinical data with their triple reuptake inhibitors DOV216303, DOV21947 (amitifadine) and DOV220075 (bicifadine). New molecules have followed such as NS2330 (tesofensine, GlaxoSmith-Kline/NeuroSearch), SEP225289 (Sepracor Inc.), CNS-1 and CNS-2 (Albany Molecular Research Institute Inc), PRC-025, PRC-050, PRC-200SS (Mayo Foundation), JNJ7925476 (Johnson & Johnson Pharmaceutical Research & Development), WF-23 (Eli Lilly), JZAD-IV-22 (PsychoGenics) and more recently TP1 (Luye Pharmaceutical Group). Others compounds will undoubtedly emerge in a near future. In 2010-2011, the structure activity relationship (SAR), of at least eleven new TRIs, has been reported (Hache et al., 2011).

4.1.1 Behavioral effects of TRIs

Behavioral data clearly demonstrated the antidepressant-like effect of TRIs that act by increasing the time of mobility and/or by reducing the time of immobility in the FST or the TST. Among the TRIs tested, JNJ7925476 appears the most potent since a low dose of this agent (0.3 mg/kg; s.c.) produced antidepressant-like effects. In term of efficacy (i.e., maximal effect), compounds such as PRC200-SS (10mg/kg; ip), D-142 or D-161 produced a greater percentage of increase in the time of mobility or decrease in the time of immobility than the others TRIs (Aluisio et al., 2008; Dutta et al., 2008; Liang et al., 2008; Dutta et al., 2011). Interestingly, JNJ7925476 and PRC200-SS display the highest affinity for SERT and NET suggesting that this double action is an important prerequisite to produce optimal behavioral responses. Since DA is known to enhance locomotor activity, the possibility cannot be excluded that TRIs increased the time of immobility in these various studies, through a psychostimulant effect. In various studies, however, TRIs did not modify locomotor activity at doses that produce antidepressant-like effects (Tian et al., 2011; Aluisio et al., 2008; Liang et al., 2008; Shaw et al., 2007; Skolnick et al., 2003), thereby ruling out the possibility that the antidepressant-like activity detected does not appear to be from "false-positive" results. An important drawback in the development of antidepressants is the fact that the new compounds are tested after acute administration in naïve, non-depressed animals. Their chronic use in animal models is more appropriate and provides more informative results to determine whether or not new pharmacological agents are worth being tested in clinical trials. A recent study in bulbectomized rats provided some interesting results. In this model, a 14-day regimen of the TRI DOV216303 normalized bulbectomy-induced hyperactivity in the open field, similar to the effect of imipramine at the same dose (Breuer et al., 2008). Inevitably, further studies in these animal models are required to determine the potential of TRIs over SSRIs and SNRIs in terms of quality of antidepressant response.

4.1.2 Neurogenic effects of TRIs

As above-mentioned (paragraph 3.4), a number of studies have demonstrated that SSRIs increase cell proliferation and neurogenesis in the DG of the hippocampus of naive (Marcussen et al., 2008; Sairanen et al., 2005; Santarelli et al., 2003; Malberg et al., 2000) or depressed rodents (David et al., 2009; Malberg and Duman, 2003). It was also reported that catecholamines (NE and DA) might stimulate this process. For example, NRIs and SNRIs have been shown to increase the local expression of neurotrophic factors including BDNF (Nibuya et al., 1995; Larsen et al., 2008; Russo-Neustadt et al., 2004) and adult hippocampus neurogenesis in the DG (Malberg et al., 2000). In a recent study aimed at comparing monoaminergic compounds with different pharmacological profiles (at doses that have been shown to produce antidepressant-like effects in behavioral models), it was demonstrated that sustained administration of the reuptake inhibitors venlafaxine and imipramine increased BDNF mRNA expression after 7 and 14 days of administration respectively, while the SSRI fluoxetine had no effect (Larsen et al., 2007). It is thus possible that the activation of the serotonergic and noradrenergic neurotransmitter system activates different downstream cascades that are both able to increase the transcription of BDNF. Whether or not this apparent effect favors antidepressant response has yet to be demonstrated. Importantly, the hippocampus receives a sparse dopaminergic innervation from the ventral tegmental area (Scatton et al., 1980), raising the possibility that DA and related receptors play a limited role in the local regulation of BDNF expression and neurogenesis. However, dopaminergic denervation in animals causes a dramatic reduction in the number of proliferating cells in the hippocampus (Hoglinger et al., 2004) while the stimulation of DA receptors with selective D2 agonists has recently been shown to enhance neurogenesis in the DG of the hippocampus (Hoglinger et al., 2004, Yang et al., 2008). In a recent series of in vivo experiments, it has been shown that the Cytokine Ciliary Neurotrophic Factor (CNTF), abundant in astrocytes close to dopaminergic terminals, constitutes an endogenous regulatory component of D2-receptor-dependent neurogenesis in DG (Yang et al., 2008; Mori et al., 2008) suggesting that TRIs might be stronger on neurotrophic factor gene expression, neural plasticity, and neurogenesis than SSRIs, NRIs and SNRIs. Using in situ hybridization, an initial study showed that treatment with the TRI NS2330 (Tesofensine), for 5 and 14 days had no effect on BDNF expression in the granular cell layer, while increasing its expression by 35 % in the CA3 after 14 days (Larsen et al., 2007). Furthermore, NS2330 stimulated the number of neuroD-positive cells after 14 days treatment and the nuclear marker of proliferation Ki67, confirming the antidepressant potential of this novel agent (Larsen et al., 2007). Although these results revealed a strong effect of NS2330, the net effect of blockade of each of the monoamine reuptake sites remains unknown. Further studies are truly necessary to dissect the contribution of each monoamine uptake target on the regulation of BDNF or others neurotrophic factors gene expression. It is possible that the stimulation of the expression of various neurotrophic factors such as BDNF and CNTF induced by the concomitant enhancement of central 5-HT, NE and DA transmission, might contribute to shorten the delay of action of traditional antidepressants drugs.

4.2 Clinical properties of TRIs

TRIs are in process of development (Millan, 2009) and most are now in Phase II clinical trials. A small citalopram-controlled trial of DOV216303 in severely depressed patients yielded significant improvements in Hamilton Depression Rating Scale (HAM-D) scores in both groups at one-week and two week time points (Skolnick et al., 2006). DOV Pharmaceutical has recently reported the results of a multi-centric, randomized, double-blind, placebo-controlled study with amitifadine (DOV21947) in 61 patients with MD (Tran et al., 2011). For the primary outcome measure, treatment with amitifadine was associated with a significantly greater improvement in the MADRS and CGI-I total score at week 6 compared with placebo. In addition, a significantly greater remission rate for the CGI-S was observed with amitifadine compared with placebo at week 6. This study also showed that amitifadine was efficacious in improving anhedonia, a core symptom of depression that is presumed to be related to a hypodopaminergia. Despite these encouraging data, it is still not clear whether non-response and/or resistance to TRIs is lower than that observed with SSRIs or SNRIs. Specific clinical trials should address this question in the future. Nevertheless, several arguments allow for optimism. 75% of patients suffering from depression are found to report somatic symptoms, including various types of pain such as headaches, stomach pain, back pain, and vague, poorly localized pain (Fava, 2003). A recent study has shown that responders who have not achieved remission have significantly more somatic symptoms than remitters following 8 weeks of treatment with fluoxetine. These data may suggest that antidepressants that are particularly effective in the treatment of pain and painful physical symptoms may yield higher remission rates in major depressive disorder (Hache et al., 2011). In addition, it has been suggested that presence of pain may be an indicator of MD that may have poorer treatment outcome with an initial SSRI (Leuchter et al., 2010). Acute and chronic pains may result from reduced levels of endogenous 5-HT, NE and DA activities, at both the spinal and supraspinal levels (Ren and Dubner, 2002). Thus, one would expect a better efficacy of dual-or triple-acting agents over selective 5-HT or NE reuptake inhibitors in analgesia (Hache et al., 2011). Several open-label randomized controlled clinical trials, meta-analyses, and systematic reviews have confirmed the clinical efficacy of selected antidepressants in persistent pain conditions (Dharmshaktu et al., 2011). Clinical studies have corroborated that bicifadine is an effective analgesic in the treatment of postoperative pain (Krieter et al., 2008). In a second study, the TRI NS7051, has shown comparable antinociceptive properties to tramadol confirming the interest of these antidepressants in the relief of pain (Munro et al., 2008). The molecule has undergone several phase II and III trials for the treatment of pain, including acute postsurgical pain and chronic low back pain, and is being evaluated for painful diabetic neuropathy (clinical trial.gov).

5. Conclusion

In summary, current antidepressant treatments are not sufficient, as many patients do not respond. Future basic and clinical research will need to take new approaches to advance the understanding and discover new methods for treatment-resistant depression. While most animal models of depression have focused on pharmacological validity, this has led to an overemphasis on mechanisms underlying currently used drugs rather than the discovery of new targets that could benefit patients suffering from treatment-resistant depression. Furthermore, using animal models will be valuable in providing a translational framework to study SSRI insensitivity, and validation of any findings in humans as potential biomarkers for treatment responsiveness will pave the way to break a tradition of using SSRI sensitive behavioral assays to interrogate novel approaches for relieving depressive phenotypes.

6. References

Akiskal HS, King D, Rosenthal TL, Robinson D and Scott-Strauss A (1981) Chronic depressions. Part 1. Clinical and familial characteristics in 137 probands. *J Affect Disord* 3(3):297-315.

Aluisio L, Lord B, Barbier AJ, Fraser IC, Wilson SJ, Boggs J, Dvorak LK, Letavic MA, Maryanoff BE, Carruthers NI, Bonaventure P and Lovenberg TW (2008) In-vitro and in-vivo characterization of JNJ-7925476, a novel triple monoamine uptake inhibitor. *Eur J Pharmacol* 587(1-3):141-146.

Ananth J (1998) Treatment-resistant depression. *Psychother Psychosom* 67(2):61-70.

Angst J and Dobler-Mikola A (1984) Do the diagnostic criteria determine the sex ratio in depression? *J Affect Disord* 7(3-4):189-198.

Antonijevic IA (2006) Depressive disorders -- is it time to endorse different pathophysiologies? *Psychoneuroendocrinology* 31(1):1-15.

Ardayfio P and Kim K-S (2006) Anxiogenic-like effect of chronic corticosterone in the light-dark emergence task in mice. *Behav Neurosci* 120(2):249-256.

Avissar S, Matuzany-Ruban A, Tzukert K and Schreiber G (2004) Beta-arrestin-1 levels: reduced in leukocytes of patients with depression and elevated by antidepressants in rat brain. *Am J Psychiatry* 161(11):2066-2072.

Bath KG, Akins MR and Lee FS (2011) BDNF control of adult SVZ neurogenesis. *Dev Psychobiol.*

Beaulieu JM, Marion S, Rodriguiz RM, Medvedev IO, Sotnikova TD, Ghisi V, Wetsel WC, Lefkowitz RJ, Gainetdinov RR and Caron MG (2008) A beta-arrestin 2 signaling complex mediates lithium action on behavior. *Cell* 132(1):125-136.

Berlim MT and Turecki G (2007a) Definition, assessment, and staging of treatment-resistant refractory major depression: a review of current concepts and methods. *Can J Psychiatry* 52(1):46-54.

Berlim MT and Turecki G (2007b) What is the meaning of treatment resistant/refractory major depression (TRD)? A systematic review of current randomized trials. *Eur Neuropsychopharmacol* 17(11):696-707.

Berton O and Nestler EJ (2006) New approaches to antidepressant drug discovery: beyond monoamines. *Nat Rev Neurosci* 7(2):137-151.

Bisgaard CF, Jayatissa MN, Enghild JJ, Sanchez C, Artemychyn R and Wiborg O (2007) Proteomic investigation of the ventral rat hippocampus links DRP-2 to escitalopram treatment resistance and SNAP to stress resilience in the chronic mild stress model of depression. *J Mol Neurosci* 32(2):132-144.

Blier P and Briley M (2011) The noradrenergic symptom cluster: clinical expression and neuropharmacology. *Neuropsychiatr Dis Treat* 7(Suppl 1):15-20.

Bloch Y, Ratzoni G, Sobol D, Mendlovic S, Gal G and Levkovitz Y (2005) Gender differences in electroconvulsive therapy: a retrospective chart review. *J Affect Disord* 84(1):99-102.

Boldrini M, Underwood MD, Hen R, Rosoklija GB, Dwork AJ, John Mann J and Arango V (2009) Antidepressants increase neural progenitor cells in the human hippocampus. *Neuropsychopharmacology* 34(11):2376-2389.

Breuer ME, Chan JS, Oosting RS, Groenink L, Korte SM, Campbell U, Schreiber R, Hanania T, Snoeren EM, Waldinger M and Olivier B (2008) The triple monoaminergic reuptake inhibitor DOV 216,303 has antidepressant effects in the rat olfactory bulbectomy model and lacks sexual side effects. *Eur Neuropsychopharmacol* 18(12):908-916.

Brown ES, Varghese FP and McEwen BS (2004) Association of depression with medical illness: does cortisol play a role? *Biol Psychiatry* 55(1):1-9.

Carroll BJ, Greden JF, Feinberg M, Lohr N, James NM, Steiner M, Haskett RF, Albala AA, DeVigne JP and Tarika J (1981) Neuroendocrine evaluation of depression in borderline patients. *Psychiatr Clin North Am* 4(1):89-99.

Clayton PJ, Grove WM, Coryell W, Keller M, Hirschfeld R and Fawcett J (1991) Follow-up and family study of anxious depression. *Am J Psychiatry* 148(11):1512-1517.

Connolly KR and Thase ME (2011) If at first you don't succeed: a review of the evidence for antidepressant augmentation, combination and switching strategies. *Drugs* 71(1):43-64.

Cooper C, Katona C, Lyketsos K, Blazer D, Brodaty H, Rabins P, de Mendonca Lima CA and Livingston G (2011) A systematic review of treatments for refractory depression in older people. *Am J Psychiatry* 168(7):681-688.

Crown WH, Finkelstein S, Berndt ER, Ling D, Poret AW, Rush AJ and Russell JM (2002) The impact of treatment-resistant depression on health care utilization and costs. *J Clin Psychiatry* 63(11):963-971.

David DJ, Samuels BA, Rainer Q, Wang JW, Marsteller D, Mendez I, Drew M, Craig DA, Guiard BP, Guilloux JP, Artymyshyn RP, Gardier AM, Gerald C, Antonijevic IA, Leonardo ED and Hen R (2009) Neurogenesis-dependent and -independent effects of fluoxetine in an animal model of anxiety/depression. *Neuron* 62(4):479-493.

de Kloet ER, Joels M and Holsboer F (2005) Stress and the brain: from adaptation to disease. *Nat Rev Neurosci* 6(6):463-475.

Dharmshaktu P, Tayal V and Kalra BS (2011) Efficacy of Antidepressants as Analgesics: A Review. *J Clin Pharmacol.*

Dudek D, Rybakowski JK, Siwek M, Pawlowski T, Lojko D, Roczen R and Kiejna A (2010) Risk factors of treatment resistance in major depression: association with bipolarity. *J Affect Disord* 126(1-2):268-271.

Duman RS, Malberg J, Nakagawa S and D'Sa C (2000) Neuronal plasticity and survival in mood disorders. *Biol Psychiatry* 48(8):732-739.

Duman RS and Monteggia LM (2006) A neurotrophic model for stress-related mood disorders. *Biol Psychiatry* 59(12):1116-1127.

Dunlop BW and Nemeroff CB (2007) The role of dopamine in the pathophysiology of depression. *Arch Gen Psychiatry* 64(3):327-337.

Dutta AK, Ghosh B, Biswas S and Reith ME (2008) D-161, a novel pyran-based triple monoamine transporter blocker: behavioral pharmacological evidence for antidepressant-like action. *Eur J Pharmacol* 589(1-3):73-79.

Dutta AK, Gopishetty B, Gogoi S, Ali S, Zhen J and Reith M (2011) The novel trisubstituted pyran derivative D-142 has triple monoamine reuptake inhibitory activity and exerts potent antidepressant-like activity in rodents. *Eur J Pharmacol.*

Emamian ES, Hall D, Birnbaum MJ, Karayiorgou M and Gogos JA (2004) Convergent evidence for impaired AKT1-GSK3beta signaling in schizophrenia. *Nat Genet* 36(2):131-137.

Fagiolini A and Kupfer DJ (2003) Is treatment-resistant depression a unique subtype of depression? *Biol Psychiatry* 53(8):640-648.

Fava M (2000) New approaches to the treatment of refractory depression. *J Clin Psychiatry* 61 Suppl 1:26-32.

Fava M (2003) Diagnosis and definition of treatment-resistant depression. *Biol Psychiatry* 53(8):649-659.

Fekadu A, Wooderson S, Donaldson C, Markopoulou K, Masterson B, Poon L and Cleare AJ (2009) A multidimensional tool to quantify treatment resistance in depression: the Maudsley staging method. *J Clin Psychiatry* 70(2):177-184.

Fekadu A, Wooderson SC, Markopoulou K and Cleare AJ (2009) The Maudsley Staging Method for treatment-resistant depression: prediction of longer-term outcome and persistence of symptoms. *J Clin Psychiatry* 70(7):952-957.

Frank E, Carpenter LL and Kupfer DJ (1988) Sex differences in recurrent depression: are there any that are significant? *Am J Psychiatry* 145(1):41-45.

Gaynes BN (2009) Identifying difficult-to-treat depression: differential diagnosis, subtypes, and comorbidities. *J Clin Psychiatry* 70 Suppl 6:10-15.

Gaynes BN, Magruder KM, Burns BJ, Wagner HR, Yarnall KS and Broadhead WE (1999) Does a coexisting anxiety disorder predict persistence of depressive illness in primary care patients with major depression? *Gen Hosp Psychiatry* 21(3):158-167.

Gaynes BN, Rush AJ, Trivedi MH, Wisniewski SR, Spencer D and Fava M (2008) The STAR*D study: treating depression in the real world. *Cleve Clin J Med* 75(1):57-66.

Goldberg D, Privett M, Ustun B, Simon G and Linden M (1998) The effects of detection and treatment on the outcome of major depression in primary care: a naturalistic study in 15 cities. *Br J Gen Pract* 48(437):1840-1844.

Gould TD, Einat H, Bhat R and Manji HK (2004) AR-A014418, a selective GSK-3 inhibitor, produces antidepressant-like effects in the forced swim test. *Int J Neuropsychopharmacol* 7(4):387-390.

Gourley SL, Wu FJ and Taylor JR (2008) Corticosterone regulates pERK1/2 map kinase in a chronic depression model. *Ann N Y Acad Sci* 1148:509-514.

Guiard BP, El Mansari M and Blier P (2009) Prospect of a dopamine contribution in the next generation of antidepressant drugs: the triple reuptake inhibitors. *Curr Drug Targets* 10(11):1069-1084.

Guiard BP, El Mansari M, Merali Z and Blier P (2008) Functional interactions between dopamine, serotonin and norepinephrine neurons: an in-vivo electrophysiological study in rats with monoaminergic lesions. *Int J Neuropsychopharmacol* 11(5):625-639.

Hache G, Coudre F, Gardier AM, Guiard BP (20011) Monoaminergic Antidepressants in the Relief of Pain: Potential Therapeutic Utility of Triple Reuptake Inhibitors (TRIs)." *Pharmaceuticals* 4(2): 285-342.

Hetrick SE, Parker AG, Hickie IB, Purcell R, Yung AR and McGorry PD (2008) Early identification and intervention in depressive disorders: towards a clinical staging model. *Psychother Psychosom* 77(5):263-270.

Hoeflich KP, Luo J, Rubie EA, Tsao MS, Jin O and Woodgett JR (2000) Requirement for glycogen synthase kinase-3beta in cell survival and NF-kappaB activation. *Nature* 406(6791):86-90.

Hoglinger GU, Rizk P, Muriel MP, Duyckaerts C, Oertel WH, Caille I and Hirsch EC (2004) Dopamine depletion impairs precursor cell proliferation in Parkinson disease. *Nat Neurosci* 7(7):726-735.

Hollon SD, Shelton RC, Wisniewski S, Warden D, Biggs MM, Friedman ES, Husain M, Kupfer DJ, Nierenberg AA, Petersen TJ, Shores-Wilson K and Rush AJ (2006) Presenting characteristics of depressed outpatients as a function of recurrence: preliminary findings from the STAR*D clinical trial. *J Psychiatr Res* 40(1):59-69.

Hoshaw BA, Malberg JE and Lucki I (2005) Central administration of IGF-I and BDNF leads to long-lasting antidepressant-like effects. *Brain Res* 1037(1-2):204-208.

Isingrini E, Camus V, Le Guisquet AM, Pingaud M, Devers S and Belzung C (2010) Association between repeated unpredictable chronic mild stress (UCMS) procedures with a high fat diet: a model of fluoxetine resistance in mice. *PLoS ONE* 5(4):e10404.

Ivanova JI, Birnbaum HG, Kidolezi Y, Subramanian G, Khan SA and Stensland MD (2010) Direct and indirect costs of employees with treatment-resistant and non-treatment-resistant major depressive disorder. *Curr Med Res Opin* 26(10):2475-2484.

Jayatissa MN, Bisgaard C, Tingstrom A, Papp M and Wiborg O (2006) Hippocampal cytogenesis correlates to escitalopram-mediated recovery in a chronic mild stress rat model of depression. *Neuropsychopharmacology* 31(11):2395-2404.

Katz RJ (1982) Animal model of depression: pharmacological sensitivity of a hedonic deficit. *Pharmacol Biochem Behav* 16(6):965-968.

Keller MB (2005) Issues in treatment-resistant depression. *J Clin Psychiatry* 66 Suppl 8:5-12.

Kessler RC, Berglund P, Demler O, Jin R, Koretz D, Merikangas KR, Rush AJ, Walters EE and Wang PS (2003) The epidemiology of major depressive disorder: results from the National Comorbidity Survey Replication (NCS-R). *JAMA* 289(23):3095-3105.

Klein DN, Schatzberg AF, McCullough JP, Keller MB, Dowling F, Goodman D, Howland RH, Markowitz JC, Smith C, Miceli R and Harrison WM (1999) Early- versus late-onset dythymic disorder: comparison in out-patients with superimposed major depressive episodes. *J Affect Disord* 52(1-3):187-196.

Kornstein SG, Schatzberg AF, Thase ME, Yonkers KA, McCullough JP, Keitner GI, Gelenberg AJ, Ryan CE, Hess AL, Harrison W, Davis SM and Keller MB (2000) Gender differences in chronic major and double depression. *J Affect Disord* 60(1):1-11.

Kornstein SG and Schneider RK (2001) Clinical features of treatment-resistant depression. *J Clin Psychiatry* 62 Suppl 16:18-25.

Kornstein SG, Wohlreich MM, Mallinckrodt CH, Watkin JG and Stewart DE (2006) Duloxetine efficacy for major depressive disorder in male vs. female patients: data from 7 randomized, double-blind, placebo-controlled trials. *J Clin Psychiatry* 67(5):761-770.

Kozisek ME, Middlemas D and Bylund DB (2008) Brain-derived neurotrophic factor and its receptor tropomyosin-related kinase B in the mechanism of action of antidepressant therapies. *Pharmacol Ther* 117(1):30-51.

Krieter PA, Gohdes M, Musick TJ, Duncanson FP and Bridson WE (2008) Pharmacokinetics, disposition, and metabolism of bicifadine in humans. *Drug Metab Dispos* 36(2):252-259.

Krishnan V, Han MH, Graham DL, Berton O, Renthal W, Russo SJ, Laplant Q, Graham A, Lutter M, Lagace DC, Ghose S, Reister R, Tannous P, Green TA, Neve RL, Chakravarty S, Kumar A, Eisch AJ, Self DW, Lee FS, Tamminga CA, Cooper DC, Gershenfeld HK and Nestler EJ (2007) Molecular adaptations underlying susceptibility and resistance to social defeat in brain reward regions. *Cell* 131(2):391-404.

Krishnan V and Nestler EJ (2008) The molecular neurobiology of depression. *Nature* 455(7215):894-902.

Kupfer DJ, Frank E, Grochocinski VJ, Cluss PA, Houck PR and Stapf DA (2002) Demographic and clinical characteristics of individuals in a bipolar disorder case registry. *J Clin Psychiatry* 63(2):120-125.

Larsen MH, Hay-Schmidt A, Ronn LC and Mikkelsen JD (2008) Temporal expression of brain-derived neurotrophic factor (BDNF) mRNA in the rat hippocampus after treatment with selective and mixed monoaminergic antidepressants. *Eur J Pharmacol* 578(2-3):114-122.

Lefkowitz RJ and Shenoy SK (2005) Transduction of receptor signals by beta-arrestins. *Science* 308(5721):512-517.

Leonardo ED and Hen R (2006) Genetics of affective and anxiety disorders. *Annu Rev Psychol* 57:117-137.

Leuchter AF, Husain MM, Cook IA, Trivedi MH, Wisniewski SR, Gilmer WS, Luther JF, Fava M and Rush AJ (2010) Painful physical symptoms and treatment outcome in major depressive disorder: a STAR*D (Sequenced Treatment Alternatives to Relieve Depression) report. *Psychol Med* 40(2):239-251.

Li X and Jope RS (2010) Is glycogen synthase kinase-3 a central modulator in mood regulation? *Neuropsychopharmacology* 35(11):2143-2154.

Li X, Rosborough KM, Friedman AB, Zhu W and Roth KA (2007) Regulation of mouse brain glycogen synthase kinase-3 by atypical antipsychotics. *Int J Neuropsychopharmacol* 10(1):7-19.

Li Y, Li H, Liu X, Bao G, Tao Y, Wu Z, Xia P, Wu C, Li B and Ma L (2009) Regulation of amygdalar PKA by beta-arrestin-2/phosphodiesterase-4 complex is critical for fear conditioning. *Proc Natl Acad Sci U S A* 106(51):21918-21923.

Liang Y, Shaw AM, Boules M, Briody S, Robinson J, Oliveros A, Blazar E, Williams K, Zhang Y, Carlier PR and Richelson E (2008) Antidepressant-like pharmacological profile of a novel triple reuptake inhibitor, (1S,2S)-3-(methylamino)-2-(naphthalen-2-yl)-1-phenylpropan-1-ol (PRC200-SS). *J Pharmacol Exp Ther* 327(2):573-583.

Liebowitz MR, Quitkin FM, Stewart JW, McGrath PJ, Harrison WM, Markowitz JS, Rabkin JG, Tricamo E, Goetz DM and Klein DF (1988) Antidepressant specificity in atypical depression. *Arch Gen Psychiatry* 45(2):129-137.

Lledo PM, Alonso M and Grubb MS (2006) Adult neurogenesis and functional plasticity in neuronal circuits. *Nat Rev Neurosci* 7(3):179-193.

Luttrell LM and Lefkowitz RJ (2002) The role of beta-arrestins in the termination and transduction of G-protein-coupled receptor signals. *J Cell Sci* 115(Pt 3):455-465.

Malberg JE and Duman RS (2003) Cell proliferation in adult hippocampus is decreased by inescapable stress: reversal by fluoxetine treatment. *Neuropsychopharmacology* 28(9):1562-1571.

Malberg JE, Eisch AJ, Nestler EJ and Duman RS (2000) Chronic antidepressant treatment increases neurogenesis in adult rat hippocampus. *J Neurosci* 20(24):9104-9110.

Marcussen AB, Flagstad P, Kristjansen PE, Johansen FF and Englund U (2008) Increase in neurogenesis and behavioural benefit after chronic fluoxetine treatment in Wistar rats. *Acta Neurol Scand* 117(2):94-100.

McGrath PJ, Khan AY, Trivedi MH, Stewart JW, Morris DW, Wisniewski SR, Miyahara S, Nierenberg AA, Fava M and Rush AJ (2008) Response to a selective serotonin reuptake inhibitor (citalopram) in major depressive disorder with melancholic features: a STAR*D report. *J Clin Psychiatry* 69(12):1847-1855.

Mori M, Jefferson JJ, Hummel M and Garbe DS (2008) CNTF: a putative link between dopamine D2 receptors and neurogenesis. *J Neurosci* 28(23):5867-5869.

Murray CJ and Lopez AD (1996) Evidence-based health policy--lessons from the Global Burden of Disease Study. *Science* 274(5288):740-743.

Murray F, Smith DW and Hutson PH (2008) Chronic low dose corticosterone exposure decreased hippocampal cell proliferation, volume and induced anxiety and depression like behaviours in mice. *Eur J Pharmacol* 583(1):115-127.

Nemeroff CB (2007) Prevalence and management of treatment-resistant depression. *J Clin Psychiatry* 68 Suppl 8:17-25.

Nemeroff CB, Widerlov E, Bissette G, Walleus H, Karlsson I, Eklund K, Kilts CD, Loosen PT and Vale W (1984) Elevated concentrations of CSF corticotropin-releasing factor-like immunoreactivity in depressed patients. *Science* 226(4680):1342-1344.

Nestler EJ, Gould E, Manji H, Buncan M, Duman RS, Greshenfeld HK, Hen R, Koester S, Lederhendler I, Meaney M, Robbins T, Winsky L and Zalcman S (2002) Preclinical models: status of basic research in depression. *Biological Psychiatry* 52(6):503-528.

Nibuya M, Morinobu S and Duman RS (1995) Regulation of BDNF and trkB mRNA in rat brain by chronic electroconvulsive seizure and antidepressant drug treatments. *J Neurosci* 15(11):7539-7547.

Nierenberg AA and DeCecco LM (2001) Definitions of antidepressant treatment response, remission, nonresponse, partial response, and other relevant outcomes: a focus on treatment-resistant depression. *J Clin Psychiatry* 62 Suppl 16:5-9.

Nutt DJ, Davidson JR, Gelenberg AJ, Higuchi T, Kanba S, Karamustafalioglu O, Papakostas GI, Sakamoto K, Terao T and Zhang M (2010) International consensus statement on major depressive disorder. *J Clin Psychiatry* 71 Suppl E1:e08.

Oquendo MA, Baca-Garcia E, Kartachov A, Khait V, Campbell CE, Richards M, Sackeim HA, Prudic J and Mann JJ (2003) A computer algorithm for calculating the adequacy of antidepressant treatment in unipolar and bipolar depression. *J Clin Psychiatry* 64(7):825-833.

Papakostas GI, Kornstein SG, Clayton AH, Soares CN, Hallett LA, Krishen A and Tucker VL (2007) Relative antidepressant efficacy of bupropion and the selective serotonin reuptake inhibitors in major depressive disorder: gender-age interactions. *Int Clin Psychopharmacol* 22(4):226-229.

Perugi G, Musetti L, Simonini E, Piagentini F, Cassano GB and Akiskal HS (1990) Gender-mediated clinical features of depressive illness. The importance of temperamental differences. *Br J Psychiatry* 157:835-841.

Quitkin FM, Stewart JW, McGrath PJ, Tricamo E, Rabkin JG, Ocepek-Welikson K, Nunes E, Harrison W and Klein DF (1993) Columbia atypical depression. A subgroup of depressives with better response to MAOI than to tricyclic antidepressants or placebo. *Br J Psychiatry Suppl*(21):30-34.

Rainer Q, Gardier AM, Hen R and David DJ (2009) [Neurogenesis-dependent and independent effects of anti-depressant drugs]. *Med Sci (Paris)* 25(10):795-798.

Ren K and Dubner R (2002) Descending modulation in persistent pain: an update. *Pain* 100(1-2):1-6.

Riso LP, Thase ME, Howland RH, Friedman ES, Simons AD and Tu XM (1997) A prospective test of criteria for response, remission, relapse, recovery, and recurrence in depressed patients treated with cognitive behavior therapy. *J Affect Disord* 43(2):131-142.

Ruhe HG, Huyser J, Swinkels JA and Schene AH (2006) Switching antidepressants after a first selective serotonin reuptake inhibitor in major depressive disorder: a systematic review. *J Clin Psychiatry* 67(12):1836-1855.

Ruhe HG, van Rooijen G, Spijker J, Peeters FP and Schene AH (2011) Staging methods for treatment resistant depression. A systematic review. *J Affect Disord*.

Rush AJ, Thase ME and Dube S (2003) Research issues in the study of difficult-to-treat depression. *Biol Psychiatry* 53(8):743-753.

Rush AJ, Trivedi MH, Wisniewski SR, Nierenberg AA, Stewart JW, Warden D, Niederehe G, Thase ME, Lavori PW, Lebowitz BD, McGrath PJ, Rosenbaum JF, Sackeim HA, Kupfer DJ, Luther J and Fava M (2006) Acute and longer-term outcomes in depressed outpatients requiring one or several treatment steps: a STAR*D report. *Am J Psychiatry* 163(11):1905-1917.

Rush AJ, Wisniewski SR, Warden D, Luther JF, Davis LL, Fava M, Nierenberg AA and Trivedi MH (2008) Selecting among second-step antidepressant medication monotherapies: predictive value of clinical, demographic, or first-step treatment features. *Arch Gen Psychiatry* 65(8):870-880.

Russo-Neustadt AA, Alejandre H, Garcia C, Ivy AS and Chen MJ (2004) Hippocampal brain-derived neurotrophic factor expression following treatment with reboxetine, citalopram, and physical exercise. *Neuropsychopharmacology* 29(12):2189-2199.

Sackeim HA (2001) The definition and meaning of treatment-resistant depression. *J Clin Psychiatry* 62 Suppl 16:10-17.

Sackeim HA, Prudic J, Devanand DP, Decina P, Kerr B and Malitz S (1990) The impact of medication resistance and continuation pharmacotherapy on relapse following response to electroconvulsive therapy in major depression. *J Clin Psychopharmacol* 10(2):96-104.

Sairanen M, Lucas G, Ernfors P, Castren M and Castren E (2005) Brain-derived neurotrophic factor and antidepressant drugs have different but coordinated effects on neuronal turnover, proliferation, and survival in the adult dentate gyrus. *J Neurosci* 25(5):1089-1094.

Samuels BA, Leonardo ED, Gadient R, Williams A, Zhou J, David DJ, Gardier AM, Wong EH and Hen R (2011) Modeling treatment-resistant depression. *Neuropharmacology.*

Santarelli L, Saxe M, Gross C, Surget A, Battaglia F, Dulawa S, Weisstaub N, Lee J, Duman R, Arancio O, Belzung C and Hen R (2003) Requirement of hippocampal neurogenesis for the behavioral effects of antidepressants. *Science* 301(5634):805-809.

Scatton B, Simon H, Le Moal M and Bischoff S (1980) Origin of dopaminergic innervation of the rat hippocampal formation. *Neurosci Lett* 18(2):125-131.

Schreiber G, Golan M and Avissar S (2009) Beta-arrestin signaling complex as a target for antidepressants and as a depression marker. *Drug News Perspect* 22(8):467-480.

Shaw AM, Boules M, Zhang Y, Williams K, Robinson J, Carlier PR and Richelson E (2007) Antidepressant-like effects of novel triple reuptake inhibitors, PRC025 and PRC050. *Eur J Pharmacol* 555(1):30-36.

Shelton RC and Tomarken AJ (2001) Can recovery from depression be achieved? *Psychiatr Serv* 52(11):1469-1478.

Shirayama Y, Chen AC, Nakagawa S, Russell DS and Duman RS (2002) Brain-derived neurotrophic factor produces antidepressant effects in behavioral models of depression. *J Neurosci* 22(8):3251-3261.

Skolnick P, Krieter P, Tizzano J, Basile A, Popik P, Czobor P and Lippa A (2006) Preclinical and clinical pharmacology of DOV 216,303, a "triple" reuptake inhibitor. *CNS Drug Rev* 12(2):123-134.

Skolnick P, Popik P, Janowsky A, Beer B and Lippa AS (2003) Antidepressant-like actions of DOV 21,947: a "triple" reuptake inhibitor. *Eur J Pharmacol* 461(2-3):99-104.

Sloan DM and Kornstein SG (2003) Gender differences in depression and response to antidepressant treatment. *Psychiatr Clin North Am* 26(3):581-594.

Sotsky SM, Glass DR, Shea MT, Pilkonis PA, Collins JF, Elkin I, Watkins JT, Imber SD, Leber WR, Moyer J and et al. (1991) Patient predictors of response to psychotherapy and pharmacotherapy: findings in the NIMH Treatment of Depression Collaborative Research Program. *Am J Psychiatry* 148(8):997-1008.

Souery D, Amsterdam J, de Montigny C, Lecrubier Y, Montgomery S, Lipp O, Racagni G, Zohar J and Mendlewicz J (1999) Treatment resistant depression: methodological overview and operational criteria. *Eur Neuropsychopharmacol* 9(1-2):83-91.

Souery D, Oswald P, Massat I, Bailer U, Bollen J, Demyttenaere K, Kasper S, Lecrubier Y, Montgomery S, Serretti A, Zohar J and Mendlewicz J (2007) Clinical factors associated with treatment resistance in major depressive disorder: results from a European multicenter study. *J Clin Psychiatry* 68(7):1062-1070.

Strohle A and Holsboer F (2003) Stress responsive neurohormones in depression and anxiety. *Pharmacopsychiatry* 36 Suppl 3:S207-214.

Surget A, Saxe M, Leman S, Ibarguen-Vargas Y, Chalon S, Griebel G, Hen R and Belzung C (2008) Drug-dependent requirement of hippocampal neurogenesis in a model of depression and of antidepressant reversal. *Biol Psychiatry* 64(4):293-301.

Thase ME (2011) Treatment-resistant depression: prevalence, risk factors, and treatment strategies. *J Clin Psychiatry* 72(5):e18.

Thase ME, Carpenter L, Kupfer DJ and Frank E (1991) Clinical significance of reversed vegetative subtypes of recurrent major depression. *Psychopharmacol Bull* 27(1):17-22.

Thase ME and Rush AJ (1997) When at first you don't succeed: sequential strategies for antidepressant nonresponders. *J Clin Psychiatry* 58 Suppl 13:23-29.

Tian JW, Jiang WL, Zhong Y, Meng Q, Gai Y, Zhu HB, Hou J, Xing Y and Li YX (2011) Preclinical pharmacology of TP1, a novel potent triple reuptake inhibitor with antidepressant properties. *Neuroscience*.

Tran P, Skolnick P, Czobor P, Huang NY, Bradshaw M, McKinney A and Fava M (2011) Efficacy and tolerability of the novel triple reuptake inhibitor amitifadine in the treatment of patients with major depressive disorder: A randomized, double-blind, placebo-controlled trial. *J Psychiatr Res*.

Tremblay P and Blier P (2006) Catecholaminergic strategies for the treatment of major depression. *Curr Drug Targets* 7(2):149-158.

Trivedi MH, Rush AJ, Wisniewski SR, Nierenberg AA, Warden D, Ritz L, Norquist G, Howland RH, Lebowitz B, McGrath PJ, Shores-Wilson K, Biggs MM, Balasubramani GK and Fava M (2006) Evaluation of outcomes with citalopram for depression using measurement-based care in STAR*D: implications for clinical practice. *Am J Psychiatry* 163(1):28-40.

Tsankova NM, Berton O, Renthal W, Kumar A, Neve RL and Nestler EJ (2006) Sustained hippocampal chromatin regulation in a mouse model of depression and antidepressant action. *Nat Neurosci* 9(4):519-525.

Vialou V, Robison AJ, Laplant QC, Covington HE, 3rd, Dietz DM, Ohnishi YN, Mouzon E, Rush AJ, 3rd, Watts EL, Wallace DL, Iniguez SD, Ohnishi YH, Steiner MA, Warren BL, Krishnan V, Bolanos CA, Neve RL, Ghose S, Berton O, Tamminga CA and Nestler EJ (2010) DeltaFosB in brain reward circuits mediates resilience to stress and antidepressant responses. *Nat Neurosci* 13(6):745-752.

Wang JW, David DJ, Monckton JE, Battaglia F and Hen R (2008) Chronic fluoxetine stimulates maturation and synaptic plasticity of adult-born hippocampal granule cells. *J Neurosci* 28(6):1374-1384.

Willner P (2005) Chronic mild stress (CMS) revisited: consistency and behavioural-neurobiological concordance in the effects of CMS. *Neuropsychobiology* 52(2):90-110.

Willner P, Towell A, Sampson D, Sophokleous S and Muscat R (1987) Reduction of sucrose preference by chronic unpredictable mild stress, and its restoration by a tricyclic antidepressant. *Psychopharmacology (Berl)* 93(3):358-364.

Wong EH, Tarazi FI and Shahid M (2010) The effectiveness of multi-target agents in schizophrenia and mood disorders: Relevance of receptor signature to clinical action. *Pharmacol Ther* 126(2):173-185.

Yang P, Arnold SA, Habas A, Hetman M and Hagg T (2008) Ciliary neurotrophic factor mediates dopamine D2 receptor-induced CNS neurogenesis in adult mice. *J Neurosci* 28(9):2231-2241.

Young MA, Fogg LF, Scheftner WA, Keller MB and Fawcett JA (1990) Sex differences in the lifetime prevalence of depression: does varying the diagnostic criteria reduce the female/male ratio? *J Affect Disord* 18(3):187-192.

Zisook S, Rush AJ, Haight BR, Clines DC and Rockett CB (2006) Use of bupropion in combination with serotonin reuptake inhibitors. *Biol Psychiatry* 59(3):203-210.

7

New Approaches for the Therapy of Treatment Refractory Depression

Oguz Mutlu, Güner Ulak, Ipek Komsuoglu Celikyurt,
Füruzan Yıldız Akar and Faruk Erden
Kocaeli University Medical Faculty, Pharmacology Department, Kocaeli
Turkey

1. Introduction

Depression is a common, chronic, recurrent and life debilitating illness with severe morbidity and increased suicide risk (Kiecolt-Glaser&Glaser, 2002). The mechanisms and brain areas underlying the pathophysiology of this disorder are not yet well understood. Treatment-resistant depression (TRD) or treatment-refractory depression is a term used in clinical psychiatry to describe cases of major depressive disorder that do not respond to adequate courses of at least two antidepressants. Clinical studies indicate elevated plasma nitrate levels and increased nitric oxide synthase (NOS) expression in the hippocampus of depressed patients (De Oliveira et al., 2008). The prevalence of depression during life is 17–19% and suicide during depression is 15% (Kessler et al., 1994). Conventional antidepressant treatment has many limitations such as some medicines are slow to take effect, side effect profile limits the success of therapy and there are also a large number of treatment resistant patients. Such a profile has necessitated new therapeutic strategies in offering faster onset of action and augmenting the therapeutic actions of currently existing antidepressants and thus getting a greater efficacy in a larger proportion of patients.

2. Pathways playing role in depression

2.1 5-hydroxytryptamine (5-HT), Noradrenaline (NA) and dopamine pathway

An important theory for the formation of depression is the monoamine hypothesis which suggests that there is a decreasing effect of biological amines like serotonin (5-HT), noradrenalin and dopamine in depression (Schildkraut, 1965). It is well known that the serotonin system plays an important role in the neural regulation of mood (Duman et al., 1997) and enhancement of 5-HT neurotransmission influences the therapeutic response to different classes of antidepressant treatment. In previous studies (Ulak et al., 2008; Yildiz et al., 2000) a SSRI fluoxetine shortened the immobility time in a forced swimming test (FST). In animal studies SSRI (selective serotonin reuptake inhibitor) drugs are believed to exert their clinical antidepressant effect by blocking the reuptake of serotonin at the synapse, resulting in an elevation of extracellular serotonin concentrations in the brain. In our previous study (Ulak et al., 2010), preadministration of parachlorophenylalanine (pCPA) to fluoxetine treated rats, significantly prolonged the immobilization time as in line with the previous studies showing that the behavioural effects of the SSRI fluoxetine in FST could be blocked by serotonin depletion (Connor et al., 2001; Zomkowski et al., 2004).

Citalopram is established to be one of the most selective of the SSRIs (Goodnick& Goldstein, 1998) and it is postulated that citalopram administration do not alter hippocampal NOS activity under basal conditions (Wegener et al., 2004). Tianeptine is an atypical antidepressant which is reported to increase serotonin re-uptake and decrease extracellular 5-HT in the brain (in contrast with most antidepressant agents) (Datla&Curzon,1993; Fattacini et al.,1990). How tianeptine exerts its effects is a question that remains. Although the neurochemical properties of tianeptine and of selective serotonin reuptake inhibitors differ, they demonstrate similar antidepressant efficacy (Wilde and Benfield, 1995). It is interesting how these two antidepressants with opposite molecular mechanisms act. The fact that both inhibitors and enhancers of the serotonin reuptake are potent antidepressants, challenges the hypothesis on the central mechanisms of actions of these drugs. Nowakowska et al. (2000) claimed that in reference spatial memory test (food finding time in a maze), tianeptine exerted no effect whereas fluoxetine caused a very marked improvement of spatial reference memory. So, besides the effects on serotonin re-uptake, other mechanisms must play an important role in the action of these drugs.

The classical antidepressant imipramine exerts its effects by inhibiting both 5-HT and noradrenalin reuptake (Carrodi&Fuxe, 1968). The novel antidepressant reboxetine is a selective noradrenalin reuptake inhibitor. It selectively inhibits the reuptake of synaptic norepinephrine with no marked affinity for other receptors or transporters (Wong et al., 2000). The antidepressant-like activity of reboxetine is described in animal models of depression like FST (Wong et al., 2000). There is a complex interaction between ventral and dorsal noradrenergic bundles projecting neurons in modulating the antidepressant-like effects of reboxetine in the forced swimming test (Cryan et al., 2002b). It is established that forced swimming test exposure increases serotonergic activity in the amygdala, frontal cortex and hippocampus and dopamine turnover in the striatum; and reboxetine attenuates forced swimming test-induced increases in amygdaloidal and cortical serotonin turnover and striatal dopamine turnover (Connor et al., 1999).The anti-immobility effects of reboxetine may be more closely related to its ability to antagonize the stressor-induced increase in dopaminergic turnover in the striatum since it is known that mesocorticolimbic dopaminergic activity may play a role in the behaviour of rats in the forced swimming test (Willner, 1995).

2.2 Role of 5-HT receptors

Studies using drugs affecting the serotonergic system do not only include the inhibition of serotonin reuptake in the synaptic terminal or inhibiting its metabolism (monoaminooxidase inhibitors); there are also antidepressants affecting 5-HT receptor subtypes and this class of antidepressants are also frequently used in the therapy of depression (Blier&Ward, 2003).

Recent studies have focused on the involvement of 5-HT1A receptors in the mechanism of action of antidepressant drugs (Blier&Ward, 2003). 5-HT1A receptor is the best known among 14 serotonergic receptor groups (Pucadyil et al., 2005) and it is important in psychiatric disorders like schizophrenia (Millan, 2000; Yasuno et al., 2004) and depression (Celada et al., 2004). The discovery of WAY 100635, the first highly selective, potent and silent 5-HT1 receptor antagonist (Forster et al., 1995), enabled further clarification on the role of 5-HT 1A receptors in the antidepressant-like effects of drugs.

Inhibition of 5-HT2A receptor releases exerts antidepressant-like effects in FST (Sibille et al., 1997). Suicide attempt in severe depressive patients due to the polymorphism in the 5-HT2 receptor gene is established (Du et al., 2000) and this supports the role of 5-HT2A receptors in depression. Inhibition of 5-HT2A/2C receptors play an important role in the antidepressant-like effects of conventional antidepressants in FST (Van Oekelen et al., 2003; Redrobe and Bourin, 1997).

It has been postulated that the inhibition of 5-HT1A receptors by WAY 100635 cause the synergic potentialization of increased extracellular 5-HT levels in serotonergic antidepressants (Romero et al., 1996). Besides, when WAY 100635 was given together with a subactive dose of fluoxetine in FST, it significantly decreased the immobility time in FST (Rocha et al., 1997).

2.3 Role of N-Methyl-D-Aspartate (NMDA) receptors

NMDA receptor activity appears to play a role in some neurophysiological phenomena and administration of NMDA antagonists exerted antidepressant-like effects in the FST in animals, a pre-clinical behavioural method used for studying the antidepressant activity of drugs (Borsini, 1995; Cryan et al., 2002a; Trullas & Skolnick, 1990). Interestingly, competitive and non-competitive NMDA receptor antagonists induce

antidepressant-like effects in animal models (Eckeli et al., 2000) and combined therapy of NMDA receptor antagonists with subactive doses of antidepressants such as fluoxetine, venlafaxine and imipramine, resulted in an antidepressant response in the FST test (Rogóz et al., 2002).

Administration of NMDA antagonists has been shown to produce antidepressant- like effects in animal models (Trullas & Skolnick, 1990). NOS inhibition may exert similar effects to that NMDA receptor antagonists. Since it has been shown that NMDA receptor antagonists augment the activity of antidepressants such as fluoxetine, venlafaxine and imipramine when given in combination (Rogoz et al., 2002), it is a fact that interruption of the NMDA-NO synthase pathway may result in antidepressant-like and/or augmented antidepressant activity (Harkin et al., 2004).

2.4 Role of Nitric Oxide (NO) pathway

NO plays an important role in the brain, and pharmacological manipulations of the NO pathway will constitute a novel approach for future therapeutic applications. In the brain, NO is synthesized from L-arginine by NOS, as a response to activation of NMDA receptors by excitatory amino acids (Garthwaite, 1991; Moncada et al., 1991). It plays an important role in regulating many behavioural, cognitive and emotional processes such as learning, aggression, locomotion, anxiety and depression (Dzoljic et al., 1997; Harkin et al., 1999; Holscher 1997; Nelson et al., 1995;Wiley et al., 1995). In recent studies, inhibition of NOS enzyme elicited antidepressant-like behavioural effects in several animal experiments (Harkin et al., 1999; Jefferys and Funder, 1996; Da Silva et al., 2000; Yildiz et al., 2000a,b) and this effect was reversed by NOS substrate L-arginine, suggesting that NO plays an important role in these behavioural responses (Harkin et al., 1999; Jefferys and Funder, 1996; Yildiz et al.,2000a,b).

A number of studies have demonstrated that NOS could modulate the release of central noradrenalin (Satoh et al., 1996), dopamine (Segieth et al., 2000; Wegener et al., 2000) and 5-HT (Smith&Whitton, 2000; Wegener et al., 2000). NOS activity is involved in the mechanism of action of several antidepressants. For example, the selective serotonin reuptake inhibitor paroxetine inhibits in vitro NOS activity and decreases plasma nitrite and nitrate levels significantly in depressed patients (Finkel et al., 1996). It is proposed that, NOS inhibitor 7-NI may increase serotonin (5- HT) levels in rat hippocampus after systemic therapy (Wegener et al., 2000), suggesting that antidepressant-like effects of NOS inhibitors can be related with the changes that occur in 5-HT levels in the brain. This is confirmed by the fact that NOS inhibition modulates central serotonin release (Kiss, 2000; Smith&Whitton, 2000; Wegener et al., 2000).

2.4.1 Effects of NOS inhibitors in depression

Various inhibitors of nitric oxide synthase (NOS) have been shown to exert antidepressant-like behavioural effect in a variety of animal models (Harkin et al., 1999; Volke et al., 2003; Yildiz et al., 2000). In previous studies, a neuronal and inducible NOS inhibitor 1-[2-(trifluoromethyl) phenyl] imidazole (TRIM) exerted an antidepressant-like effect in the FST (Borsini, 1995; Cryan et al., 2002; Trullas & Skolnick, 1990; Ulak et al., 2008; Volke et al., 2003) and in the unpredictable chronic mild stress (UCMS) model (Mutlu et al., 2009) in animals. UCMS model is a promising and valuable animal model of depression which shows similar features to the depressive symptoms seen in human. This stres model consists from repeated mild physical and psychological stressors. Mice were subjected several times a day for 7 weeks to different kinds of stressors in a chronic, inevitable and unpredictable way.

In a previous study (Mutlu et al., 2009) we showed that UCMS regimen induced a coat state degradation and this effect was reversed by a selective neuronal and inducible nitric oxide synthase inhibitor TRIM as well as by fluoxetine. Interestingly, the onset of this action was faster after TRIM compared to fluoxetine (Fig 1a). Indeed, coat state improvement occurred 3 weeks after TRIM treatment whereas 5 weeks therapy was necessary to observe fluoxetine's action. Similar effects were also observed in the splash test (Fig. 1b). Moreover, in the resident–intruder test, stressed mice demonstrated a larger degree of aggressivity, an effect abolished by both drugs (Fig. 1c). These results cannot be attributed to the effects of the drugs on activity since both TRIM and fluoxetine had no effect on locomotor activity.

It is proposed that, a NOS inhibitor 7-Nitroindazol (7-NI) may increase serotonin (5-HT) levels in rat hippocampus after systemic therapy (Wegener et al., 2000), suggesting that antidepressant-like effects of NOS inhibitor can be related to the changes that occur in 5-HT levels in the brain. This is confirmed by the fact that NOS inhibition modulates central serotonin release (Kiss, 2000; Smith&Whitton, 2000; Wegener et al., 2000). In rats exposed to chronic mild stress, 5-HT and 5-HIAA (5-hydroxy indol acetic acid) levels decreased significantly in many brain regions, compared to nonstressed animals (Li et al., 2003; Vancassel et al., 2008). Therefore, it can be the fact that effects of TRIM might be explained by its ability to reverse the UCMS-induced alteration of 5-HT.

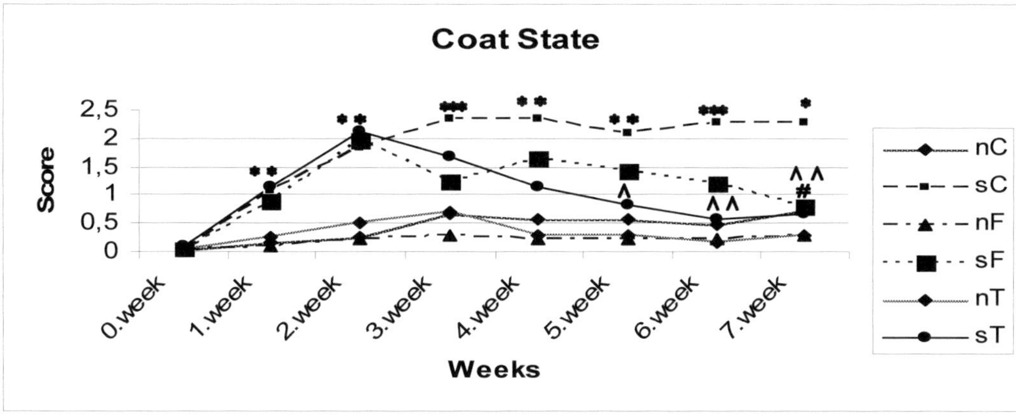

Fig. 1a. Effects of fluoxetine (15 mg/kg, i.p.) and TRIM (30 mg/kg, i.p.) given for 35 days on coat state in non-stressed and stressed groups during UCMS. All of the treatments begun after 2 weeks of stress regimen and were administered during 5 weeks. Data are means±SEM. *p<0.05, **p<0.01, ***p<0.001, difference between stressed and non stressed vehicle; ^p<0.05, ^^p<0.01 difference between stressed TRIM and stressed vehicle. # p<0.05, difference between stressed and non stressed fluoxetine group. nC = nonstressed control(vehicle) group, nF = nonstressed fluoxetine group, nT =nonstressed TRIM group, sC = stressed control (vehicle) group, sF = stressed fluoxetine group, and sT = stressed TRIM group.

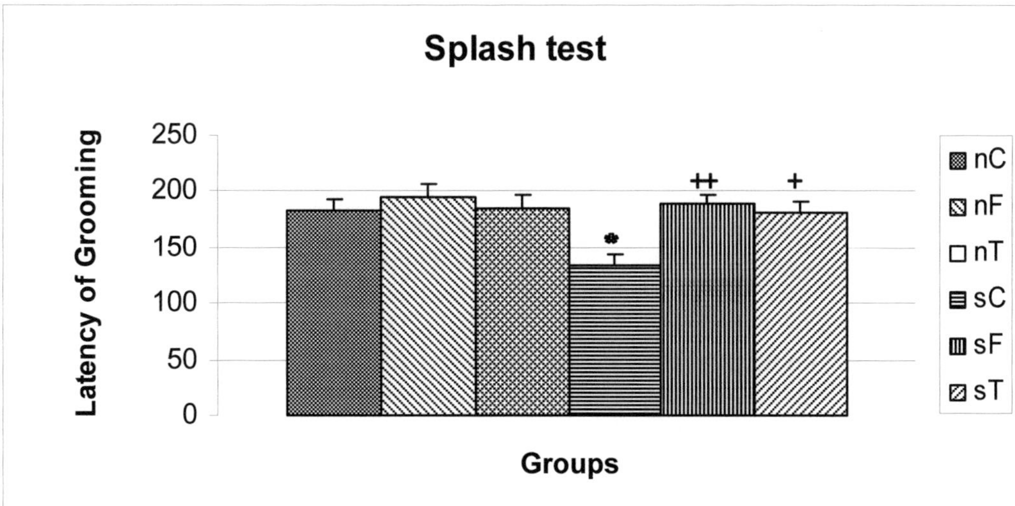

Fig. 1b. Effects of fluoxetine (15 mg/kg, i.p.) and TRIM (30 mg/kg, i.p.) given for 35 days on total time of grooming in the splash test in the end of the unpredictable chronic mild stress regimen. Data are means±SEM. *p<0.01, compared to non-stressed vehicle group, +p<0.05, ++p<0.01, compared to the stressed vehicle group. nC = nonstressed control (vehicle) group, nF = nonstressed fluoxetine group, nT = nonstressed TRIM group, sC = stressed control (vehicle) group, sF = stressed fluoxetine group, and sT = stressed TRIM group.

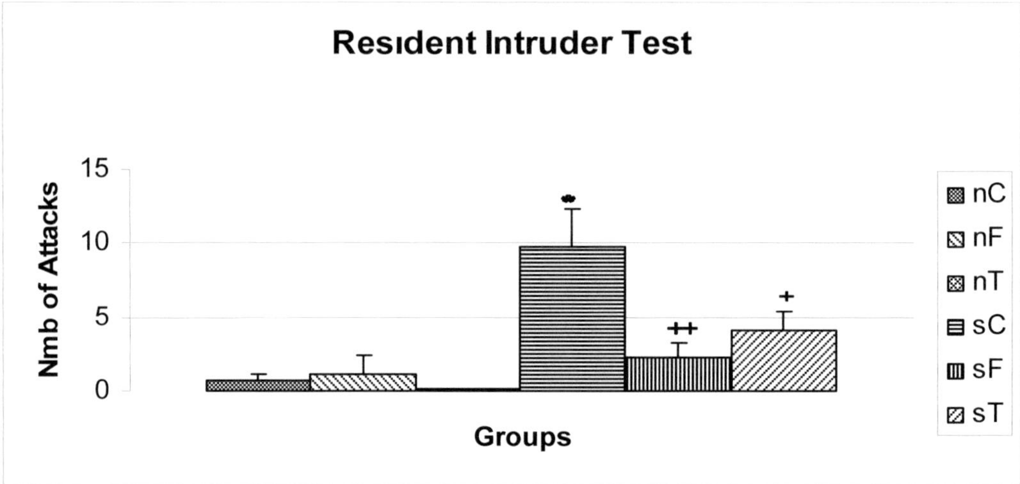

Fig. 1c. Effects of fluoxetine (15mg/kg, i.p/day, 35 days) and TRIM(30 mg/kg, i.p./day, 35 days) on attack frequency in the resident-intruder test after UCMS. Data are means±SEM. *p<0.0001, compared to the non-stressed vehicle group, +p<0.05, ++p<0.01, compared to the stressed vehicle group. nC = nonstressed control (vehicle) group, nF = nonstressed fluoxetine group, nT = nonstressed TRIM group, sC = stressed control (vehicle) group, sF = stressed fluoxetine group, and sT = stressed TRIM group.

Indeed inhibition of NO synthesis may exert similar effects to the NMDA receptor antagonists (Wiley et al.,1995) and it can be suggested that NOS inhibition can have antidepressant effects similar to NMDA receptor antagonists.

Recent studies postulated that various inhibitors of NOS such as competitive nonspecific NOS inhibitor NG-nitro-Larginine methyl ester (L-NAME), NG-nitro-L-arginine (L-NA), selective neuronal NOS (nNOS) inhibitors 7-nitroindazole (7-NI) and NW-propyl-L-arginine (L-NPA) possess antidepressant-like properties in animal models (Ghasemi et al., 2008; Harkin et al., 2004; Volke et al., 2003; Yildiz et al., 2000a,b). It is suggested that nNOS plays a key role in the antidepressant- like effects of NOS inhibitors (Volke et al., 2003). This is in line with the observation that nNOS mRNA release increases after stress in several brain regions (De Oliveira et al., 2000) and that CMS exposure regulates nNOS expression selectively in hippocampus while it doesn't change inducible NOS (iNOS) and endothelial NOS (eNOS) expressions (Zhou et al., 2007). Furthermore, over-expression of nNOS suppresses hippocampal neurogenesis in the hippocampus of animals exposed to chronic stress while nNOS inhibition preserves and reverses CMS induced effects by promoting hippocampal neurogenesis (Zhou et al., 2007). Zhou et al. (2007) showed that CMS-induced behavioural despair and hippocampal neurogenesis impairment were prevented and reversed in mice receiving a nNOS inhibitor 7-NI. TRIM had different pharmacokinetic and pharmacodynamic features when compared with 7-NI and controversial results exist for the selectivity on nNOS inhibition of these two compounds (Fidecka, 2003; Handy et al., 1995; Volke et al., 2003). TRIM at 50 mg/kg doses inhibits nNOS and clearly exerts antidepressive and anxiolytic effects although it also inhibits locomotion and motor activity at this dose (Volke et al., 2003).

2.4.2 Effects of the concurrent administration of NOS inhibitors and antidepressants on depression

Noradrenalin and serotonin are two neurotransmitters widely reported to be involved in the mechanism of action of antidepressants and the development of drugs selectively affecting these transmitters has provided the opportunity to determine the role of these transmitter systems, alone and in combination, in an antidepressant response. NOS activity is involved in the mechanism of action of several antidepressants. For example, the selective serotonin reuptake inhibitor paroxetine inhibits in vitro NOS activity and decreases plasma nitrite and nitrate levels significantly in depressed patients (Finkel et al., 1996), whereas chronic therapy with imipramine or citalopram did not change NOS activity in the examined brain regions (cortex, hippocampus or cerebellum) (Jopek et al., 1999). Furthermore, Wegener et al. (2003) showed that, serotonergic antidepressants paroxetine, citalopram and tianeptine and mixed serotonergic–noradrenergic antidepressant imipramine decreased hippocampal NOS activity in vitro in rats although they don't have direct effects on NOS under clinically relevant conditions. It seems that there are controversial results for the effects of different antidepressants on NOS activity but the actions on NOS are common to a variety of structurally dissimilar serotonergic antidepressants.

Ulak et al., (2008) examined the effects of a selective nNOS inhibitor TRIM, a 5-HT/NA reuptake inhibitor imipramine, SSRIs (selective serotonine reuptake inhibitors) citalopram and fluoxetine, serotonin reuptake enhancer tianeptine or selective NA reuptake inhibitor reboxetine alone or in combination in the FST in rats. TRIM decreased the immobility time at 50 mg/kg dose in the FST in rats. When given alone TRIM, imipramine, citalopram, fluoxetine, tianeptine and reboxetine did not shorten the immobility time of rats. The higher doses of these drugs, except citalopram produced a significant reduction in the immobility of rats. Coadministration subeffective doses of TRIM and reboxetine did not affect the behavior of rats in the FST whereas subeffective dose of TRIM given in combination with imipramine, citalopram, fluoxetine and tianeptine significantly reduced the immobility time of rats in the FST (Fig 2, 3, 4, 5, 6). Thus the pharmacological mechanism seems to be more due to serotonergic than adrenergic neurotransmission and co-administration of antidepressants acting via serotonergic system by TRIM may enhance beneficial effects in therapy-resistant depression and thus represent a potential source of novel drugs for antidepressant therapy.

Moreover the ability of TRIM to potentiate the behavioural activity of antidepressants acting via serotonergic system in the FST is not attributed to a nonspecific locomotor stimulant effect of these drugs.

Following reasons can be suggested to explain the augmentation of the effects of antidepressant drugs acting via the serotonergic system by nNOS inhibitor TRIM in the FST in rats: One is that activation of NMDA receptors result in the formation of NO and increases cyclic guanosine monophosphate (cGMP) levels (East and Garthwaite, 1991). Consistent with our findings, Harkin et al. (2004) showed that NO synthase inhibitor NGnitro- L-arginine (L-NA) augmented the effects of imipramine, fluoxetine, sertraline and citalopram but not reboxetine in the mouse FST; moreover this synergistic effect was also tested between 7-nitroindazole and imipramine or fluoxetine. Thus it was claimed that NOS inhibitors augment the effects of serotonin reuptake inhibitors in the FST. Moreover it has been shown that L-NA and 7-NI exert similar antidepressant-like behavioural profiles as SSRI in FST in rats. Although it is not clear whether NMDA receptor antagonists exert antidepressant- like effects in the FST via the serotonergic mechanism, it has been postulated that this antidepressant-like behaviour of L-NA and 7-NI is endogen serotonin dependent (Harkin et al., 2003). So it is postulated that the antidepressant augmenting effects of NOS inhibitors may be attributed to the modulation of serotonin release (Harkin et al., 2004). Since it has been demonstrated that inhibition of NOS can modulate the release of central serotonin (Kiss, 2000;Wegener et al., 2000), this may be the point of view.

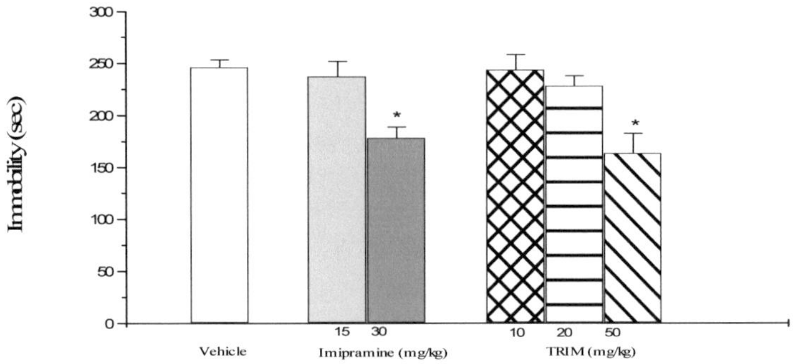

a

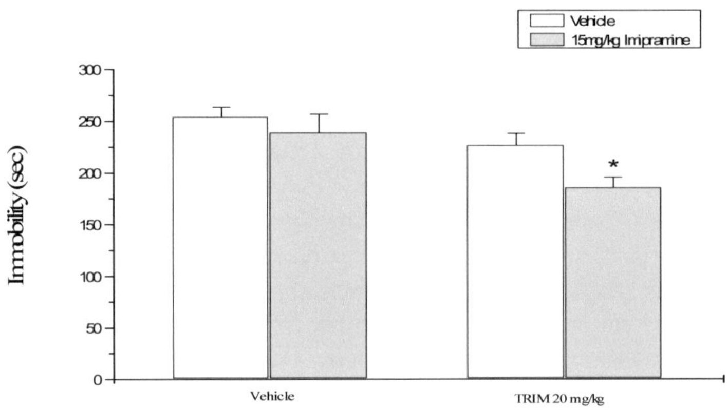

b

Fig. 2. (a). Effects of imipramine and TRIM on the immobility time in the rat FST. Each column represents the mean±SEM of 7–14 animals.*p<0.001 compared to vehicle control (Tukey test). (b). TRIM potentiates the activity of imipramine in the rat FST. Each column represents the mean±SEM of 7–10 animals.*p=0.011 compared to vehicle imipramine (15 mg/kg) (Dunnet test).

A second explanation for this result is that paroxetine, a selective serotonin reuptake inhibitor, is also a potent inhibitor of NOS enzyme activity (Finkel et al., 1996). Later, Wegener et al. (2003) showed that serotonergic antidepressants paroxetine, citalopram and tianeptine and the mixed serotonergic–noradrenergic antidepressant imipramine decrease NOS activity in vivo suggesting that actions on NOS are common to a variety of structurally dissimilar serotonergic antidepressants. From this point of view, it may be speculated that,

NOS inhibition in the brain plays some role in the antidepressant effect of drugs acting via serotonergic system. Since NMDA receptors play an important role in brain NOS activation, these effects may be due to secondary inhibitory effects on NMDA receptors.

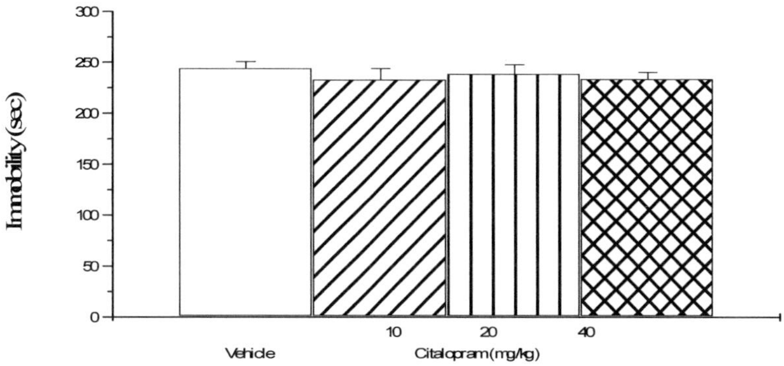

a

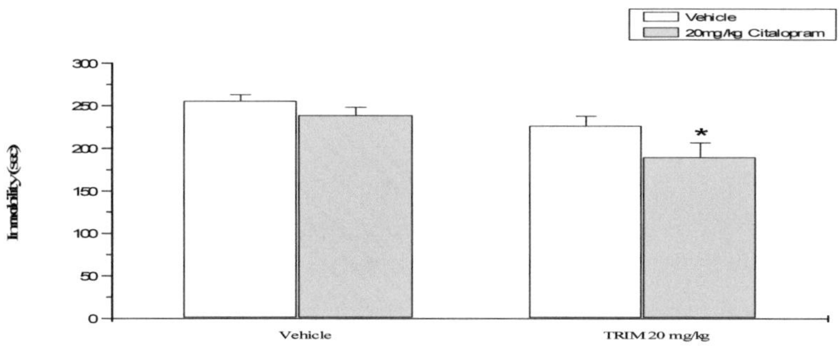

b

Fig. 3. (a). Effects of citalopram on the immobility time in the rat FST. Each column represents the mean±SEM of 7-9 animals. Citalopram failed to shorten the immobility time in the FST in rats. (b).TRIM (20 mg/kg) augments the activity of citalopram in the rat FST. Each column represents the mean±SEM of 7-9 animals.*p=0.017 compared to vehicle citalopram (Dunnet test).

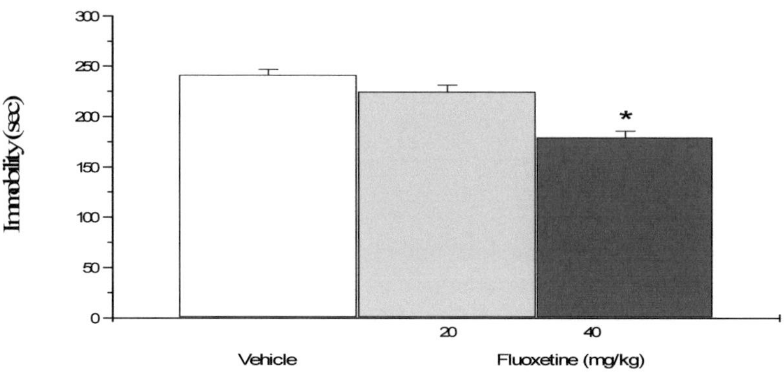

a

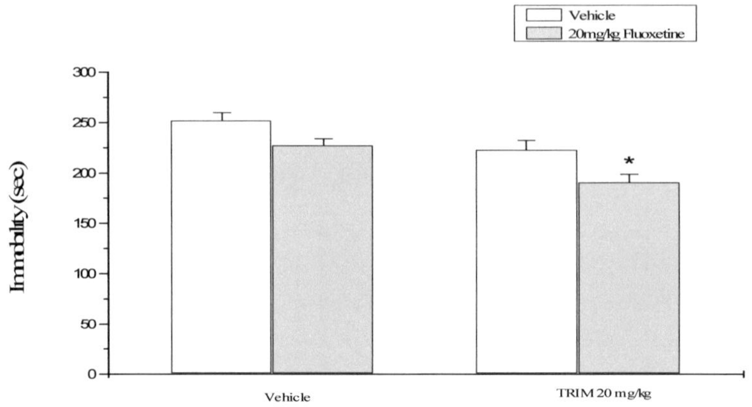

Fig. 4. (a). Effects of fluoxetine on the immobility time in the rat FST. Each column represents the mean±SEM of 7 animals. *p<0. 001 compared to vehicle control (Tukey test). (b).TRIM (20 mg/kg) augments the activity of fluoxetine in the rat FST. Each column represents the mean±SEM of 6-10 animals.*p=0.01 compared to vehicle fluoxetine (Dunnet test).

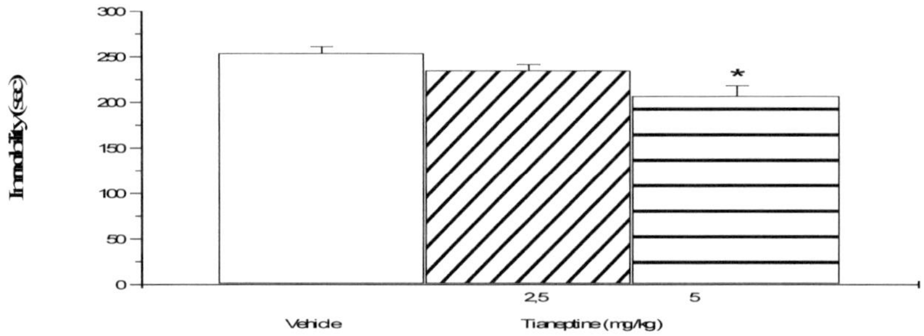

a

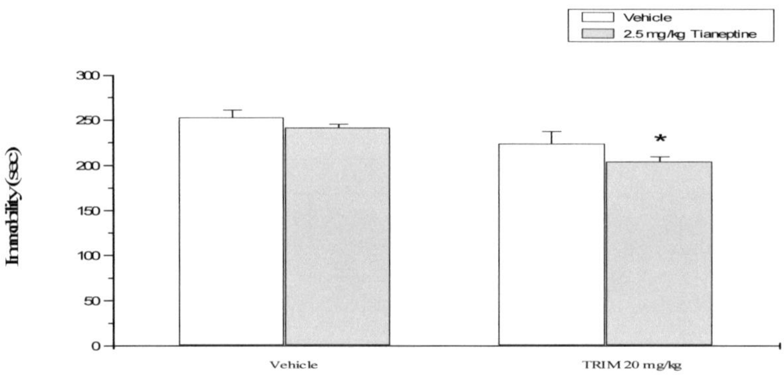

b

Fig. 5. (a). Effects of tianeptine on the immobility time in the rat FST. Each column represents the mean±SEM of 6–7 animals.*p<0.01 compared to vehicle control (Tukey test). (b). TRIM (20 mg/kg) augments the activity of tianeptine in the rat FST. Each column represents the mean±SEM of 6–9 animals.*p=0.015 compared to vehicle tianeptine (Dunnet test).

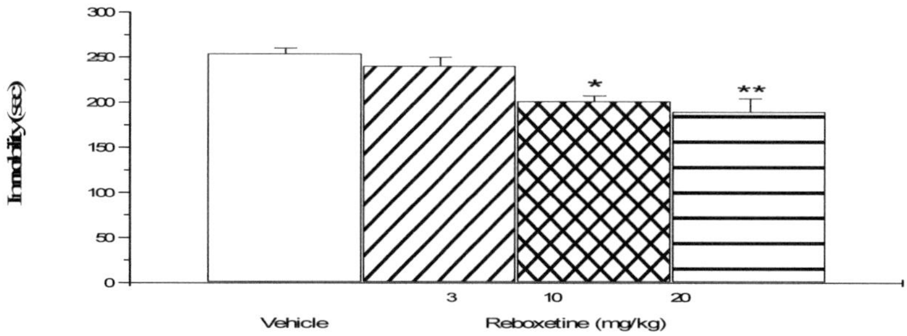

a

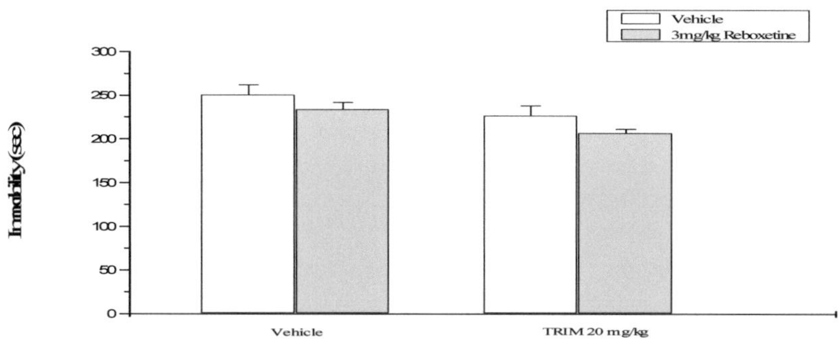

b

Fig. 6. (a). Effects of reboxetine on the immobility time in the rat FST. Each column represents the mean±SEM of 7-9 animals.*p<0.01,**p<0.001 compared to vehicle control (Tukey test). (b).TRIM (20 mg/kg) failed to augment the activity of reboxetine in the rat FST. Each column represents the mean±SEM of 8-12 animals. Reboxetine+TRIM combined group compared to vehicle reboxetine group (p=0.066, Dunnet test).

Thus the pharmacological mechanism seems to be more due to serotonergic than adrenergic neurotransmission and co-administration of antidepressants acting via the serotonergic system by TRIM, a selective nNOS inhibitor may enhance beneficial effects in therapy-resistant depression and thus represent a potential source of novel drugs for antidepressant therapy.

2.4.3 Effects of the coadministration of NOS inhibitors and 5-HT receptor antagonists on depression

In a previous study in our laboratory (Ulak et al., 2010), the involvement of the serotonergic system in the antidepressant-like effect of TRIM in the FST in rats was studied by depleting endogenous 5-HT with the tryptophan hydroxylase inhibitor pCPA (Connor et al., 2001; Page et al., 1999) and by using 5-HT1 and 5-HT2 receptor antagonists to investigate the behavioural responses to TRIM in the FST since it is well known that that these receptors play an important role in mood disorders (Clenet et al., 2001; Gardier et al., 1996; O'Neill and Conway, 2001; Redrobe et al., 1996; Redrobe and Bourin, 1998). This study extended the previous data of us, which had shown that TRIM augmented the effect of antidepressants acting via serotonergic system in the FST in rats (Ulak et al., 2008). In this study, TRIM exerted antidepressant-like activity comparable to that of the tricyclic antidepressant imipramine. Pretreatment of rats with WAY 100635, a selective 5-HT1A receptor antagonist, or with GR127935, a selective 5-HT1B/1D receptor antagonist) slightly reversed the immobility-reducing effect of TRIM, but this failed to reach a statistically significant level; while alone they had no effect in the rat FST (Fig 8). Pretreatment with methiothepin (a non-selective 5-HT receptor antagonist), cyproheptadine (a 5-HT2 receptor antagonist) or ketanserin (a 5HT2A/2C receptor antagonist) prevented the effect of TRIM in the FST (Fig 7, 9). So further experiments are needed to clarify the involvement of 5-HT1 receptors in the antidepressant-like effect of TRIM.

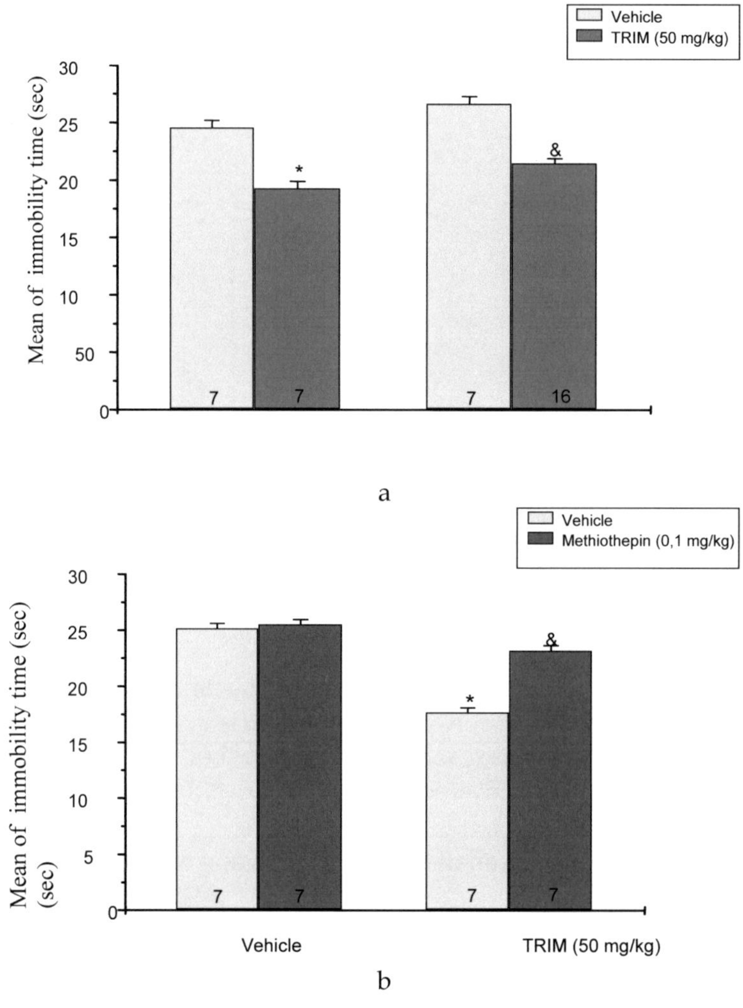

Fig. 7. a: Effects of the pretreatment of animals with pCPA on TRIM-induced reductions on immobility time in the rat FST. The number of animals per group is shown in the columns. Results are expressed as mean±SEM *p<0.001 compared to control (Tukey's test), &pb0.05 compared to pCPA untreated TRIM group (Tukey's test). b: Effects of pretreatment of animals with methiothepine on TRIM-induced reductions on immobility time in the rat FST. The number of animals per group is shown in the columns. Results are expressed as mean±SEM *p<0.001 compared to control (Tukey's test), &pb0.001 compared to methiothepine untreated TRIM group (Tukey's test).

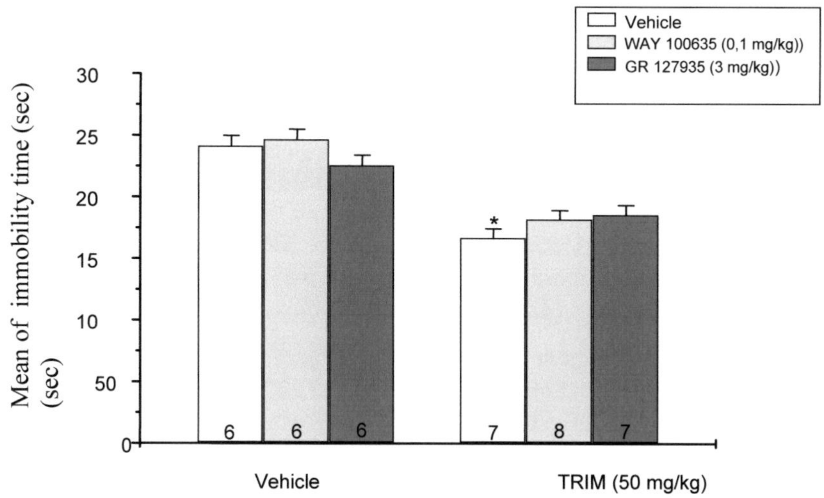

Fig. 8. Effects of pretreatment of animals with: WAY 100635, (b) GR 127935 on TRIM-induced reductions in immobility time in the rat FST. The number of animals per group is shown in the columns. Results are expressed as mean±SEM. *p<0.001 compared to control (Tukey's test).

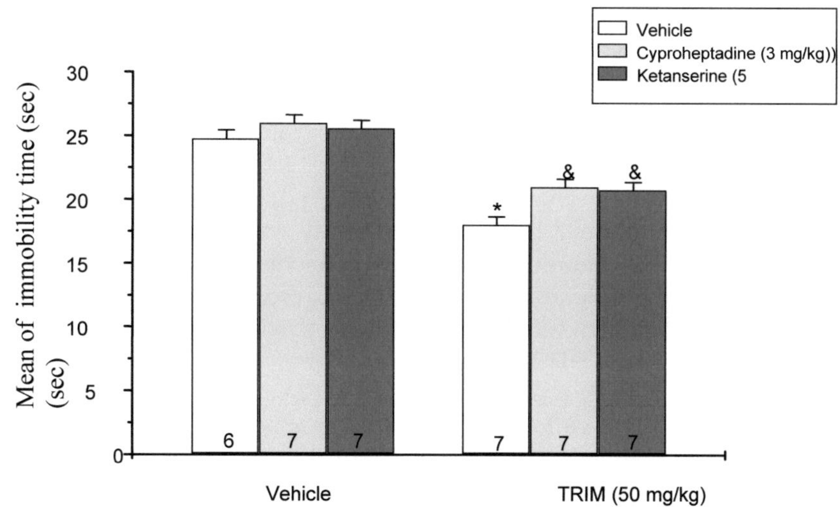

Fig. 9. The effect of pretreatment of animals with cyproheptadine or ketanserine on TRIM-induced reductions in immobility time in the rat FST. The number of animals per group is shown in the columns. Results are expressed as mean±SEM. *p<0.001 compared to control (Tukey's test), &p<0.05 compared to TRIM+vehicle administered group (Tukey's test).

The results of our previous study reveal that TRIM-induced reduction of immobility time in the FST was partially attenuated by pretreatment with the 5-HT depleting agent pCPA in rats. The treatment regimen of pCPA used in this study produced a greater than 90% depletion of cortical 5-HTconcentration in the rat but had no effect on cortical dopamine and noradrenalin concentrations (Connor et al., 2001; Harkin et al., 2003). Pretreatment with pCPA did not alter the immobility time of control animals but attenuated the anti-immobility effect of TRIM. Thus the results of our study suggested that endogenous 5-HT is involved in the antidepressant-like effect of TRIM. In line with our findings, serotonin depletion with pCPA prevented the antidepressant-like effect of the NOS inhibitors 7-NI and NG-nitro-,L-arginine in FST (Harkin et al., 2003; Yildiz et al., 2000). The antidepressant-like effect of NOS inhibitors in the FST is dependent on NOS and NMDA receptor inhibition (Mutlu et al., 2009; Wiley et al., 1995;). So reversal of the TRIM-induced antidepressant-like effect by pCPA treatment might be due to activation of 5-HT resulting from NOS inhibition and blockade of NMDA receptors (Zomkowski et al., 2002).

While methiothepin, a non-selective 5-HT receptor antagonist had no effect on immobility time in FST in our study and other studies (Buckley et al., 2004; Zomkowski et al., 2004), the reversal of antidepressant-like effect of TRIM by pretreatment of rats with methiothepin, reinforces the idea that 5-HT is involved in the action of TRIM in the FST. There are few studies investigating the interaction between the antidepressants and 5-HT receptor subtype affecting substances in animal depression models. Tatarczynska et al., (2004) suggested that pretreatment of rats with 5-HT1A receptor antagonist and with 5-HT1B/1D receptor antagonist reversed the immobility-reducing effect of TRIM, in the rat FST. 5-HT1B receptor antagonists were also reported to reverse the antidepressant-like effect of paroxetine and imipramine (Gardier et al., 2003; O'Neill and Conway, 2001). The results of our study revealed that pretreatment of rats with WAY 100635, a selective 5-HT1A receptor antagonist or with GR127935, a selective 5-HT1B/1D receptor antagonist) slightly reversed the immobility-reducing effect of TRIM, but this failed to reach a statistically significant level; while on its own, they had no effect in the rat FST.

Although the role of 5-HT2 receptors on the effect of antidepressants was investigated before (Middlemiss et al., 2002; Redrobe and Bourin, 1998), there is no study about the interaction of 5-HT2 receptor antagonists and nNOS inhibitors in animal models of depression. So another important finding of our study was that, the antidepressant-like effect of TRIM in the FST was prevented by pretreatment with cyproheptadine, a 5-HT2 receptor antagonist and with ketanserin, a 5HT2A/2C receptor antagonist having higher affinity for 5HT2A receptors than for 5HT2C receptors (Van Oekelen et al., 2003). TRIM may interact with both 5HT2A and 5HT2C receptors which are also reported to play role in the action of antidepressants (Clenet et al., 2001). Thus 5-HT2A receptors, at least partially, have a role on the antidepressant-like effect of TRIM. It is reported that NOS inhibitors increased the release of 5-HT in prefrontal cortex (Smith and Whitton, 2000). Therefore, it could be postulated that TRIM affects 5-HT2A receptors by increasing 5-HT level in the synaptic terminal.

3. Novel antidepressants

In current studies (unpublished data) in our laboratory we investigated the effect of tianeptine (5 mg/kg, 35 days) and olanzapine (2.5 mg/kg, 35 days), in (UCMS exposed mice when compared with the ones of the widely used selective serotonine reuptake antidepressant drug fluoxetine (15 mg/kg/day, 35 days). We revealed that olanzapine also has significant antidepressant like effects in the UCMS test which supports the efficacy of atypical antipsychotics as antidepressants in unipolar major depression and in treatment-resistant unipolar depression. A significant difference between the coat state score of non-stressed and UCMS-exposed groups was observed (unpublished data). Both fluoxetine and olanzapine significantly reversed the UCMS-induced degradation in the coat state. Both olanzapine and fluoxetine blocked the stress-induced deficit in total latency of grooming in the splash test, decreased the attack frequency in the resident intruder test, decreased the immobility time in the tail suspension test. No significant effect was observed between stressed and nonstressed animals in the novelty suppressed feeding test. There was no significant difference between the body weight and locomotion of the animals at the end of UCMS regimen. Both olanzapine and fluoxetine decreased enhanced levels of plasma ACTH, cortisol and IL-6 while only fluoxetine reversed stress-induced increasement of TNF-α levels in mice. Olanzapine had anxiolytic-like effects both in stressed and nonstressed mice in the open field test (unpublished data). Recent studies also showed that a new atypical antipychotic asenapine reversed UCMS induced effects in rodents (Marston et al., 2010).

A large number of novel serotonin targets are in a testing phase. One particularly interesting novel serotonin target is the 5HT2C receptor. Blockade of 5HT2C receptors causes release of both norepinephrine and dopamine and these agents can be called norepinephrine dopamine disinhibitors or NDDIs. A novel antidepressant agomelatine combines this property of 5HT2C antagonism and thus NDDI actions with additional agonist actions at melatonin receptors (MT1 and MT2). Agomelatin also has 5HT2B antagonist properties. This portfolio of pharmacological actions predicts not only antidepressant actions due to the NDDI mechanism of 5HT2C antagonism but also sleep-enhancing properties due to MT1 and MT2 agonist actions. Another NDDI with 5HT2C antagonist properties is flibanserin. This agent also has 5HT2A antagonist and 5HT1A agonist properties and, because of its robust NDDI properties, it is under investigation for sexual dysfunction linked to deficient dopamine activity, including conditions such as hypoactive sexual desire disorder (HSDD). Triple reuptake inhibitors (TRIs) or serotonin-norepinephrine-dopamine-reuptake inhibitors (SNDRIs), beta 3 receptor agonists, glucocorticoid antagonists, corticotrophin releasing factor 1 (CRF 1) antagonists, vasopressin 1B antagonists, and neurokinin antagonists are examined for depression. TRIs or SNDRIs combinations are applied in order to examine the idea that if one mechanism is good (i.e., SSRI) and two mechanisms are better (i.e., SNRI), then maybe targeting all three mechanisms of the trimonoamine neurotransmitter system would be the best in terms of efficacy. The question for TRIs is how much blockade of each monoamine transporter is desired, especially for the dopamine transporter or DAT. Too much dopamine activity can lead to drug abuse, not enough means that the agent is essentially an SNRI. Perhaps the desirable doses is robust inhibition of the serotonin transporter and substantial inhibition of the norepinephrine transporter, like the known SNRI, plus %10 to%25 inhibition of DAT. Some experiments suggest that DRI action also increases acetylcholine release, so TRIs may modulate a fourth neurotransmitter system and act as multitransmitter modulators(new study?). Further testing will determine whether the available TRIs will represent an advance over SSRIs or SNRIs in the treatment of depression. A very novel mechanism for an antidepressant is posed by amibegron, an agonist of beta 3 receptors. The role of beta 3 receptors in the brain is still being clarified, but it appears that they may be localized in high density in the amygdala, where they may regulate neuronal activity in ventromedial prefrontal cortex and thereby exert their antidepressant actions. Extensive testing reference? in animal models of depression demonstrates the antidepressant actions of amibegron, and human testing is currently in progress. Glucocorticoid antagonists, corticotrophin releasing factor 1 (CRF 1) antagonists and vasopressin 1B antagonists will be further examined not only for depression but also for various stress-related conditions. Nemifitide is itself a novel pentapeptide modeled on the structure of melanocyte inhibitory factor (MIF-1), a tripeptide shown to be active in animal models of depression and in small clinical studies of depressed patients reference? MIF-1 (also known as L-prolyl-L-leucy-L-glycinamide, or PLG) is also the tripeptide tail of oxytocin and its precursor neurophysin. Nemifitide is a pentapeptide analog not only of the tripeptide MIF-1 but also of the tripeptide tail of vasopressin. Nemifitide is administered by subcutaneous injection and has been shown to be active in animal models of depression; it is prelimary results of experiments with depressed patients, that early findings suggest possible efficacy with rapid onset, including effectiveness in treatment-resistant patientsreference?. Further testing in patients with major depressive episodes is ongoing (Stahl, 2010).

Another class of peptide antagonists is the neurokinin antagonists. Neurokinins belong to the family of peptides known as tachykinins. Tachykinins include not only neurokinins but also newly discovered endokinins and tachykinin gene-related peptides that act mostly outside the brain but at the same receptors where the tachykinins act (especially the NK1 receptor). Low-molecular-weight antagonists have been identified for each of the three known neurokinin receptors, NK1, NK2, and NK3. NK1 antagonists, also known as substance P antagonists, have been hotly pursued for many years as treatments not only for depression but also for pain, schizophrenia, and other psychiatric disorders. To date, the clinical results with substance P antagonists, from studies on major depression and in pain-related conditions, have been disappointing. However, recent evidencereference? suggests that saredutant, an NK2 antagonist, may be effective not only in animal models of depression but also in patients with major depressive episodes. Hypothetically, conditions associated with excessive release of endogenous NKA (or its extended or shortened versions), especially under conditions of stress or major depression, benefit from the blocking of NK2 receptors; that could explain why this mechanism may produce an antidepressant effect. NK3 antagonists are also tested for various psychiatric disorders (Stahl, 2010).

4. Conclusion

In conclusion, NOS inhibitors can be a novel approach for antidepressant therapy, exerting their effect possibly on neuronal NOS and TRIM, by the selective inhibition of both nNOS and iNOS. The antidepressant-like effect of TRIM in the FST seems to be mediated, at least in part, by an interaction with 5-HT2 receptors, while non-significant effects were obtained with 5-HT1 receptors. Further studies are needed to enlighten whether the antidepressant-like effect of NOS inhibitors are dependent on endogene serotonin and to know how these serotonin receptors are playing a role in this effect. Besides, the potentiation of the antidepressant-like effect of fluoxetine by TRIM might have a therapeutic value for NOS inhibitors and form a new treatment strategy to increase the clinical effect of antidepressants. A large number of novel serotonin targets are in a testing phase for the treatment of depression. Norepinephrine dopamine disinhibitors or NDDIs, agomelatine, flibanserin, triple reuptake inhibitors (TRIs) or serotonin-norepinephrine-dopamine-reuptake inhibitors (SNDRIs), beta 3 receptor agonists, glucocorticoid antagonists, corticotrophin releasing factor 1 (CRF 1) antagonists, vasopressin 1B antagonists, and neurokinin antagonists are further examined for the treatment of depression.

5. Acknowledgements

We would like to thank to Mrs. Catherine Belzung (Université François Rabelais, Faculté des Sciences et Techniques, Tours, France) for helpful comments about our studies.

6. References

Blier, P.&Ward, N.M. (2003). Is there a role for 5-HT1A agonists in the treatment of depression? *Biol Psychiatry*;53:193–203.

Borsini, F. (1995). Role of the serotonergic system in the forced swimming test. *Neurosci Biobehav Rev*;19:377–95.

Buckley, M.J.; Surowy, C.; Meyer, M.& Curzon, P. (2004). Mechanism of action of A-85380 in an animal model of depression. *Neuropsychopharmacol Biol Psychiatry*;28(4): 723–30.

Carrodi, H.& Fuxe, K. (1968). The effects of imipramine on central monoamine neurones. *J Pharm Pharmacol*;20:230–1.

Celada, P., Puig, M., Amargos-Bosch, M., Adell, A.& Artigas, F. (2004). The therapeutic role of 5-HT1A and 5-HT2A receptors in depression. *J Psychiatry Neurosci*;29(4):252–65.

Clenet, F.; De Vos, A.& Bourin, M. (2001). Involvement of 5-HT(2C) receptors in the anti-immobility effects of antidepressants in the forced swimming test in mice. *Eur Neuropsychopharm*;11:145–52.

Connor, T.J.; Dennedy, M.C.; Harkin, A.&Kelly, J.P. (2001). Methylenedioxymethamphetamine induced suppression of interleukin-1beta and tumour necrosis factor-alpha is not mediated by serotonin. *Eur J Pharmacol*;418:147–52.

Connor, T.J.; Kelliher, P.; Harkin, A.; Kelly, J.P.& Leonard, B.E. (1999). Reboxetine attenuates forced swim test -induced behavioral and neurochemical alterations in the rat. *Eur J Pharmacol*;379:125–33.

Cryan, J.F.; Markou, A.& Lucki, I. (2002a). Assessing antidepressant activity in rodents: recent developments and future needs. *Trends Pharmacol Sci*;23:238–45.

Cryan, J.F.; Page, M.E.& Lucki, I. (2002b). Noradrenergic lesions differentially alter the antidepressantlike effects of reboxetine in a modified forced swim test. *Eur J Pharmacol*;436: 197–205.

Datla, K.P.& Curzon, G. (1993). Behavioural and neurochemical evidence for the decrease of brain extracellular 5-HT by the antidepressant drug tianeptine. *Neuropharmacology*;32:839–45.

De Oliveira, R.M.W.; Guimarães, F.S.& Deakin, J.F.W. (2008). Expression of neuronal nitric oxide synthase in the hippocampal formation in affective disorders. *Braz J Med Biol Res*;41(4):333–41.

Dhir, A.& Kulkarni, S.K. (2007). Effect of addition of yohimbine (alpha-2-receptor antagonist) to the antidepressant activity of fluoxetine or venlafaxine in the mouse forced swim test. *Pharmacology*;80:239–43.

Du, L., Bakish, D.; Lapierre, Y.D.; Ravindran, A.V.& Hrdina, P.D. (2000). Association of polymorphism of serotonine 2A receptor gene with suicidal ideation in major depressive disorder. *Am J Med Genet*;96:56–60.

Duman, R.S.; Heninger, O.R.& Nestler, E.L. (1997). A molecular and cellular theory of depression. *Arch Gen Psychiatry*;54:597–606.

Dzoljic, E., De Vries, R.& Dzoljic, M.R. (1997). New and potent inhibitors of nitric oxide synthase reduce motor activity in mice. *Behav Brain Res*;87(2):209–12.

East, S.J.& Garthwaite, J. (1991). NMDA receptor activation in rat hippocampus induces cyclic GMP formation through the L-arginine-nitric oxide pathway. *Neurosci Lett*; 123:17–9.

Fattacini, C.M.& Bolanos-Jimenez, F.& Gozlan, H.& Hamon, M. (1990). Tianeptine stimulates uptake of 5-hydroxytryptamine in vivo in the rat brain. *Neuropharmacology*;29:1–8.

Fidecka, S. (2003). Study on the influence of potent inhibitors of neuronal nitric oxide synthase on the antinociceptive and anticonvulsant activity of benzodiazepines in mice. *Pol J Pharmacol*;55:193–201.

Finkel, M.S.; Laghrissi-Thode, F.; Pollock, B.G.& Rong, J. (1996). Paroxetine is a novel nitric oxide synthase inhibitor. *Psychopharmacol Bull*;32:653–8.

Forster, E.A.; Cliffe, I.A.; Bill, D.J.; Dover, G.M.; Jones, D., Reilly, Y.&Fletcher, A. (1995). A pharmacological profile of the selective silent 5-HT1A receptor antagonist, WAY 100635. *Eur J Pharmacol*;281:81–8.

Gardier, A.M.; David, D.J.; Jego, G.; Przybylski, C.; Jacquot, C.& Durier, S., Gruwez, B.; Douvier, E.; Beauverie, P.; Poisson, N.; Hen, R.& Bourin, M. (2003). Effects of chronic paroxetine treatment on diaysate serotonin in 5-HT1B receptor knockout mice. *J Neurochem*;86(1):13–24.

Gardier, A.M.; Malagie, I.; Trillat, A.C.; Jacquot, C.& Artigas, F. (1996). Role of 5-HT1A autoreceptors in the mechanism of action of serotoninergic antidepressant drugs: recent findings from in vivo microdialysis studies. *Fundam Clin Pharmacol*;10(1):16–27.

Garthwaite, J. (1991). Glutamate, nitric oxide and cell–cell signalling in the nervous system. *Trends Neurosci*;14:60–7.

Ghasemi, M.; Sadeghipour, H.; Mosleh, A.; Sadeghipour, H.R.; Mani, A.R.; Dehpour, A.R. (2008). Nitric oxide involvement in the antidepressant-like effects of acute lithium administration in the mouse forced swimming test. *Eur Neuropsychopharmacol*;18:323–32.

Goodnick, P.J.& Goldstein, B.J. (1998). Selective serotonin reuptake inhibitors in affective disorders: I. Basic pharmacology. *J Psychopharmacol*;12(3suppl):S5–S20.

Handy, R.L.C.;Wallace, P.; Gaffen, Z.A.; Whitehead, K.J.& Moore, P.K. (1995). The antinociceptive effect of 1-(2 trifluoromethylphenyl)imidazole (TRIM), a potent inhibitor of neuronal nitric oxide synthase in vitro, in the mouse. *Br J Pharmacol*;116:2349–50.

Harkin, A.; Connor, T.J.; Burns, M.P.& Kelly, J.P. (2004). Nitric oxide synthase inhibitors augment the effects of serotonin re-uptake inhibitors in the forced swimming test. *Eur Neuropsychopharmacol*;14(4):274–81.

Harkin, A.; Connor, T.J.; Walsh, M.; St. Jonh, N.& Kelly, J.P. (2003). Serotonergic mediation of the antidepressant-like effects of nitric oxide synthase inhibitors. *Neuropharmacology*;44:616–23.

Harkin, A.J.; Bruce, K.H.; Craft, B.& Paul, I.A. (1999). Nitric oxide synthase inhibitors have antidepressant-like properties in mice. 1. Acute treatments are active in the forced swim test. *Eur J Pharmacol*;372(3):207–13.

Holscher, C. (1997). Nitric oxide, the enigmatic neuronal messenger: its role in synaptic plasticity. *Trends Neurosci*;20:298–303.

Jefferys, D.&Funder, J. (1996). Nitric oxide modulates retention of immobility in the forced swimming test in rats. *Eur J Pharmacol*;295:131–5.

Jopek, R.; Kata, M.& Nowak, G. (1999). The activity of rat brain nitric oxide synthase following chronic antidepressant treatment. *Acta Pol Pharm*;56(4):307–10.

Kessler, R.C.; Mc Gonagle, K.A.; Nelson, C.B.; Hughes, M.; Swartz, M.& Blazer, D.G. (1994). Sex and depression in the national comorbidity Survey II: Cohort effects. *J Affect Disord*;30(1):15–26.

Kiecolt-Glaser, J.& Glaser, R. (2002). Depression and immune function. Central pathways to morbidity and mortality. *J Psychosom Res*;53:873.

Kiss, J.P. (2000). Role of nitric oxide in the regulation of monoaminergic neurotransmission. *Brain Res Bull*;52:459–66.

Li, J.M.; Kong, L.D.; Wang, Y.M.; Cheng, C.H.K.; Zhang, W.Y.& Tan, W.Z. (2003). Behavioral and biochemical studies on chronic mild stress models in rats treated with a Chinese traditional prescription Banxia-houpu decoction. *Life Sci*;74:55–73.

Marston, H.M.; Martin, F.D.; Papp, M.; Gold, L.; Wong, E.H.& Shahid, M. (2010). Attenuation of chronic mild stress-induced 'anhedonia' by asenapine is not associated with a 'hedonic' profile in intracranial self-stimulation. *J Psychopharmacol*; Aug 10. [Epub ahead of print]

Middlemiss, D.N.; Price, G.W.& Watson, J.M. (2002). Serotonergic targets in depression. Curr Opin Pharmacol;2:18–22. Millan MJ. Improving the treatment of schizophrenia: focus on serotonin (5-HT)(1A) receptors. *J Pharmacol Exp Ther* 2000;295(3):853–61.

Moncada, S.; Palmer, R.M.J.& Higgs, E.A. (1991). Nitric oxide: physiology, pathophysiology and pharmacology. *Pharmacol Rev*;43:109–42.

Mutlu, O.; Ulak, G.; Laugeray, A.& Belzung, C. (2009). Effects of neuronal and inducible NOS inhibitor 1-[2 (trifluoromethyl) phenyl] imidazole (TRIM) in unpredictable chronic mild stress procedure in mice. *Pharmacol Biochem Behav* 92(1):82-7.

Nelson, R.J.; Demas, G.E.; Huang, P.L.; Fishman, M.C.; Dawson, V.L.; Dawson, T.M.&Snyder, S.E. (1995). Behavioural abnormalities in male mice lacking neuronal nitric oxide synthase. *Nature*;378:383–6.

Nowakowska, E.; Kus, K.; Chodera, A.& Rybakowski, J. (2000). Behavioural effects of fluoxetine and tianeptine, two antidepressants with opposite action mechanisms, in rats. *Arzneimittelforschung*;50(1):5–10.

O'Neill, M.F.& Conway, M.W. (2001). Role of 5-HT1A and 5-HT1B receptors in themediation of behavior in the forced swim test in mice. *Neuropsychopharmacology*;24:391–8.

Pucadyil, T.J.; Kalipatnapu, S.& Chattopadhyay, A. (2005). The serotonin 1A receptor: a representative member of serotonin receptor family. *Cell Mol Neurobiol*;25(3–4): 553–80.

Redrobe, J.P.& Bourin, M. (1998). Clonidine potentiates the effects of 5-HT, 5-HT2A/2C and 5-HT1A/1B antagonists and 8-OH-DPAT in the mouse forced swimming test. *Eur Neuropsychopharmacol*;8:169–73.

Redrobe, J.P.& Bourin, M. (1997). Partial role of 5-HT2 and 5-HT3 receptors in the activity of antidepressants in the mouse forced swimming test. *Eur J Pharmacol*;325: 129–35.

Redrobe, J.P., MacSweeny, C.P.& Bourin, M. (1996). The role of 5-HT1A and 5-HT1B receptors in antidepressant drug actions in mouse forced swimming test. *Eur J Pharmacol*;318:213–20.

Rocha, M.A.; Puech, A.J.& Thiebot, M.H. (1997). Influence of anxiolytic drugs on the effects of specific serotonin reuptake inhibitors in the forced swimming test in mice. *J Psychopharmacol*;11:218–21.

Rogoz, Z.; Skuza, G.; Maj, J.& Danysz, W. (2002). Synergistic effect of uncompetitive NMDA receptor antagonists and antidepressant drugs in the forced swimming test in rats. *Neuropharmacology*;42:1024–30.

Romero, L., Hervas, I.& Artigas, F. (1996). The 5-HT1A antagonist WAY 100635 selectively potentiates the presynaptic effects of serotonergic antidepressants in the rat brain. *Neurosci Lett*;219:123–6.

Satoh, S.; Murayama, T.& Nomura, Y. (1996). Sodium nitroprusside stimulates noradrenaline release from rat hippocampal slices in the presence of dithiothreitol. *Brain Res*;733:167–74.

Schildkraut, J.J. (1965). The catecholamine hypothesis of affective disorders:a review of supporting evidence. *Am J Psychiatry*;122(5):509–22.

Segieth, J., Fowler, L., Whitton, P.& Pearce, B. (2000). Nitric oxide-mediated regulation of dopamine release in the hippocampus in vivo. *Neuropharmacology*;39(4):571–7.

Sibille, E.; Sarnyai, Z.; Benjamin, D.; Gal, J.; Baker, H.& Toth, M. (1997). Antisense inhibition of 5-hydroxytriptamine 2A receptor induces an antidepressant-like effect in mice. *Mol Pharmacol*;52:1056–63.

Smith, J.C.& Whitton, P.S. (2000). Nitric oxide modulates N-methyl-D-aspartate evoked serotonine release in the raphe nuclei and frontal cortex of the freely moving rat. *Neurosci Lett*;291(1):5–8.

Stahl, S.M. (2008). *Stahl's Essential Psychopharmacology:Neuroscientific Basis and Practical Applications* (Third Edition). Cambridge University Press, ISBN 978-0-521-85702-4, USA

Tatarczynska, E.; Klodzinska, A.; Stachowicz, K.&Chojnacka-Wojcik, E. (2004). Effect of combined administration of 5HT1A or HT1B/1D receptor antagonists and antidepressants in the forced swimming test. *Eur J Pharmacol*;487:133–42.

Trullas, R.& Skolnick, P. (1990). Functional antagonists at the NMDA receptor complex exhibit antidepressant action. *Eur J Pharmacol*;185:1-10.

Ulak, G.; Mutlu, O.; Tanyeri, P.; Komsuoglu, F.I.; Yıldız Akar, F.& Erden, B.F. (2010). Involvement of serotonin receptor subtypes in the antidepressant-like effect of trim in the rat forced swimming test. *Pharmacol Biochem Behav*;; 95:308–314.

Ulak, G.; Mutlu, O.; Yıldız Akar, F.; Komsuoğlu, F.I.; Tanyeri, P.& Erden, B.F. (2008). Neuronal NOS inhibitor 1-(2-trifluoromethylphenyl)-imidazole augment the effects of antidepressants acting via serotonergic system in the forced swimming test in rats. *Pharmacol Biochem Behav*;90(4):563–8.

Van Oekelen, D.; Luyten, W.H.M.L.&Leysen, J.E. (2003). 5-HT2A and 5-HT2C receptors and their atypical regulation properties. *Life Sci*;72:2429–49.

Vancassel, S.; Leman, S., Hanonick, L.; Denis, S.; Roger, J.; Nollet, M.; Bodard, S.; Kousignian, I.; Belzung, C.& Chalon, S. (2008). n-3 polyunsaturated fatty acid supplementation reverses stress-induced modifications on brain monoamine levels in mice. *J Lipid Res*;49(2):340–8.

Volke, V.; Wegener, G.; Bourin, M.& Vasar, E. (2003). Antidepressant- and anxiolytic-like effects of selective neuronal NOS inhibitor 1-(2-trifluoromethylphenyl)-imidazole in mice. *Behav Brain Res*;140:141–7.

Wegener, G.; Bandpey, Z.; Heiberg, I.L.; Volke, V.; Trabace, L.& Rosenberg R.& Harvey, B.H. (2004). Combined chronic treatment with citalopram and lithium does not modify the regional neurochemistry of nitric oxide in rats brain. *J Physiol Pharmacol*;55(3):575–86.

Wegener, G.; Volke, V.; Harvey, B.H.& Rosenberg, R. (2003). Local, but not systemic administration of serotonergic antidepressants decreases hippocampal nitric oxide synthase activity. *Brain Res*;959:128–34.

Wegener, G.; Volke, V.& Rosenberg, R. (2000). Endogenous nitric oxide decreases hippocampal levels of serotonin and dopamine in vivo. *Br J Pharmacol*;130:575–80.

Wilde, M.I.; Benfield, P. (1995). Tianeptine. A review of its pharmacodynamic and pharmacokinetic properties, and therapeutic efficacy in depression and coexisting anxiety and depression. *Drugs*;49:411–39.

Wiley, J.L.; Cristello, A.F.& Balster, R.L. (1995). Effects of site-selective NMDA receptor antagonists in an elevated plus-maze model of anxiety in mice. *Eur J Pharmacol*;294:101–7.

Willner, P. (1995). Dopaminergic mechanisms in depression and mania. In: Bloom FE, Kupfer DJ, editors. *Psychopharmacology*: the Fourth Generation of Progress. New York: Raven Press; p. 921–31.

Wong, E.H.; Sonders, M.S.; Amara, S.G.; Tinholt, P.M.; Piercey, M.F.; Hoffmann, W.P., Hyslop, D.K.; Franklin, S.; Porsolt, R.D.; Bonsignori, A.; Carfagna, N.& McArthur, RA. (2000). Reboxetine: a pharmacologically potent, selective, and specific norepinephrine reuptake inhibitor. *Biol Psychiatry*;47:818–29.

Yasuno, F.; Suhara, T.; Ichimiya, T.; Takano, A.; Ando, T.& Okubo, Y. (2004). Decreased 5-HT1A receptor binding in amygdala of schizophrenia. *Biol Psychiatry*;55(5):439–44.

Yildiz, F.; Erden, B.F.; Ulak, G.; Utkan, T.& Gacar, N. (2000). Antidepressant-like effect of 7-nitroindazole in the forced swimming test in rats. *Psychopharmacology* (Berl);149:41–4.

Yildiz, F.; Ulak, G.; Erden, B.F.& Gacar, N. (2000) Anxiolytic-like effects of 7-nitroindazole in the rat plus-maze test. *Pharmacol Biochem Behav*;65:199–202.

Zhou, Q.; Hu, Y.; Hua, Y.; Mei, H.; Luo, C.& Han, X. (2007). Neuronal nitric oxide synthase contributes to chronic stress-induced depression by suppressing hippocampal neurogenesis. *J Neurochem*;103(5):1843–54.

Zomkowski, A.D.E.; Hammes, L.; Lin, J.; Calixto, J.B.; Santos, A.R.S.& Rodriques, A.L.S. (2002). Agmatine produces antidepressant-like effects in two models of depression in mice. *NeuroReport*;13:387–91.

Zomkowski, A.D.E.; Rosa, A.O.; Lin, J.; Santos, A.R.S.; Calixto, J.B.& Rodrigues, A.L.S. (2004). Evidence for serotonine suptypes involvement in agmatine antidepressant-like effect in the mouse forced swimming test. *Brain Res*;1023:253–63.

Section 4

Personality Psychology

8

Does Personality Affect Compulsive Buying? An Application of the Big Five Personality Model

Kalina Mikołajczak-Degrauwe, Malaika Brengman, Birgit Wauters and Gina Rossi
Vrije Universiteit Brussel
Belgium

1. Introduction

Compulsive Buying (CB) is 'a consumer's tendency to be preoccupied with buying that is revealed through repetitive buying and a lack of impulse control' (Ridgway et al., 2008). Although Kraepelin (1915) and Bleuler (1976) described this phenomenon many years ago, it was the study of Faber et al. (1987) which increased the interest in that topic. For more than 20 years empirical studies have been conducted to increase our knowledge about this maladaptive consumer behavior. The main focus of these studies has been on identifying the antecedents and consequences of CB. First of all, CB is viewed as a method of coping with life's challenges (Scherhorn, 1990), low self-esteem (d'Astous et al., 1990; Hanley & Wilhelm, 1992; O'Guinn & Faber, 1989) and/or internal psychological tension (Valence et al., 1988). It is also seen as a process whereby the consumer wants to escape from negative feelings, stress and anxiety (Edwards, 1993; Ergin, 2010; O'Guinn & Faber, 1989). Buying a product causes release of the internal tension. At the same time however feelings of guilt and frustration appear as the person could not control the inner drive to buy an unneeded product. The consumer is caught in a vicious circle.

O'Guinn and Faber (1989) argued that there is no single factor but it is a combination of psychological, physiological, genetic, social and cultural factors that can explain the etiology of CB. This is confirmed in a large number of studies revealing numerous factors differentiating compulsive from non-compulsive buyers. Among them: *'dependence'* (DeSarbo & Edwards, 1996; O'Guinn & Faber, 1989; Valence et al., 1988), *'tendency to fantasize'* (O'Guinn & Faber, 1989), *'psychasthenia'* (Scherhorn, 1990), *'compulsiveness'* (Balabanis, 2001; O'Guinn & Faber, 1989), *'perfectionism'* (DeSarbo & Edwards, 1996; Kyrios et al., 2004; O'Guinn & Faber, 1989), *'materialism'* (DeSarbo & Edwards, 1996; Johnson & Attmann, 2009; O'Guinn & Faber, 1989; Rose, 2007), *'money attitudes'* (Dongijn et al., 2009; Hanley & Wilhelm, 1992), *'impulsiveness'* (Christenson et al., 1994; DeSarbo & Edwards, 1996; Rose, 2007), *'denial'* (DeSarbo & Edwards, 1996), *'excitement seeking'* (DeSarbo & Edwards, 1996), *'obsessive thoughts'* (Kwak et al., 2004), *'risk-taking tendencies'* (Kwak et al., 2004), *'narcissism'* (Rose, 2007), *'external locus of control'* (Watson, 2009), *'self-control'* (Sneath et al., 2009), *'depression'* (Ergin, 2010; Sneath et al., 2009), *'concern for store return policies'* (Hassay &

Smith, 1998), *'concern with immediate consequences'* (Joireman et al., 2010) and *'credit card abuse'* (Faber & O'Guinn, 1988). CB has also been associated with specific early developmental experiences and the family environment (DeSarbo & Edwards, 1996; Faber & O'Guinn, 1988; McElroy et al., 1994; Scherhorn, 1990; Valence et al., 1988). Some researchers argue that CB is an attempt to compensate for a distortion of autonomy incurred in childhood (Scherhorn, 1990). It is believed that knowing the history of consumer's early experiences helps to understand why some people are more prone to develop this maladaptive consumer behavior.

Despite its negative consequences and a high comorbidity with mood, substance use and eating disorders (McElroy et al., 1994; Schlosser et al., 1994), CB is not officially recognized as a mental disorder (American Psychiatric Association [APA], 2000). Moreover, there is a disagreement about the nosology of CB: some researchers consider CB as an addictive disorder (Scherhorn, 1990), others as an obsessive-compulsive disorder (Ridgway et al., 2008). Nonetheless, there exist criteria for compulsive buying disorder (CBD), widely accepted by the researchers in the domain: 1) frequent preoccupation with shopping or irresistible buying impulses; 2) buying more than is needed or/and can be afforded; 3) distress related to buying behavior; 4) significant interference with work or social areas of functioning (McElroy et al., 1994). Currently CB is most often diagnosed as 'Impulse Control Disorder Not Otherwise Specified'.

Though no consensus about the classification of CB as a mental disorder was yet found there is no doubt that CB is a serious psychological problem which causes significant impairments in financial, legal, social and occupational areas of functioning of an affected person. Therefore it is of major importance to investigate the nature of CB and its antecedents in more detail. Knowing which variables significantly influence CB will help clinicians and affected persons to understand what the 'driving force' behind this maladaptive behavior is and to address the potential source of the problem during the therapy.

Because of their stability, personality traits are considered very useful in predicting behaviour. Although few studies were conducted in order to find the link between CB and personality (eg., Mowen & Spears, 1999; Balabanis, 2001; Wang & Yang, 2008), the inconsistent results prevent from drawing reliable conclusions. The aim of the current study is to explore the causes of these inconsistencies and to give an ultimate answer to the question whether Big Five personality traits differentiate compulsive and non-compulsive buyers.

2. Compulsive buying and the Big Five

'Personality' is 'the set of psychological traits and mechanisms within the individual that are organized and relatively enduring and that influence his or her interactions with, and adaptations to, the intrapsychic, physical, and social environments' (Larsen & Buss, 2010, p. 4). For many years efforts in research on personality have been focused on identifying the elemental personality traits. In 1934 Thurstone suggested that there are five independent common factors underlying personality, a notion further supported by Fiske (1949), Tupes & Christal (1961) and a host of other researchers (e.g., Costa & McCrae, 1985; John, 1999; Goldberg, 1992; Wiggins, 1996). The Five Factor model of personality, also known as the Big

Five (Goldberg, 1992) consists of five broad personality dimensions: *Extraversion*, *Agreeableness*, *Conscientiousness*, *Neuroticism* (or Emotional Instability) and *Intellect/Imagination* (or Openness to Experience). *Extravert* people are social, active and have a tendency to experience positive emotions whereas individuals scoring high on *Agreeableness* are sympathetic, trusting and cooperative. *Conscientious* people are well-organized and scrupulous while those scoring high on *Intellect* are open to new experiences, intellectually curious and imaginative. The last dimension - *Neuroticism* represents a tendency to experience psychological distress and emotional instability (Costa and McCrae, 1992).

Since the Big Five has achieved the greatest degree of consensus of all trait taxonomies (Larsen & Buss, 2010), it has been used to explain individual differences in a large amount of research (e.g., Endler & Spear, 1998). Although the first attempts to understand and predict consumer behavior through the use of personality variables have yielded disappointing results (Kassarjian, 1971), there has recently been a growing interest in personality influences in consumer research (e.g., Egan & Taylor, 2010; Lin, 2010; Mowen, 2000). The first attempt to identify a link between personality and compulsive buying behaviour was made by Mowen and Spears (1999). They employed Allport's hierarchical approach where surface traits are explained by central traits which are predicted by cardinal psychological traits. With regard to this approach the Five Factor Model of personality was used to explain materialism and the needs for arousal, which in turn predict compulsive buying behaviour. With respect to personality traits the results showed that low *Conscientiousness*, high *Agreeableness* and low *Stability* predict compulsive buying directly.

A similar approach was applied in two studies by Mowen (2000) with *impulsiveness* and *compulsiveness* as central traits. When data were analyzed excluding mediators from the model, only two personality traits - *Neuroticism* and *Agreeableness*, appeared to be significant predictors of compulsive buying.

Also Balabanis (2001) used the Five Factor Personality Model to explain compulsive buying behaviour. The results indicated that *Extraversion* and *Intellect*, the two factors which did not appear to directly influence compulsive buying in previous studies, were found to be related to buying compulsiveness in lottery tickets and scratch-cards. *Extraversion* was positively and *Intellect* negatively related to compulsive buying behaviour. Surprisingly, in contradiction to the findings by Mowen and Spears (1999), Balabanis (2001) found a negative correlation between *Agreeableness* and CB.

A few years later Wang and Yang (2008) published their paper on the influence of personality and compulsive buying in an online shopping context. In accordance with the findings of Mowen and Spears (1999), the researchers found *Stability* to be negatively correlated with compulsiveness in buying. With regard to the other Big Five personality traits no significant differences between compulsive and non-compulsive buyers were found.

It is important to notice that also Schlosser et al. (1994) and Mueller et al. (2010) were interested in personality influences on CB. However since their studies were conducted in clinical samples, their aim was not to compare compulsive with non-compulsive buyers in a general consumer population but to 'assess the overall life-style and problems of subjects already *recognised as compulsive shoppers*' (Schlosser et al., 1994, p. 205) or 'identify personality prototypes in *treatment seeking patients* with CB' (Mueller et al., 2010, p. 930).

Study	Extraversion	Agreeableness	Conscientiousness	Neuroticism	Intellect
Mowen and Spears, 1999	ns.*	+	-	+	ns.
Mowen, 2000	ns.	+	ns.	+	ns.
Balabanis, 2001	+	-	ns.	+	-
Wang and Yang, 2008	ns.	ns.	ns.	+	ns.

*ns. - not significant

Table 1. Relationship between CB and the Big Five Personality Traits: the Overview of Previous Research Results

As demonstrated above, with the exception of *Neuroticism,* no consistent conclusions can be drawn from the previous research on the relationship between compulsive buying behavior and personality (see Table 1). This can be due to the fact that these studies were investigating CB behavior in different buying contexts. For example Balabanis (2001) focused on scratch-cards and lottery tickets buying behavior whereas other studies examined compulsive buying behavior in general. A second ground for the inconsistent results might be due to the different samples investigated. The majority of above mentioned studies neglect to reveal the percentage of compulsive buyers in their sample. It is therefore possible that the authors were investigating the (direct or indirect) link between (compulsive) buying tendency (measured on a continuum basis) and personality with a very limited amount of actual compulsive buyers in their sample. Furthermore, all research samples of above mentioned studies under consideration consisted of only students. Although research based on student samples might be a useful source of information, it cannot be generalized to the buying population.

As a result the question about the relationship between CB and personality still remains unresolved. Taking into account the generally established significance of personality in determining consumer behavior (Haugtvedt et al., 1992; Kassarjian, 1971), the objective of the current study is to explore personality differences between consumers with and without compulsive buying tendency. In this study the above mentioned shortcomings of previous research will be addressed and the prevalence of compulsive buyers in the general (not exceptionally student) consumer population in Flanders will be revealed.

3. Statement of hypotheses

'Extraversion' implies a more impulsive person with lower self-control (Eysenck & Eysenck, 1985). Since compulsive buying is positively related to impulsiveness (Christenson et al., 1994; DeSarbo & Edwards, 1996; Rose, 2007) and low self-control (Sneath et al., 2009) we expect that:

H1: Compulsive buyers score higher on '*Extraversion*' than non-compulsive buyers.

'Agreeableness' involves trust, sympathy and altruism (Costa & McCrae, 1992). It deals with motives for maintaining positive relations with others (Jensen-Campbell & Graziano, 2001). The fact that compulsive buying is not a socially desirable behavior and therefore can prevent maintaining positive relations with others leads to the development of the second hypothesis:

H2: Compulsive buyers score lower on '*Agreeableness*' than non-compulsive buyers.

'*Conscientiousness*' refers to responsibility, precision and discipline (Costa & McCrae, 1992). People scoring high on '*Conscientiousness*' are well-organized and consider the consequences of their actions carefully. Since compulsive buying behavior is an impulsive, irresponsible act we expect that:

H3: Compulsive buyers score lower on '*Conscientiousness*' than non-compulsive buyers.

Individuals scoring high on '*Neuroticism*' tend to have low self-esteem and high levels of anxiety and depression (Costa & McCrae, 1985). Each of these variables has been associated with compulsive buying (Edwards, 1993; Ergin, 2010; O'Guinn & Faber, 1989), hence we hypothesize that:

H4: Compulsive buyers score higher on '*Neuroticism*' than non-compulsive buyers.

'*Intellect*' is characterized by original, imaginative and broad interests (McCrae & Costa, 1985). Since people scoring high on this trait are intellectually curious and have a better perception of reality, we do not expect them to engage in compulsive buying behavior. Therefore we presume that:

H5: Compulsive buyers score lower on '*Intellect*' than non-compulsive buyers.

4. Method

4.1 Participants and procedure

Data for the current study were collected over a three-month period in the beginning of 2010 in Flanders, the Dutch speaking part of Belgium. To obtain a representative sample of the Flemish consumer population we have used several ways to spread our online questionnaire. First of all we used invitations on online forums such as Flair and Libelle (women magazines popular in Belgium), a forum for shopping addicts (http://www.yes.nl/cafe/) and a forum for seniors (http://www.seniorennet.be/forum/). We have advertised the survey in our university newsletter and asked colleagues and friends to forward the questionnaire. To encourage potential respondents we promised an incentive of €100 for one randomly chosen respondent.

A total number of 2298 respondents actually participated in the study. After a careful data cleaning procedure (only Flemish adults, aged 18 years or older, who answered all the questions within a reasonable time frame, were taken into account), 1522 participants were retained from the primary dataset serving as the basis for the further analyses. The sample was clearly dominated by female participants (72,6%). Approximately 80% of the respondents was younger than 30 years with 21-24 years old participants being represented most (42%). Taking into account the focus of our study (general consumer population) and the fact that young females do the majority of shopping, this does not affect the representativity of our sample.

4.2 Measures

Although the majority of the researchers in the domain use the clinical screener of Faber and O'Guinn (1992) to measure *compulsive buying tendency*, Ridgway et al. (2008) identified two major shortcomings of this scale. First of all, it does not measure the obsessive-compulsive dimension of buying, since all the items focus on the impulse control aspect. Secondly, items concerning income and financial consequences prevent consumers with higher incomes from being recognized as compulsive buyers, as they can afford their unusual spending habits. Ridgway et al. (2008, p. 625) conclude that 'unless consumers have already been identified with a buying disorder, the clinical screener may misclassify some of them as compulsive buyers, because of its dependence on income-related items and the weights assigned to those items in the scoring algorithm'. Moreover, according to Ridgway et al. (2008), compulsive buying measurements should not focus on identifying consequences of maladaptive consumer behaviour, but on the underlying behavioural tendencies.

Therefore we opted to measure *compulsive buying tendency* with the 6-item scale developed by Ridgway et al. (2008). This scale does not include items concerning income and financial consequences, it incorporates both characteristics of obsessive-compulsive behaviour as well as the impulse-control dimensions of buying and is the first to appropriately assess the extent of *compulsive buying tendency* in the general population of consumers. Four items are measured on 7-point Likert scale from 'strongly disagree' to 'strongly agree' (*'My closet has unopened shopping bags in it'*, *'Others might consider me a shopaholic'*, *'Much of my life centers around buying things'* and *'I consider myself an impulse purchaser'*) and two items are measured on a 7-point scale from 'never' to 'very often' (*'I buy things I don't need'* and *'I buy things I did not plan to buy'*) (all items translated to Dutch with back-translation following international guidelines on test translation[1]). According to the guidelines provided by Ridgway et al. (2008), respondents who obtained a score of 25 or more points are considered compulsive buyers.

The Mini-IPIP measure of personality (Donnellan et al., 2006) was used to assess the respondents' Big Five personality traits. The scale consists of 20 items and is a short form of the 50-item International Personality Item Pool-Five-Factor Model measure (Goldberg, 1999). With 4 items per trait (items translated to Dutch with back-translation following international guidelines on test translation), the scale assesses the Big Five personality dimensions namely *Extraversion, Agreeableness, Conscientiousness, Neuroticism* and *Imagination/Intellect*. Confirmatory factor analysis performed in AMOS 18.0 revealed an acceptable goodness of fit and composite reliability (CR) of the scale in the current study.

5. Results

5.1 Confirmatory factor analysis of the Big Five measure

The goodness of fit of the Big Five model of Donnellan et al. (2006) was verified in our sample. Though all items loaded sufficiently on their scales (see Graph 1), the initial model indicated a poor fit.

Therefore three changes were entered in the model. Firstly, one item of *Neuroticism* (*'I am relaxed most of the time'*) was deleted, since it seemed to load not only on the latent variable *Neuroticism* but also on *Extraversion*. Secondly, the necessity of the introduction of 3 paths of covariance between two error terms of *Conscientiousness*, two error terms of *Agreeableness* and

[1] International Test Commission: http://www.intestcom.org/guidelines/index.php

two of *Intellect* were indicated by the modification indices[2]. Finally the error terms of one item of *Neuroticism* and one of *Intellect* were linked. This lead to an acceptable goodness of fit: χ^2 (df=138)= 994; GFI= .932; AGFI= .907 and RMSEA= .064. Since χ^2 statics are influenced by the sample size (Dickey, 1996) other test statistics were taken into consideration when evaluating the model fit. The Goodness of Fit Index and the Adjusted Goodness of Fit Index well exceed the required minimum levels of respectively .85 and .80. Also the Root Mean Square error of approximation was below the cut-off value of .08 (Brown & Cudeck, 1993).

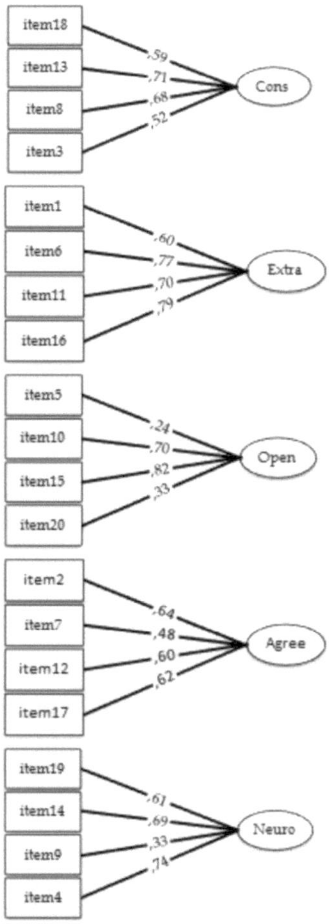

Graph 1. Conirmatory Factor Analysis with SEM: Item-Scale Loadings.

The scales' reliabilities were tested by verifying the composite reliabilities (ρ_c)[3]. *Conscientiousness* had a ρ_c of .74, *Extraversion:* ρ_c=.81, *Neuroticism*: ρ_c=.72; *Agreeableness*: ρ_c=.66 and *Intellect*: ρ_c=.78. All reliabilities exceed the minimum level of .60 (Höck & Ringel, 2006), indicating a good scale reliability (Bagozzi & Yi, 1988).

[2] Error terms can be correlated when several observed variables, which are supposed to be indicators of one latent construct, have some systematic error. Detailed discussions on correlating errors are given by Cote et al. (2001, 87-89).

[3] Composite reliability (ρ_c) is a SEM approach for the reliability estimate of the latent variable.

5.2 Differences between compulsive and non-compulsive buyers

Using the cut-off point of 25 validated by Ridgway et al. (2008, see measurements for further explanation), 93 out of 1522 respondents (6,1%) were classified as compulsive buyers (see Table 2). There were significantly more women in the compulsive buying group than in the non-compulsive buying group (Chi^2= 23,771; p<,001). There were also significant differences in *age* between both groups (Chi^2= 16,710; p=,005). Compulsive buyers seem to be younger than other consumers (average age 22years for compulsive and 26years for non-compulsive buyers, the difference is significant at p<.000). With regard to *education* (Chi^2= 3,385; p=,336) and *income* (Chi^2= 1,719; p=,887) no significant differences between compulsive and non-compulsive buyers were found.

	Total		Non-Compulsive		Compulsive	
	n	%	*n*	%	*n*	%
Gender						
Male	433	28,4	429	30,0	4	4,3
Female	1089	71,6	1000	70,0	89	95,7
Total	1522	100,0	1429	100,0	93	100,0
Age						
18-20 years	408	26,8	370	25,9	38	40,9
21-24 years	637	41,9	596	41,7	41	44,1
25-29 years	191	12,5	181	12,7	10	10,8
30-39 years	121	8,0	118	8,3	3	3,2
40-49 years	83	5,5	82	5,7	1	1,1
50 years or older	82	5,4	82	5,7	0	,0
Total	1522	100,0	1429	100,0	93	100,0
Education						
High school degree	686	45,1	639	44,7	47	50,5
Bachelor degree	315	20,7	294	20,6	21	22,6
Master degree	461	30,3	436	30,5	25	26,9
Post-Master degree	60	3,9	60	4,2	0	,0
Total	1522	100,0	1429	100,0	93	100,0
Income						
Less than 1500€	261	17,1	248	17,4	13	14,0
1501-2500€	222	14,6	212	14,8	10	10,8
2501-3500€	152	10,0	141	9,9	11	11,8
3500€ or over	220	14,5	203	14,2	17	18,3
No idea	520	34,2	487	34,1	33	35,5
I'd rather not say	147	9,7	138	9,7	9	9,7
Total	1522	100,0	1429	100,0	93	100,0

Table 2. Socio-Demographic Profile of the Respondents

Independent sample t-tests were conducted between compulsive and non-compulsive buyers regarding their personality traits (see Table 3). Compulsive buyers appeared to be significantly more *Extravert* (p<.001, *d*=.50), *Neurotic* (p<.001, *d*=.36) and *Agreeable* (p=.003, *d*=.35) in comparison to non-compulsive consumers. On the other hand, non-compulsive buyers scored higher on the trait *Intellect* ($p<.001$, d=.35) when compared to compulsive buyers. No significant difference between both groups could be revealed with regard to the trait *Conscientiousness* (p= .089, d=.20).

	Non-Compulsive Buyers		Compulsive Buyers		Cohen's d
	M	*SD*	*M*	*SD*	
Extraversion	3,35	0,77	3,72	0,72	0,497**
Agreeableness	4,01	0,53	4,17	0,41	0,348*
Conscientiousness	3,4	0,74	3,24	0,88	0,197
Intellect	3,74	0,64	3,52	0,63	0,348**
Neuroticism	2,83	0,81	3,13	0,86	0,36**

*p ≤.01; **p ≤ .001

Table 3. Differences in the Average Scores on the Big Five Personality Measure between Compulsive and Non-Compulsive Buyers

6. Conclusion

Since no consistent findings could be drawn from previous research on the relationship between CB and personality, the aim of this study was to put the findings of the respective studies into perspective and to repeat the research on a large sample and with a reliable measure of compulsive buying behaviour in the general buying population. In the sample of 1522 respondents, 93 (6,1%) were classified as compulsive buyers. This is in line with previous research on the topic (e.g., Black, 2007; Koran et al., 2006). The research revealed significant demographical differences between compulsive and non-compulsive buyers, with young women having the most chance to buy compulsively. This tendency can be due to fact, that emotional and identity-related dimensions of shopping are more important for women than for men (Babin et al., 1994; Dittmar et al., 2004) and reflect the developmental needs of young people to explore consumer activities or to establish an adult identity by material goods (Dittmar, 2005).

The findings of the current study confirm the utility of the personality approach to comprehend consumer behaviour and extend our understanding of compulsive buying behaviour. The study provides strong empirical support that personality does have an impact on CB. First of all, the results confirm H1, meaning that outgoing, sociable, active people are more prone to buy compulsively. Opposite to what we expected (H2), the t-test results showed that compulsive buyers score higher on *Agreeableness* as compared to non-compulsive buyers. This effect deserves extra attention and can explain why Balabanis (2001) found a negative relation between these two variables. If we think of compulsive buying as a not socially desirable behaviour we expect *Agreeable* people to score lower on CB since they are highly motivated to maintain positive relations with others (Jensen-Campbell & Graziano, 2001). For scratch-cards and lottery ticket buyers this appeared to be true (Balabanis, 2001) but not in our research where a general tendency to buy was measured. This is an important finding as it shows that *Agreeableness* can be sensitive to the retail context under investigation and might point out, that excessive buying does not always have to be considered as socially undesirable.

Also H4 and H5 were confirmed by the study. As expected, *Neuroticism* was positively related to CB. Emotional unstable people who often experience a variety of negative feelings, such as anxiety, depression, anger or embarrassment (McCrae & Costa, 1985) are more prone to buy compulsively. On the other hand, *Intellect* was negatively related to CB which means that the more imaginative, daring, reasonable a person is, the lower tendency she or he has to buy compulsively. Finally, the results didn't confirm H3 meaning that the trait *Conscientiousness* does not differentiate between compulsive and non-compulsive buyers. This means that responsibility, precision and self-discipline are characteristic which neither prevent nor make people more prone to engage in excessive buying behavior.

Some limitations of the current study have to be reported. First of all in any given Internet community, there are some individuals who are more likely than others to complete an online survey. This tendency can lead to a systematic bias known as self-selection bias (Thompson et al., 2003). Secondly, the focus of the current study was an investigation of the differences between compulsive and non-compulsive buyers with regard to the Big Five personality traits. It would be interesting to see whether different, more specific measures of personality could predict CB better (eg., Personality Adjective Check List, Strack ,1991). Furthermore, since our study didn't focus on a particular retail context, it would be interesting to investigate whether the prevalence of CB and the personality of compulsive buyers differ depending on the shopping context. Finally, with online shopping gaining in importance, additional studies on online compulsive buying behaviour should be undertaken.

The current research provides strong empirical evidence that compulsive buying is very present in the Flemish consumer population. Based on the representative consumer sample this study revealed that some specific inner characteristics of a consumer can make a person more prone to CB. How individuals seek reinforcement is valuable information for the affected individuals and their families, and can be taken into account by clinicians working with consumers seeking help. It is important to realize that the consumers' personality will influence help-seeking behaviour and also responses to treatment of compulsive buying.

7. Acknowledgement

The authors would like to thank Ching-Man Tang and Sara Lesage, both Master students at the VUB who devoted their Master thesis to the subject of Compulsive Buying, for their collaboration in this research project.

8. References

Association, A. P. (2000). Diagnostic and Statistical Manual of Mental Disorders. 4th, Text Revision. Date of access 20.05.2011, Available from: http://www.psychiatryonline.com/resourceTOC.aspx?resourceID=1

Babin, B. J., Darden, W. R., & Griffin, M. (1994). Work and/or fun: Measuring hedonic and utilitarian shopping value. *Journal of Consumer Research,* Vol.20, No. 4, pp. 644-656, ISSN 0093-5301

Bagozzi, R. P., & Youjare, Y. (1988). On the Evaluation of Structural Equation Models. *Journal of the Academy of Marketing Science,* Vol. 16, No.1, pp. 74-94 ISSN 1552- 7824.

Balabanis, G. (2001). The relationship between lottery ticket and scratch-card buying behaviour, personality and other compulsive behaviors. *Journal of Consumer Behavior,* Vol.2, No.1, pp. 7-22, ISSN 1470-2398

Black, D. W. (2007). A review of compulsive buying disorder. *World Psychiatry,* Vol.6, No.1, pp. 14–18, ISSN 1723-8617

Bleuler, E. (1976). *Textbook of psychiatry,* Arno Press, ISBN 0-405-074107, New York, New York, USA

Brown, M., & Cudeck, R. (1993). Alternative Ways of Assesing Model Fit. In: *Testing Structural Equation Models,* A. B. Kenneth & J. S. Long, (Eds.), 445-455, Sage Publications, ISBN 978-080-3945-07-4, Newbury Park, California, USA

Christenson, G. A., Faber, R. J., de Zwaan, M., & Raymond, N. C. (1994). Compulsive buying: Descriptive characteristics and psychiatric comorbidity. *Journal of Clinical Psychiatry,* Vol. 5, No.1, pp. 5-11, ISSN 1555-2101

Costa, P. T., & McCrae, R. R. (1985). *The NEO Personality Inventory,* Psychological Assessment Resources, Odessa, Florida, USA

Costa, P. T., & McCrae, R. R. (1992). Normal personality assessment in clinical practice: The NEO personality inventory. *Psychological Assessment,* Vol.4, No.1, pp. 5-13, ISSN 1040-3590

Cote, J., Netemeyer, R. & Bentler, P. (2001). Structural equation modeling: improving model fit by correlating errors. *Journal of Consumer Psychology,* Vol.10, No.2, pp. 87-88, ISSN 1532-7663

d'Astous, A. (1990). An inquiry into the compulsive side of normal consumers. *Journal of Consumer Policy,* Vol.13, No.1, pp. 15-31, ISSN 1573-0700

DeSarbo, W. S., & Edwards, E. A. (1996). Typologies of compulsive buying behavior: a constrained clusterwise regression approach. *Journal of Consumer Psychology,* Vol.5, No. 3, pp. 231-262, ISSN 1532-7663

Dickey, D. (1996). Testing the fit of our models of psychological dynamics using confirmatory method, In: *Advances in social science methodology,* B. Thompson, (Ed.), 219-227, JAI Press, ISBN 9781559387729, Greenwich, Connecticut, USA

Dittmar, H. (2005). Compulsive buying – a growing concern? An examination of gender, age, and endorsement of materialistic values as predictors. *British Journal of Psychology,* Vol.96, No. 4, pp. 467–491, ISSN 2044-8295

Dittmar, H., Long, K., & Meek, R. (2004). Buying on the internet: Gender differences in online and conventional buying motivations. *Sex Roles,* Vol.50, No.5-6, pp. 423-444, ISSN 1573-2762

Dongijn, L., Ying, J., Shenhui, A., Zhe, S., & Wenji, J. (2009). The influence of money attitudes on young Chinese consumers' compulsive buying. *Young Consumers: Insight and Ideas for Responsible Marketers,* Vol.10, No.2, pp. 98-109, ISSN 1747-3616

Donnellan, M. B., Oswald, F. L., Baird, B. M., & Lucas, R. E. (2006). The Mini-IPIP scales: Tiny-yet-effective measures of the Big Five factors of personality. *Psychological Assessment,* Vol.18, No.2, pp. 192–203, ISSN 1040-3590

Edwards, E. A. (1993). Development of a new scale for measuring compulsive buying behavior. *Financial Counseling and Planning,* Vol.4, No. 1, pp. 67-84, ISSN 1052-3073

Egan, V., & Taylor, D. (2010). Shoplifting, unethical consumer behaviour, and personality. *Personality and Individual Differences,* Vol.48, No. 8, pp. 878-884, ISSN 0191-8869

Endler, N. S., & Speer, R. L. (1998). Personality Psychology: Research Trends for 1993-1995. *Journal of Personality,* Vol.66, No. 5, pp. 621-669, ISSN 1467-6494

Ergin, E. A. (2010). Compulsive buying behavior tendencies: The case of Turkish consumers. *African Journal of Business Management,* Vol.4, No.3, pp. 333-338, ISSN 1993-8233

Eysenck, H. J., & Eysenck, M. W. (1985). *Personality and individual differences: a natural science approach.* New York: Plenum Press.

Faber, R. J., & O'Guinn, T. C. (1988). Compulsive consumption and credit abuse. *Journal of Consumer Policy,* Vol.11, No. 1, pp. 97-109, ISSN 1573-0700

Faber, R. J., & O'Guinn, T. C. (1992). A clinical screener for compulsive buying. *Journal of Consumer Research,* Vol. 19, No.3, pp. 459-469, ISSN 0093-5301

Faber, R. J., O'Guinn, T. C., & Krych, R. (1987). Compulsive consumption, In: *Advances in Consumer Research,* M. Wallendorf & P. Anderson, (Eds.), The Association for Consumer Research, ISBN 978-091-5552-19-1, 132-135, Provo, Utah, USA

Fiske, D. W. (1949). Consistency of the Factorial Structures of Personality Ratings from Different Sources. *Journal of Abnormal and Social Psychology,* Vol.44, No.3, pp. 329-344, ISSN 0096-851X

Goldberg, L. R. (1992). The development of markers for the Big-Five factor structure. *Psychological Assessment,* Vol.4, No.1, pp. 26-42, ISSN 1040-3590

Goldberg, L. R. (1999). A broad-bandwidth, public-domain, personality inventory measuring the lower-level facets of several five-factor models, In: *Personality Psychology in Europe,* I. Mervielde, I. Deary, F. De Fruyt & F. Ostendorf, (Eds.), Tilburg University Press, ISBN 90-361-9929-8, 7-28, Tilburg, The Netherlands

Hanley, A., & Wilhelm, M. S. (1992). Compulsive buying: An exploration into self-esteem and money attitudes. *Journal of Economic Psychology,* Vol.13, No.1, pp. 5-18, ISSN 0167-4870

Hassay, D. N., & Smith, M. C. (1998). Compulsive buying: An examination of the consumption motive. *Psychology and Marketing,* Vol.13, No.8, pp. 741 - 752, ISSN 1520-6793

Haugtvedt, C. P., Petty, R. E., & Cacioppo, J. T. (1992). Need for cognition and advertising: Understanding the role of personality variables in consumer behavior. *Journal of Consumer Psychology,* Vol.7, No.3, pp. 239-260, ISSN 1532-7663

Höck, M., & Ringle, C. M. (2006). Strategic networks in the software industry: an empirical analysis of the value continuum, *IFSAM VIIIth World Congress,* 28.10.2010, Available from http://www.fim-unihh.de/IFSAM06.pdf

Jensen-Campbell, L. A., & Graziano, W. G. (2001). Agreeableness as a moderator of interpersonal conflict. *Journal of Personality,* Vol.69, No.2, pp. 323 - 362, ISSN 1467-6494

John, O. P. (1999). The "Big Five" Factor Taxonomy: Dimensions of Personality in the Natural Language and Questionnaires, In: *Handbook of Personality: Theory and Research,* O.P. John & L. A. Pervin, (Eds.), Guilford Press, 978-157-2306-95-0 66-100, New York, New York, USA

Johnson, T., & Attmann, J. (2009). Compulsive buying in a product specific context: clothing. *Journal of Fashion Marketing and Management,* Vol.13, No.3, pp. 394-405, ISSN 1361-2026

Joireman, J., Kees, J., & Sprott, D. (2010). Concern with immediate consequences magnifies the impact of compulsive buying tendencies on college students' credit card debt. *Journal of Consumer Affairs,* Vol.44, No.1, pp. 155-178, ISSN 1745-6606

Kassarjian, H. H. (1971). Personality and consumer behavior: A review. *Journal of Marketing Research,* Vol. 8, No.11, pp. 409-418, ISSN 1547-7193

Koran, L. M., Faber, R. J., Aboujaoude, E., Large, M. D., & Serpe, R. T. (2006). Estimated prevalence of compulsive buying behavior in the United States. *The American Journal of Psychiatry,* Vol.163, No.10, pp. 1806-1812, ISSN 1535-7228

Kraepelin, E. (1915). *Psychiatrie* (8th ed.). Leipzig: Barth.

Kwak, H., Zinkjan, G. M., & Lester-Roushanzamir, E. P. (2004). Compulsive comorbidity and its psychological antecedents: a cross-cultural comparison between the US and South Korea. *Journal of Consumer Marketing,* Vol.21, No.6, pp. 418-434, ISSN 0736-3761

Kyrios, M., Frost, R. O., & Steketee, G. S. (2004). Cognitions in compulsive buying and acquisition. *Cognitive Therapy and Research,* Vol.*28,* No.2, pp. 241-258, ISSN 1573-2819

Larsen, R. J., & Buss, D. M. (2010). *Personality Psychology: Domains of Knowledge About Human Nature,* McGraw Hill Higher Education, ISBN 978-007-0164-99-4, London, England

Lin, L.-Y. (2010). The relationship of consumer personality trait, brand personality and brand loyalty: an empirical study of toys and video games buyers. *Journal of Product and Brand Management,* Vol.19, No.1, pp. 4-18, ISSN 1061-0421

McCrae, R. R., & Costa, P. T., Jr. (1985). Openness to experience. In: *Perspectives in personality,* R. Hogan & W. H. Jones, (Eds.), 145–172, JAI Press, ISBN 089232547X, Greenwich, Connecticut, USA

McElroy, S. L., Keck, P. E., Pope Jr., H. G., Smith, J. M. R., & Strakowski, S. M. (1994). Compulsive buying: A report of 20 cases. *Journal of Clinical Psychiatry,* Vol.55, No.6, pp. 242-248, ISSN 1555-2101

Mowen, J. (2000). *The 3M model of motivation and personality: Theory and empirical applications to consumer behavior.* Boston, Dordrecht, London: Kluwer Academic Publishers.

Mowen, J. C., & Spears, N. (1999). Understanding compulsive buying among college students: A hierarchical approach. *Journal of Consumer Psychology,* Vol.8, No.4, pp. 407-430, ISSN 1532-7663

Mueller, A., Claes, L., Mitchell, J. E., Wonderlich, S. A., Crosby, R. D., & de Zwaan, M. (2010). Personality prototypes in individuals with compulsive buying based on the Big Five Model. *Behaviour Research and Therapy,* Vol.48, No.9, pp. 930-935, ISSN 0005-7967

O'Guinn, T. C., & Faber, R. J. (1989). Compulsive buying: A phenomenological exploration. *Journal of Consumer Research,* Vol.16, No.2, pp. 147-157, ISSN 0093-5301

Ridgway, N. M., Kukar-Kinney, M., & Monroe, K. B. (2008). An expanded conceptualization and a new measure of compulsive buying. *Journal of Consumer Research,* Vol.35, No.4, pp. 622-639, ISSN 0093-5301

Rose, P. (2007). Mediators of the association between narcissism and compulsive buying: The roles of materialism and impulse control. *Psychology of Addictive Behaviors,* Vol.21, No.4, pp. 576-581, ISSN 0893-164X

Scherhorn, G. (1990). The addictive trait in buying behaviour. *Journal of Consumer Policy,* Vol.13, No.1, pp. 33-51, ISSN 1573-0700

Schlosser, S., Black, D. W., Repertinger, S., & Freet, D. (1994). Compulsive buying: Demography, phenomenology, and comorbidity in 46 subjects. *General Hospital Psychiatry,* Vol.16, No.3, pp. 205-212, ISSN 0163-8343

Sneath, J. Z., Lacey, R., & Kennett-Hensel, P. A. (2009). Coping with a natural disaster: Losses, emotions, and impulsive and compulsive buying. *Marketing Letters,* Vol. 20, No.1, pp. 45-60, ISSN 1573-059X

Strack, S. 1991. *Manual for the Personality Adjective Check List (PACL),* 21st Century Assessment, Southern Pasadena, California, USA

Thompson, L. F., Surface, E. A., Martin, D. L., & Sanders, M. G. (2003). From paper to pixels: Moving personnel surveys to the Web. *Personnel Psychology,* Vol. 56, No.1, pp. 197-227, ISSN 1744-6570

Thurstone, L. L. (1934). The vectors of mind. *Psychological Review,* Vol.41, No.1, pp. 1-32, ISSN 0033-295X

Tupes, E. C., & Christal, R. E. (1961). Recurrent Personality Factors Based on Trait Ratings. Lackland Air Force Base, TX: Personnel Laboratory, Air Force Systems Command

Valence, G., d'Astous, A., & Fortier, L. (1988). Compulsive buying: Concept and measurement. *Journal of Consumer Policy,* Vol.11, No.4, pp. 419-433, ISSN 1573-0700

Wang, C.-C., & Yang, H.-W. (2008). Passion for online shopping: the influance of personality and compulsive buying. *Social Behavior and Personality,* Vol.36, No.5, pp. 693-706, ISSN 0301-2212

Watson, S. (2009). Credit card misuse, money attitudes, and compulsive buying behaviors: A comparison of internal and external locus of control (LOC) consumers. *College Student Journal,* Vol. 43, No.2, pp. 268-275, ISSN 0146-3934

Wiggins, J. S. (1996). *The Five-Factor Model of Personality: Theoretical Perspectives,* Guilford Press, ISBN 978-157-2300-68-2, New York, NewYork, USA

The Bar-On Emotional Quotient Inventory (EQ-i): Evaluation of Psychometric Aspects in the Dutch Speaking Part of Belgium

Mercedes De Weerdt and Gina Rossi
Vrije Universiteit Brussel (VUB)
Belgium

1. Introduction

Psychology in the 20th century has been dominated by the importance given to cognitive intelligence. It has become increasingly clear however, that IQ-scores are not always good predictors of academic or professional success (McClelland, 1973; Goleman, 1995). The apparent inability of traditional measures of cognitive intelligence (e.g. IQ) to predict success in life, led to the development of the concept of emotional intelligence (EI), first labelled as such by Salovey and Mayer (1990). The idea itself however was not new.

In order to find an answer to the question "*why do some people succeed in possessing better emotional well-being than others* ?", and expanding into "*why are some individuals more able to succeed in life than others* ?", Bar-On started his research in 1980 with a systematic review of variables (i.e. abilities, competencies, skills) which he believed to be responsible for success in general (Bar-On, 1997a). He defined the concept of EI as "*an array of personal, emotional and social competencies and skills that influence one's ability to succeed in coping with environmental demands and pressures*" (Bar-On, 1997, p14). The general idea is that a large part of success seems to be determined by non-IQ factors and that emotional intelligence can be seen as a meta-ability, comprising an important set of those factors (such as motivation, impulse-control, mood-regulation, empathy, …), which determine how well we use other abilities, such as cognitive intelligence.

However, there are arguments that the concept of EI is not clearly defined, that different definitions and tests are being used - not always including the same aspects, and that many of the measures are neither reliable nor valid (Ciarrochi, Chan & Caputi, 2000). In essence there are two views on EI (Hedlund & Sternberg, 2000): some argue that emotional intelligence includes everything that is not measured by IQ but instead is related to success (Bar-On, 1997; Goleman, 1995); others advocate an ability model of emotional intelligence, that measures the ability to perceive and understand emotional information (Mayer, Caruso & Salovey, 2000). According to Petrides and Furham (2001) it would be more beneficial to describe trait EI and ability EI as two separate constructs instead of one being measured in two different ways. Some researchers even questioned whether emotional intelligence is anything more than a set of personality variables for which adequate measures already exist (Davies, Stankov & Roberts, 1998). Although the definitions of EI may differ among the many researchers, instead of being contradictory to one another, they appear to be complementary and they all share a common purpose which is to extend the traditional view of intelligence by underlining the importance of social, emotional and personal factors regarding intelligent behaviour (Dawda & Hart, 2000).

Furthermore, some of the developed measures for EI (Bar-On, 1997; Schutte, Malouff, Hall, Haggerty, Cooper, Golden & Dornheim, 1998; Mayer, Caruso & Salovey, 1999) do include extensive reliability and validity studies, showing reasonable to good psychometric properties for these tests. Over the last years a growing number of scientific articles on emotional intelligence and its measures have been published (e.g. Armstrong, Galligan & Critchley, 2011; Davis & Humphrey, 2012; Qualter, Gardner, Pope, Hutchinson & Whiteley, 2011; Schutte & Malouff, 2011; Zeidner, Shani-Zinovich, Matthews & Roberts, 2005), showing not only a growing interest in this concept, but also providing scientific support for some of its measures (e.g. EQ-i - Bar-on Emotional Quotient Inventory (1997a, 1997); MSCEIT - Mayer-Salovey - Caruso Emotional Intelligence Test, 2002).

In this article we focus on the Bar-on Emotional Quotient Inventory (EQ-i; Bar-on, 1997a, 1997), one of the first scientific developed measures that attempts to assess EI. Bar-on worked extensively on developing a multi factorial and theoretically eclectic measure for EI, the Bar-on EQ-i, which measures the *potential* to succeed rather than the success itself (Bar-On, 1997). According to Bar-On the core of emotional intelligence is 'understanding oneself and others, being able to relate to people and possessing the ability to adapt and cope with one's surroundings' which in term will increase one's chances of success when dealing with environmental demands. Because EI renders the way in which someone applies his knowledge to certain situations, it can also help to predict future success. (Bar-on, 1997a). An extensive body of reliability and validity research, demonstrated with samples from several different countries over a period of 17 years, was published in the technical manual (Bar-on, 1997). We restrict ourselves to an overview of the most important results and we refer to the manual for more details.

The reliability studies included the investigation of the internal consistency and test-retest reliability and showed good reliability. For all the subscales, the internal consistency coefficients were high, ranging from a .69 (Social Responsibility) to .86 (Self-Regard), with an overall average internal consistency coefficient of .76 and thus indicating a very good homogeneity. Results for the test-retest reliability in a South African sample showed an average coefficient of .85 after one month and .75 after four months. Subscales Self-Regard, Happiness and Impulse Control appeared to be more stable over time in comparison to the other subscales. (Bar-On, 1997).

A principal component factor analysis was carried out by Bar-On (1997) to examine factorial validity. He used the criteria of eigenvalues greater than one to determine that a 13 factor solution 'afforded the greatest interpretability' (p99), but of this 13 factors only the first five factors each explained more than 2.25% of variance (Bar-On, 1997). However, results of a study conducted by Palmer and colleagues (2001) did not support this 13 factor structure. Instead they found a six factor solution by performing a principal axis factoring on a normal population sample of 337 participants, using parallel analysis (Horn, 1965) and the scree test (Cattell, 1966) to determining the best factor solution.

Dawda & Hart (2000) examined the reliability and validity of the EQ-i in a sample of 243 university students. Their results supported overall good reliability and validity of the EQ-i and further promoted the EQ-i as a broad measure of emotional intelligence. Nevertheless, they also suggested a limited usefulness of the intermediate EQ composite scales, due to the fact that the Interpersonal, Adaptation and Stress Management EQ scales contain subscales that display considerable different convergent and discriminant validity indexes. Therefore, when assessing more specific aspects of emotional intelligence, the use of the EQ subscale scores (which are mostly more internally consistent) would be more appropriate. Although the EQ-i scores did not seem to be affected by response or gender bias, they considered further research necessary.

In order to examine Bar-On's (1997) suggestion that emotional intelligence is an important factor in predicting academic success, Newsome et al (2000) tried to determine the relationship between academic achievement and emotional intelligence, personality and cognitive ability in a sample of university students. They found evidence that academic achievement could be predicted by cognitive ability and personality measures (extraversion and self-control), but their results provided no support for the incremental validity of emotional intelligence in predicting academic achievement. Instead of rejecting the construct or hypothesis, the authors attributed the failure to establish conclusive findings to the lack of consensus on a definition of emotional intelligence and how it should be measured. Parker et al (2004) argued that a number of methodological problems more precisely the fact that Newsome used a heterogeneous group of students, could have been the reason for not finding a relationship between academic success and emotional intelligence. O'Connor and Little (2003) investigated whether academic success could be predicted by emotional intelligence and found EI not to be a valid predictor. Other researchers however where in line with Bar-On's findings (1997) and stated that emotional intelligence could indeed be considered to be a valid predictor for academic performance (Khajehpour, 2011; Parker, Creque, Barnhart, Harris, Majeski, Wood, Bond & Hogan, 2004; Parker, Summerfeldt, Hogan & Majeski, 2004; Parker, Hogan, Eastabrook, Oke & Wood, 2006; Qualter et al., 2011; Van der Zee, Thijs & Schakel, 2002).

Numerous studies have also showed that higher levels of emotional intelligence were associated with a better subjective well-being and with greater life satisfaction and positive affect (Austin, Saklofske & Egan, 2005; Gallagher & Vella-Brodrick, 2008; Schutte, Malouff, Simunek, McKenley & Hollander, 2002; Schutte et al., 2011). Furthermore emotional intelligence also appeared to be negatively associated with stressful events and distress. People scoring high on EI were more successful in dealing with negative life event stress (Armstrong et al., 2011). A meta-analytic study of 44 effect sizes done by Schutte, Malouff, Thorsteinsson, Bhullar & Rooke (2007) on a sample of 7898 participants showed a strong association between emotional intelligence and mental health. Martins, Ramalho & Morin (2010) confirmed these results in their comprehensive meta-analysis based on 105 effect sizes and 19.815 participants. Ciarrochi, Dean & Anderson (2002) investigated whether EI moderated the relationship between stress and mental health variables such as depression, hopelessness and suicidal ideation. They used emotion perception (EP) and managing other's emotion (MOE) as EI variables. Results of their study showed that both EP and MOE moderated the link between stress and mental health. Moreover, EP and MOE proved to be distinct of other measures (e.g. the big five personality factors, self-esteem, trait anxiety), implying that emotional intelligence ought to be considered as a separate construct. Their study also demonstrated the importance of EI in understanding the connection between mental health and stress.

The construct of alexithymia (i.e. inability to express feelings with words; from Greek, namely a=lack, lexis=word and thymos=emotion) was first introduced in the seventies by Nemiah and collegues (1970) and appears to be inversely related to the construct of emotional intelligence. Parker, Taylor and Bagby (2001) confirmed the relationship between those two constructs in a community sample of adults, using the Twenty-Item Toronto Alexithymia Scale (TAS-20) and the EQ-i. Also contrary to the conclusion (that EQ-i appears to be an unreliable self-report measurement) of Davies et al. (1998), Parker and colleagues (2001) corroborated the findings of Bar-On (1997a) and found acceptable levels of internal consistency for all EQ-i scales. Similar studies have also demonstrated negative correlations between emotional intelligence and alexithymia (Austin et al., 2005; Karimi & Besharat, 2010). Finally, when exploring the relationship between emotional intelligence and the severity of social anxiety in patients with generalised social phobia, Jacobs et al (2008) concluded that there was indeed a significant correlation between both variables.

The above mentioned authors started important validation work, however, there is still a need for more independent studies as many researchers pointed out, to further examine the construct validity of the measure and the relationship between emotional intelligence and other related constructs are still considered interesting topics of research (Ciarrochi et al., 2000; Hedlund et al., 2000; Bar-On, 2000; Reiff, Hatzes, Bramel & Gibbon, 2001; Derksen, Kramer & Katzko, 2002). We therefore evaluate the psychometric properties of the Dutch version of the EQ-i (Derksen, Jeuken & Klein-Herenbrink, 1997) in a Flemish population (Flanders is the Dutch speaking part of Belgium). For this purpose the EQ-i and Minnesota Multiphasic Personality Inventory - 2 (MMPI-2; Derksen, de Mey, Sloore, & Hellenbosch, 2006) were administered to a non-clinical Flemish sample. Basic reliability was tested by Cronbach Alpha and an exporatory factor analysis was carried out to examine the factorial validity. Convergent and divergent validity of the EQ-i with the MMPI-2 was evaluated and some demographic aspects were used to test the EQ-i's discriminative power between the possible subgroups. Finally a regression analysis was used to investigate which MMPI-2 variable would best predict EQ-i scores. Departing from the collected demographic data we assumed that if the EQ-i is a good measure of emotional intelligence, we should be able to see this in the relationship between EQ-i scores and respectively educational level, employment status and degree of psychopathology (i.e. MMPI-2 profile).

Research generally revealed a relationship between emotional intelligence and academic success, using grade point averages as a measure of academic success (Schutte et al., 1998; Reiff, 2001; Van Der Zee et al., 2002). A study of the incremental validity of emotional intelligence in predicting academic and social success beyond personality and academic intelligence done by Van Der Zee and collegues (2002) demonstrated that emotional intelligence could indeed account for the additional variance. Swart's (1996) study of academic success in first-year students in South-Africa showed significant differences in EQ-i mean scores between academically successful and unsuccessful students, proving that academically successful people score significantly higher on the EQ-i (Swart 1996, in Bar-On, 1997). We wanted to test if we could replicate these findings. Because grade points averages are only one way of labelling academic success and since their usefulness in comparing different levels of education is questionable, we opted to use amount of education (i.e. highest level of education) as a possible measure of academic success. Moreover we expected emotional intelligence to be positive related with the general level of education, as described by Sjöberg (2001). With regard to the relationship between emotional intelligence and academic success as well as occupational success we were especially interested in which of the EQ-i subscales contributed to this relationship. Several authors (Emmons & Kaiser, 1996; Parker et al., 2004; Reiff, 2001; Zeidner, Matthews & Roberts, 2009) pointed for example to interpersonal skills, self-esteem, goal orientation, adaptability and optimism as important factors in relation to academic achievement and employment status, and consequently to mental health. Therefore we expected EQ-i subscales analogous to these concepts, such as self-regard, self-actualization, stress-tolerance, flexibility and optimism to be of particular importance as aspects of emotional intelligence contributing to educational level and employment status.

With regards to emotional well-being we hypothesized that people who experience none or a few emotional problems or disorders would score higher on emotional intelligence than people with emotional problems or disorders. Considering the inverse relationship between emotional intelligence and alexithymia and the findings of Parker et al (2001) that suggested that high emotional intelligence might be a possible protective factor for mental (and physical) health, we assumed some of the EQ-i subscales such as self-regard, interpersonal relationship, stress tolerance and optimism will be good predictors.

2. Method

2.1 Procedure

All the data for this study was collected by third year psychology students who received course credits in return. They administered both tests (EQ-i and MMPI-2) to non-clinical volunteers. An informed consent was signed by all participants. The assessment measures are described in more detail below. In addition some biographic and demographic data was also collected (such as information on gender, age, education, etc.). Our sample was very heterogeneous with regard to geographic location, education level and occupation.

We first discuss results of an unpublished study into the general reliability of the EQ-i, performed in an earlier stage of data collection. In that study we investigated internal consistency using Cronbach Alpha comparing results with the original study done by Bar-On (1997). Furthermore we did a principal axis factor analysis (Direct Oblimin with Kaiser Normalisation) and performed parallel analysis (Horn, 1965; O'Connor, 2000) to determine which factor solution would best represent our data. In this procedure eigenvalues were extracted from random data sets which had the same number of cases and variables and were therefore similar to the actual dataset. When the eigenvalue of the real data set was larger than the mean eigenvalue from the random data set, the factor was retained (O'Connor, 2000).

On the complete sample, general statistics for the EQ-i results were calculated, and a comparative analysis of EQ-i profiles was performed for different groups (i.e. gender, education level and occupational status). Significant differences that reached at least a medium (.40) effect size (cohen's *d*, 1988) were interpreted. In the second part of our research divergent validity between the EQ-i and the MMPI-2 was evaluated using Pearson correlations coefficients. Because multiple comparisons were made, a Bonferroni correction was applied to determine significance. The conventional .05 was divided by the amount of tests (e.g. for the validity and clinical scales .05 was divided by the number of analysis; 21x13= 273, .05/273=.00018). Correlations were transformed into Fisher Z-scores using the transformation tables (Cohen, 1988). Only a large (z=.50) effect sizes was interpreted. Finally using regression analysis we investigated which MMPI-2 variables would best predict EQ-i scores.

2.2 Participants

The sample used for general reliability analyses consisted of 187 valid EQ-i protocols (82 men, 105 women) with participants ranging in age between 18 and 85 and a mean age of 36.73 (SD= 18,14).

Our final sample consisted of 967 participants (415 men, 552 women), between the age of 18 and 81 years old with a mean age of 41.05 (SD =13.12). Biographical data showed that 55% of our population was either married or living together, whereas 21% was not involved in a serious relationship at the time of the assessment. Furthermore, 55% had a university or college education, another 21% finished high school, indicating that our population had a relatively high educational level. Our sample consisted of students (11 %), 58% was employed and another 15% was either unemployed or retired. These data indicate some biases: e.g. a large amount of the sample has a university or college degree and a higher number of women (57%) was present. As such our sample might not be completely representative for the total population.

2.3 Measures

2.3.1 EQ-i

The EQ-i (Bar-On, 1997) was used to assess emotional intelligence. This is a 133-item self-report inventory, where respondents indicate on a 5-point Likert scale (1= "Very seldom or not true of me"; 5="Very often true of me") how representative the statements are for themselves. Standard scores are calculated, in accordance with IQ-scores, with a mean score of 100 and a standard deviation of 15. Test scores include a Total EQ-score, five Composite Scale scores, and 15 Content Scale scores (see Table 1). In addition the EQ-i also contains some scales that assess response style and validity: Positive Impression scale, Negative Impression scale, Omission Rate and Inconsistency Index. In accordance to the Bar-On EQ-i technical manual (p.41-42) EQ-i profiles with an Inconsistency Index score higher than 12, an Omission Rate higher than 6% and scores of 130 or more on the Positive and Negative Impression Scale were considered invalid. Protocols containing a response of "2 "(Seldom true of me) or "1" (Very seldom or Not true of me) on item 133 "I responded openly and honestly to the above sentences", and thus rendering the results invalid, were also left out of our analysis.

The Dutch version of the EQ-i (Derksen et al, 1997) was administered using the standard instructions and computer-scoring by the test publisher for The Netherlands and Belgium, Pen Tests Publisher (PEN).

2.3.2 MMPI-2

The Dutch version of the Minnesota Multiphasic Personality Inventory-2 (MMPI-2; Derksen et al., 2006) - one of the most widely used self-report personality inventories (Butcher,

Derksen, Sloore & Sirigatti, 2003) - was used as an external criterion to evaluate the EQ-i. Currently, the MMPI-2 is predominantly used to evaluate psychopathology in a variety of populations and to assess aspects of personality in both clinical and non-clinical populations. Subjects obtain T-scores on 7 validity, 10 basic clinical scales and 15 content scales. The Dutch version of the MMPI-2 was administered according to the standard instructions. All MMPI-2 profiles met the following inclusion criteria: Cannot Say raw scores < 30, VRIN and TRIN T-score < 80, L scale T-score < 80, K scale T-score < 75, F scale and Fb scale T-score < 110 (Derksen et al., 2006, p70 - 77).

3. Results and discussion

3.1 Reliability of EQ-i scales

3.1.1 Internal consistency

The internal consistency was evaluated by examining Cronbach alpha's for each scale (table 1). The coefficients range from average α=.66 (Reality testing) to high α= .87 (Self regard). When comparing our results to the Bar-On study (1997) we found our coefficients to be slightly lower than the US-study with the exception of Emotional Self-Awareness (ES), Interpersonal Relationship (IR) and Social Responsibility (RE). Overall our results showed a very good reliability.

EQ-i	Belgium N=187	USA N=3931
ES	.83	.80
AS	.76	.81
SR	.87	.89
SA	.67	.80
IN	.76	.79
EM	.75	.75
IR	.80	.77
RE	.72	.70
PS	.77	.80
RT	.66	.75
FL	.71	.77
ST	.79	.84
IC	.78	.79
HA	.78	.81
OP	.77	.82

Note: ES = Emotional Self-Awareness, AS = Assertiveness, SR = Self-Regard, SA = Self-Actualisation, IN = Independence, EM = Empathy, IR = Interpersonal Relationship, RE = Social Responsibility, PS = Problem Solving, RT = Reality Testing, FL = Flexibility, ST = Stress Tolerance, IC = Impulse Control, HA = Happiness, OP = Optimism

Table 1. Internal consistency

3.1.2 Exploratory factor analysis

A Principal axis factor analysis was carried out on the 117 items of the 15 subscales, to examine the factorial structure of the EQ-i. The 15 items of the validity scales and item 133 were not used. A parallel analyses yielded 7 factors accounting for 38.8% of the total variance (15.2%, 6.3%, 5.2%, 3.9%, 3.1%, 2.7%, 2.4%). In line with previous research (Bar-On, 1997a; Palmer et al., 2003) we looked at items loading ≥.40. Results are shown in table 2.

	Item nr.	Factor 1	Factor 2	Factor 3	Factor 4	Factor 5	Factor 6	Factor 7
SR	11*	**.558**				**.524**		
	24	**.646**				**.576**		
	40	**.472**	.144		.239	.284	-.152	.144
	56	**.596**		.202		.399	-.124	.243
	70	**.651**		.129		**.429**		.289
	85	**.744**	.137		.291	.357		.212
	100	**.717**					-.152	
	114	**.740**				.123	-.191	
	129	**.615**	.131		.251	.244	-.263	.116
RE	16		.386		.122	-.171		.386
	30	-.285	.225	**.435**		-.107		
	46		.215	.204		.102		.337
	61*		.301	-.164	.383			.246
	72*		**.526**	.114	**.422**			.229
	76		.275	**.545**	.128			
	90	.125	.267	.124	.248			**.412**
	98*	-.197	**.556**	.205	.392	-.120		.170
	104	.141	.177	.364	.262	-.213		
	119*	-.129	.261	.100	.313	-.155	.207	.129
IC	13	.151		**.566**			-.268	
	27		-.375	.224	-.112		-.198	
	42		.112	**.674**	.140			.144
	58			.235		-.110	-.204	
	73			**.470**	.137		-.291	
	86			**.733**				
	102			**.624**	.315			
	117	.156		**.656**			-.120	
	130	.153		**.639**			-.177	.118
PS	1	.123		.128	**.448**	.107	-.111	
	15			.112	**.583**			
	29		.103	.180	**.623**	.178		
	45	.162			**.739**	.100	-.116	
	60		.155		**.700**		-.102	
	75	.297				**.586**	-.178	
	89		.175		**.722**	.122	-.157	.137

	Item nr.	Factor 1	Factor 2	Factor 3	Factor 4	Factor 5	Factor 6	Factor 7
	118	.249				**.530**	-.116	.148
ES	7	.131	**.783**					.107
	9		**.669**		.237		-.101	
	23*	.155	**.686**			.122	-.129	.244
	35*	.359	**.459**	.235		.310	-.211	.159
	52	.126	**.713**				-.151	.177
	63	.378	.371		.257	.160		
	88*	.274	.333	.169	.349	.252	-.223	
	116	.150	**.692**			.234	-.141	.240
AS	22		.278		.117	**.452**		.149
	37	.238	.334			.335	-.216	
	67	.249	.205	-.242	.287	**.421**	-.192	
	82	.322				**.458**	-.317	
	96	.344	**.488**	-.169	.225	.319		.169
	111	.289	.233	-.396	.140	**.472**		.100
	126	.291	.271	-.155	.153	**.658**		.162
	3		.100			**.401**	-.289	.117
	19	.269		-.153		**.608**		
	32			-.107	.217	**.587**	-.266	
IN	48	.214			.156	**.669**	-.202	
	92	.168	.146	-.269	.240	**.570**	-.231	.101
	107			.208		**.454**	-.292	-.167
	121	.105		.233		**.522**	-.234	-.105
	14	.357	.126	-.164		.396	**-.416**	.357
	28		.328	.225	.311	.147	**-.459**	.251
	43		.185	.152			-.321	
FL	59	.289		-.102		.128	**-.425**	**.411**
	74	.114	.213		.292	.133	**-.439**	.251
	87	.227	.109			.193	**-.467**	**.460**
	103	.239	.121	.225		.176	**-.643**	.259
	131			-.185	-.105	.179	**-.492**	
	4	.250	.261	.174	.258	.265	**-.437**	
	20*	.113	.174		.283	.302	**-.532**	
	33	**.420**				.305	**-.581**	
	49	**.422**		.109		.344	**-.601**	.194
ST	64	**.421**		.184		**.451**	-.265	.199
	78	.339		.297	.165	.170	**-.585**	
	93			.123		.295	**-.487**	
	108*	.375	.299		**.451**	**.472**	-.310	.148
	122	**.447**			.137	.501	-.260	.133
IR	10		**.517**	.103			.113	.320
	23*	.155	**.686**			.122	-.129	.244

	Item nr.	Factor 1	Factor 2	Factor 3	Factor 4	Factor 5	Factor 6	Factor 7
	31*	**.456**	.395	-.114	.259	.210		.306
	39	.294	.355	-.385	.113	.187	-.178	.201
	55*		**.413**	-.199	.238		-.105	.150
	62*	.393	.331	-.229	.251	.174		.334
	69	.164	.390		.207	.305		**.508**
	84	.149	**.551**		.240		-.105	.287
	99	.295	**.424**		.358		-.228	**.408**
	113	.337	**.419**	-213	.287	.117		.247
	128	.238	.264	-.108	.194	.220	-.107	**.466**
EM	18	-.136	.385		.118	.132		.322
	44		**.601**		.259		-.136	.156
	55*		**.413**	-.199	.238		-.105	.150
	61*		.301	-.164	.383			.246
	72*		**.526**	.144	**.422**			.229
	98*	-.197	**.556**	.205	.392	-.120		.170
	119*	-.129	.261	.100	.313	-.155	.207	.129
	124		.218		.399	-.260	.212	.117
RT	8	.285	.170		.331	.212		
	35*	.359	**.459**	.235		.310	-.211	.159
	38	.120	.226	.227		.111		.237
	53	.200	.301	.276		.169	-.133	.386
	68	.202	.336	.369		.366		**.427**
	83			.248		.220	.169	
	88*	.274	.333	.169	.346	.252	-.223	
	97			**.513**	.172	.146		
	112	.196	.148		.387	.221	-.194	
	127	.284		.167	.228	**.497**	-.225	.381
OP	11*	**.558**				**.524**	-.323	
	20*	.113	.174		.283	.302	**-.532**	
	26	**.483**	.156		.124	.116	**-.496**	.235
	54	**.470**	.118		.161		-.234	.175
	80	.274	.291		.269	.284	-.381	.315
	106	**.413**	.195		.206		-.378	.228
	108*	.375	.299		**.451**	**.472**	-.310	.148
	132	**.575**	.106			**.403**	-.257	.235
HA	2	**.409**		.110			-.168	**.476**
	17	.119	.239					**.412**
	31*	**.456**	.395	-.114	.259	.210		.306
	47	**.615**	.197	.103			-.316	.382
	62*	.393	.331	-.229	.251	.174		.334
	77	**.437**		.131	-.167	.278	-.324	**.434**
	91	**.623**	.202	.152			-.258	**.575**

	Item nr.	Factor 1	Factor 2	Factor 3	Factor 4	Factor 5	Factor 6	Factor 7
	105	.341	.150	.146	.322		-.118	.218
	120	**.478**	.231	-.185	.283			.318
SA	6	.268	**.418**	.151	.296	.139	-.276	.256
	21	.398	.217			**.417**	-.338	.160
	36	.337	.149	.292		.273	-.201	.315
	51	.286	.135		.129	.162	-.273	**.572**
	66					.217	-.200	**.512**
	81	.251	.392		.390	.186	-.359	**.421**
	95	.253			.286		-101	**.448**
	110	.157		-.133	.301			.217
	125	.375	.333	.137		.343	-.169	.165

All factor loadings >.40 are in bold face, item loadings <.10 have been omitted. * Items used in different subscales.
Note: ES = Emotional Self-Awareness, AS = Assertiveness, SR = Self-Regard, SA = Self-Actualisation, IN = Independence, EM = Empathy, IR = Interpersonal Relationship, RE = Social Responsibility, PS = Problem Solving, RT = Reality Testing, FL = Flexibility, ST = Stress Tolerance, IC = Impulse Control, HA = Happiness, OP = Optimism

Table 2. Factor loading for EQ-i , subscales (direct-oblim).

The first factor we identified contained high loadings (≥.40) from all items of Self-Regard, the majority of items from Optimism and Happiness and half the items from Stress Tolerance. Contrary to Palmer (2003) and Bar-On (1997) we didn't find items above .40 of the subscale Self Actualisation on factor 1, but only moderate loadings >.25. Other than that our results are similar to the findings of Bar-On (1997) and Palmer et al. (2003). This factor was named 'Self-Contentment' by Bar-on (1997) because items 'relate to contentment with oneself and one's life' (p.100). Palmer et al. preferred the term 'Emotional Disposition' which is a name we also favour. We found high item loadings (≥.40) from subscales Interpersonal Relationship, Empathy and Emotional Self-Awareness on factor 2. Unlike Palmer et al. items from the subscale Social Responsibility didn't show high loadings with this factor but instead we found the items of Emotional Self-Awareness to load highly onto this second factor. Palmer et al. labelled this factor 'Interpersonal EQ'. Our third and fourth factor appeared to be very similar to factor 3 and 4 of the Palmer et al. study. Our third factor consisted almost entirely of Impulse Control items and one or two items from Social Responsibility and Reality Testing. This factor is therefore named 'Impulse Control'. The fourth factor that emerged had high item loadings from the subscale Problem Solving and two items shared by subscales Social Responsibility and Empathy and another two shared by Stress Tolerance and Optimism, this factor was labelled 'Problem Solving'. Contrary to findings of Palmer et al., we did not find the factor which he called 'Character', consisting mainly of high item loadings from subscales Flexibility and Independence. Instead we found two separate factors for Palmer et al.'s sixth factor: our fifth factor containing high item loadings from most items of subscales Independence and Assertiveness and a few items from Self-Regard, Problem Solving and Stress Tolerance, and a sixth factor including high item loadings from most items of Flexibility and Stress Tolerance. Our results are more in line with the findings of Bar-On (1997) who also found a (sixth) factor containing items from subscales Assertiveness and Independence. We labelled our fifth factor

'Independence/Assertiveness and our sixth factor 'Flexibility/Stress Tolerance'. Finally the seventh factor included items from Self-Actualisation, Interpersonal Relationships, two items from Happiness and Flexibility and one item from Reality Testing and was named 'Interpersonal Adaptation/Self Actualisation'. Palmer's et al.'s last factor was labelled Emotional Self-Awareness pertaining most items from subscale Emotional Self-Awareness, this was contrary to our findings.

3.2 General EQ-i profile

Table 3 shows the mean EQ-i profile of our sample of 967 participants. For the overall sample the total EQ (102.34), as well as the specific scale scores (ranging from 99.78 on Self Regard to 105.74 on Emotional Self-Awareness) can be considered as average scores. This is in accordance with earlier research on normal samples (Bar-on, 1997), although our scores are sometimes slightly lower.

	MEAN N=967	Men N=415	Women N=552
Total EQ-Score	*102.34*	*102.69*	*102.08*
Intrapersonal*	101.94	103.22	100.98
ES***	105.74	103.02	107.79
AS*	101.81	103.22	100.74
SR***	98.78	100.99	97.12
SA	101.38	102.09	100.85
IN***	100.16	103.45	97.68
Interpersonal***	102.35	**97.61**	**105.91**
EM***	104.58	**99.32**	**108.54**
IR***	102.93	100.47	104.78
RE***	100.34	**94.84**	**104.47**
Adaptability	104.00	104.98	103.26
PS***	103.64	105.82	101.99
RT*	104.67	103.40	105.62
FL*	100.78	102.35	99.60
Stress Management***	99.62	102.12	97.75
ST***	99.23	**103.39**	**96.11**
IC	99.91	99.87	99.94
General Mood	101.25	102.17	100.56
HA	100.52	100.59	100.47
OP**	101.92	103.66	100.61

Differences significant at *p≤.05;**p ≤.01;***p≤.0008
Effect sizes (cohen's *d*, 1988): small (>.20), **medium (>. 40)**, *large (>.80)*
Note: ES = Emotional Self-Awareness, AS = Assertiveness, SR = Self-Regard, SA = Self-Actualisation, IN = Independence, EM = Empathy, IR = Interpersonal Relationship, RE = Social Responsibility, PS = Problem Solving, RT = Reality Testing, FL = Flexibility, ST = Stress Tolerance, IC = Impulse Control, HA = Happiness, OP = Optimism

Table 3. Comparison of mean profiles

With regard to gender differences (table 3), our results confirm the findings reported by Bar-on (1997): although no significant difference is seen between males and females in total EQ-score, several gender differences do exist with respect to some factorial components. When considering small (>.20) and medium effect (>.40) sizes, women seem to have better interpersonal skills (i.e. empathy, interpersonal relationship, social responsibility) than men, while the latter seem to have a higher self-regard, are more independent and better in problem solving, can cope better with stress and are more flexible. Although differences between men and women are small they are consistent and seem to compensate each other in overall EI. A study from Dawda et al. (2000) on 243 university students also showed no significant difference between EQ Total score but contrary to our findings they only found men to score significantly higher than women on independence and optimism and lower on social responsibility. Reiff et al (2001) on the other hand did find that the female students in his sample of 128 college students, scored significantly higher on interpersonal skills than their male fellow students.

3.3 Level of education

Looking at education level as a measure for academic success, we divided our subjects into three groups: **Group 1** (N=84) did not complete high-school; **Group 2** (N=198) has successfully finished high-school; and **Group 3** (N=531) has a college or university education. By means of a one-way ANOVA we evaluated whether EQ-i scores could discriminate between these groups. Results (table 4) show that overall EQ-scores increase with level of education.

Cohen's d effect sizes (Cohen, 1988) were calculated to further analyse these differences and results (table 5) showed that: EQ-scores especially seemed to differentiate the group that did not finish high-school from the group with a college education (almost all medium effect sizes >.40). Differences between the high school and no education group and between the high school and the college group were less distinctive, with only small effect sizes. Our results regarding academic success were mostly consistent with the findings reported by Swart (1996, in Bar-On, 1997), who compared successful and unsuccessful university students (based on their grades). Although we found a higher number and more significant differences, this was probably due to the fact that our groups were much more distinctive from each other as far as level of academic success was concerned. This confirms that EI is indeed linked to academic success (measured by education level).

3.4 Employment status

By means of a one-way ANOVA we compared the EQ-i profiles of students, employed or unemployed (i.e. unemployed, housewife or retired) individuals. Scores of the student and the unemployed populations are generally slightly lower than those of the working groups (table 6).

To analyse the differences we calculated Cohen's *d* effect sizes. Results presented in table 7 show that there were only two medium effects (>.40, for social responsibility (RE)) meaning that both the working and the unemployed population can cooperate with others and are more responsible and dependable than the student group. Other effects were only small (>.20) and appeared to differentiate the working group from the two other groups, the working group scored significantly higher on: Total EQ, Intrapersonal, Self-Actualisation, Adaptability and Optimism. The group of the unemployed scored significantly lower as compared to the remaining groups on: flexibility, stress management and happiness. As for the student group, they only scored significantly lower on problem solving than the two other groups. The working group score higher on reality testing than the students furthermore they have a better general mood and are more flexible than the unemployed. Both working group and students can cope better with stress than the unemployed.

	No HS N=84	High school N=198	College N=531
*Total EQ-Score****	95.48	99.35	104.56
Intrapersonal***	97.06	99.28	103.76
ES***	99.27	103.96	107.28
AS**	98.50	99.09	103.39
SR	96.64	97.14	99.93
SA***	95.58	98.82	103.37
IN	98.69	98.41	100.99
Interpersonal**	96.67	101.30	103.4
EM**	100.54	103.55	105.22
IR***	96.98	101.31	104.35
RE	97.61	100.88	100.29
Adaptability***	96.70	101.08	106.22
PS**	98.81	101.88	105.32
RT*	100.50	103.89	105.69
FL***	93.23	96.53	103.19
Stress Management***	93.93	96.56	101.79
ST***	93.11	96.70	101.36
IC*	96.90	97.59	101.25
General Mood**	96.26	99.22	102.94
HA**	95.76	98.83	102.12
OP*	97.92	100.08	103.28

Differences significant at *$p \leq .05$;**$p \leq .01$;***p≤..0008

Note: ES = Emotional Self-Awareness, AS = Assertiveness, SR = Self-Regard, SA = Self-Actualisation, IN = Independence, EM = Empathy, IR = Interpersonal Relationship, RE = Social Responsibility, PS = Problem Solving, RT = Reality Testing, FL = Flexibility, ST = Stress Tolerance, IC = Impulse Control, HA = Happiness, OP = Optimism

Table 4. Profiles according to level of education

	No HS vs HS	No HS vs College	HS vs College
*Total EQ-Score****	<u>.25</u>	**.58**	<u>.34</u>
Intrapersonal***	<u>.15</u>	**.45**	<u>.31</u>
ES***	<u>.32</u>	**.55**	<u>.22</u>
AS**	.04	<u>.32</u>	<u>.27</u>
SA***	<u>.21</u>	**.49**	<u>.32</u>
Interpersonal**	<u>.31</u>	**.42**	.14
EM**	<u>.22</u>	<u>.33</u>	.12
IR***	<u>.28</u>	**.46**	<u>.21</u>
Adaptability***	<u>.27</u>	**.60**	<u>.32</u>
PS**	.18	**.40**	<u>.21</u>
RT*	<u>.22</u>	<u>.33</u>	.12
FL***	<u>.20</u>	**.60**	**.41**
Stress Management***	.15	**.46**	<u>.32</u>
ST***	<u>.24</u>	**.55**	<u>.30</u>
IC*	.04	<u>.25</u>	<u>.23</u>
General Mood**	.19	**.41**	<u>.25</u>
HA**	.19	<u>.39</u>	<u>.23</u>
OP*	.14	<u>.34</u>	<u>.20</u>

Differences significant at *p≤.05;**p ≤.01;***p≤..0008
Effect size (Cohen's *d*, 1988): <u>small</u> (>.20), **medium** (>.40), *large* (>.80)
Note: ES = Emotional Self-Awareness, AS = Assertiveness, SA = Self-Actualisation, EM = Empathy, IR = Interpersonal Relationship, ;PS = Problem Solving, RT = Reality Testing, FL = Flexibility, ST = Stress Tolerance, IC = Impulse Control, HA = Happiness, OP = Optimism

Table 5. Effect sizes according to level of education

	Student N=109	Working N=561	Unemployed N=150
*Total EQ-Score**	99.78	103.50	99.76
Intrapersonal*	99.72	103.04	99.54
ES	104.06	106.17	104.71
AS	102.94	102.11	100.07
SR	95.99	99.83	97.52
SA ***	98.32	102.92	97.94
IN	98.20	101.09	98.09
Interpersonal	99.77	102.38	103.14
EM	102.83	104.23	105.51
IR	104.04	102.96	101.51
RE***	93.70	100.31	104.15
Adaptability*	101.09	105.26	101.27
PS*	99.76	104.74	103.11
RT*	100.87	105.84	103.45
FL**	102.00	101.30	96.45
Stress Management*	99.19	100.67	96.02
ST***	98.29	100.82	94.39
IC	100.18	100.03	98.89
General Mood*	99.63	102.46	98.45
HA*	101.54	101.38	97.61
OP**	97.50	103.26	99.97

Differences significant at *$p \leq .05$;**$p \leq .01$;***$p \leq ..0008$
Note: ES = Emotional Self-Awareness, AS = Assertiveness, SR = Self-Regard, SA = Self-Actualisation, IN = Independence, EM = Empathy, IR = Interpersonal Relationship, RE = Social Responsibility, PS = Problem Solving, RT = Reality Testing, FL = Flexibility, ST = Stress Tolerance, IC = Impulse Control, HA = Happiness, OP = Optimism

Table 6. Profiles according to working status

	Student vs working	Working vs unemployed	Student vs unemployed
*Total EQ-Score**	.24	.24	.00
Intrapersonal*	.22	.24	.01
SA ***	.29	.32	.02
RE***	.40	.25	.66
Adaptability*	.26	.24	.01
PS*	.32	.10	.21
RT*	.31	.16	.16
FL**	.04	.26	.32
Stress Management*	.09	.27	.19
ST***	.16	.09	.24
General Mood*	.17	.26	.07
HA*	.01	.24	.25
OP**	.34	.21	.14

Differences significant at *p≤.05;**p ≤.01;***p≤..0008
Effect size (Cohen's *d*, 1988): small (>.20), **medium** (>.40), *large* (>.80)
Note: ES = Emotional Self-Awareness, AS = Assertiveness, SR = Self-Regard, SA = Self-Actualisation, IN = Independence, EM = Empathy, IR = Interpersonal Relationship, RE = Social Responsibility, PS = Problem Solving, RT = Reality Testing, FL = Flexibility, ST = Stress Tolerance, IC = Impulse Control, HA = Happiness, OP = Optimism

Table 7. Effect sizes according to working status

These differences are comparable with those presented in Bar-On's manual (1997), although they are less extreme. This is logical however, since Bar-On compared two groups that were at the opposite end of the continuum of occupational success (i.e. unemployed versus top leadership positions). Our employed group on the other hand is a mixed group, making the scores more average and the differences with the unemployed group less extreme. This indicates that differences in occupational success are indeed linked to differences in EQ-i scores

3.5 Concurrent validity of the EQ-i

The calculated correlations between the different EQ-i scales and the MMPI-2 Clinical and Content Scales were transformed into Fisher's z-scores. Results displayed in tables 8a and 8b show that overall EQ-i scores tend to correlate negatively with MMPI-2 scores, indicating that people high on emotional intelligence factors show less behavioural and personality problems and psychopathology (as measured by the MMPI-2) than people scoring low on emotional intelligence.

Looking more specifically at the highest correlations with a large effect size (.50), we see that people who score high on (clinical) depression (scale 2D and Dep of the MMPI-2) – seem to have little self-regard (SR: -.55 and -.66), feel unhappy (HA: -.60 and -.74) and pessimistic

(OP: -.50 and -.55) and have a low general mood (-.62 and -.76). Those who are socially introverted (0Si) and uncomfortable (Sod) have EQ-i scores that indicate they are not very assertive (-.63 and -.50) and are unhappy about their interpersonal relationships (IR: -.65) and their life in general (general mood: -.60 and -.52). They have a low total EQ (-.63 and -.52), and low intrapersonal scores (-.66 and -.52).

	L	F	K	Hs	D	Hy	Pd	Mf	Pa	Pt	Sc	Ma	Si
TotalEQ-score	**.31**	**-.45**	.55	-.11	-.54		-.20	-.10	-.18	**-.49**	-.28		-.63
Intrapersonal	.22	**-.35**	**.42**		-.54		-.15	-.10	-.13	**-.47**	-.23	.16	-.66
ES	.11	-.22	.29		-.25					-.20	-.14	.10	-.40
AS	.11	-.21	**.30**		**-.38**			-.12		**-.32**	-.12	.18	-.63
SR	.25	**-.37**	**.40**	-.11	-.55		-.27	-.17	-.23	-.51	-.26	.11	-.52
SA	.13	**-.33**	.28	-.11	**-.44**		-.21		-.12	**-.37**	-.21	.13	**-.44**
IN	.21	-.16	.28		**-.32**					**-.33**			**-.41**
Interpersonal	.20	**-.38**	**.33**		-.23		-.11			-.20	-.20		**-.46**
EM		-.18	.14										-.18
IR		**-.34**	**.32**		**-.39**					-.27	-.18	.19	-.65
RE	.27	-.29	.21				-.12						
Adaptability	.28	**-.35**	**.46**		**-.38**		-.16		-.15	**-.40**	-.26		-.10
PS	.19	-.17	.17		-.20		-.12			-.25	-.18		-.19
RT	**.31**	**-.41**	**.46**		-.27		-.25	-.12	-.23	**-.38**	**-.33**	-.16	-.25
FL	.13	-.21	**.38**		**-.35**					-.26		.14	**-.47**
Stress Management	**.30**	-.28	.52		-.29		-.14		-.19	-.28	-.13	-.14	-.27
ST	.21	-.27	**.42**	-.12	**-.45**			-.11	-.16	**-.40**	-.13		**-.46**
IC	.26	-.20	**.40**				-.13		-.15			-.28	
General Mood	.19	**-.42**	**.40**	-.15	-.62	-.11	-.29	-.13	-.25	-.55	**-.30**	.14	-.60
HA	.13	**-.42**	**.35**	-.17	-.60	-.15	**-.33**	-.11	-.27	**-.47**	**-.32**		-.55
OP	.21	**-.31**	**.33**		-.50		-.18	-.12	-.16	**-.47**	-.20	.16	-.50

Fisher z-scores: small (z=.10), **medium (z=.30),** large (z=.50) and all significant at p≤.0001

Note: ES = Emotional Self-Awareness, AS = Assertiveness, SR = Self-Regard, SA = Self-Actualisation, IN = Independence, EM = Empathy, IR = Interpersonal Relationship, RE = Social Responsibility, PS = Problem Solving, RT = Reality Testing, FL = Flexibility, ST = Stress Tolerance, IC = Impulse Control, HA = Happiness, OP = Optimism, F = Infrequency, L = Lie, K = Correction, Hs = Hypochondriasis, D = Depression, Hy = Hysteria, Pd = Psychopathic Deviate, Mf = Masculinity-Femininity, Pa = Paranoia, Pt = Psychastenia, Sc = Schizophrenia, Ma = Hypomania, Si = Social Introversion

Table 8a. Correlation matrix EQ-i - MMPI-2 (validity and clinical scales) in Fisher z-scores

	Anx	Frs	Obs	Dep	Hea	Biz	Ang	Cyn	Asp	Tpa	Lse	Sod	Fam	Wrk	Trt
TotalEQ-score	-.59	-.28	-.68	-.73	**-.34**	-.25	**-.39**	**-.31**	-.25	-.29	-.73	-.52	**-.39**	-.74	-.69
Intrapersonal	**-.49**	-.21	-.60	-.63	-.28	-.14	-.20	-.23	-.15	-.13	-.78	-.52	**-.30**	-.66	-.65
ES	-.21	-.13	**-.30**	**-.31**	-.17		-.18	-.17	-.13	-.17	**-.37**	**-.37**	-.18	**-.31**	**-.43**
AS	**-.31**	-.18	**-.42**	**-.38**	-.20			-.20	-.10		-.58	-.50	-.19	-.50	**-.45**
SR	-.54	-.16	-.54	-.66	-.28	-.17	-.26	-.17	-.10	-.15	-.66	-.42	**-.32**	-.62	-.54
SA	**-.34**	-.13	**-.40**	-.56	-.19	-.11	-.14	-.18	-.11		**-.49**	**-.38**	-.23	**-.46**	-.51
IN	**-.32**	-.19	-.50	**-.37**	-.16		-.10	-.15	-.12		-.56	-.25	-.16	-.50	**-.39**
Interpersonal	-.21	-.20	-.29	**-.42**	-.17	-.17	-.27	-.21	**-.35**	-.22	**-.34**	**-.46**	-.21	**-.35**	**-.39**
EM							-.13	-.13	-.14	-.11	-.10	-.17		-.10	-.18
IR	-.28	-.12	**-.33**	**-.42**	-.19	-.12	-.21	-.20	-.12	-.17	**-.44**	-.65	-.20	**-.39**	**-.44**
RE	-.10		-.14	-.19		-.16	-.21	-.13	-.29	-.19	-.15	-.17	-.16	-.22	-.20
Adaptability	-.50	-.29	-.58	-.55	**-.30**	-.27	**-.35**	-.28	-.22	-.27	-.55	**-.33**	**-.32**	-.60	-.54
PS	-.23	-.10	-.25	-.27	-.11		-.17				**-.31**	-.11	-.15	**-.33**	-.26
RT	**-.45**	-.23	-.54	-.51	**-.30**	**-.39**	**-.39**	**-.30**	-.26	**-.30**	**-.46**	-.21	**-.39**	-.54	**-.46**
FL	**-.40**	-.29	**-.47**	**-.41**	-.25	-.13	-.25	-.25	-.15	-.23	**-.42**	**-.41**	-.17	**-.42**	**-.47**
Stress Manag	-.58	-.29	-.55	**-.46**	**-.33**	-.27	-.59	**-.31**	-.27	**-.45**	**-.42**	-.18	**-.36**	-.51	**-.41**
ST	-.56	**-.32**	-.59	**-.49**	**-.31**	-.15	**-.31**	-.23	-.16	-.22	-.54	**-.33**	-.27	-.59	**-.47**
IC	**-.37**	-.16	**-.31**	-.27	-.22	-.27	-.62	-.26	-.26	**-.47**	-.19		**-.31**	-.27	-28
General Mood	-.56	-.19	-.55	-.76	**-.30**	-.16	-.27	-.20	-.12	-.15	-.60	-.52	**-.32**	-.62	-.59
HA	-.51	-.14	**-.45**	-.74	**-.31**	-.16	-.25	-.20	-.11	-.16	**-.47**	-.52	**-.33**	-.50	-.54
OP	**-.46**	-.20	-.51	-.55	-.22	-.12	-.21	-.16		-.11	-.59	**-.39**	-.22	-.59	-.50

Fisher z-scores: small (z=.10), **medium (z=.30)**, large (z=.50) and all significant at p≤.0001
Note: ES = Emotional Self-Awareness, AS = Assertiveness, SR = Self-Regard, SA = Self-Actualisation, IN = Independence, EM = Empathy, IR = Interpersonal Relationship, RE = Social Responsibility, PS = Problem Solving, RT = Reality Testing, FL = Flexibility, ST = Stress Tolerance, IC = Impulse Control, HA = Happiness, OP = Optimism, ANX = Anxiety, FRS = Fears, OBS = Obsessiveness, DEP = Depression, HEA = Health Concerns, BIZ = Bizarre Mentation, ANG = Anger, CYN = Cynicism, ASP = Antisocial Practices, TPA = Type A, LSE = Low Self-Esteem, SOD = Social Discomfort, FAM = Family Problems, WRK = Work Interference, TRT = Negative Treatment Indicators.

Table 8b. Correlation matrix EQ-i – MMPI-2 (Content scales) in Fisher z-scores

Low Self-Esteem (Lse), as can be expected, has a strong negative correlation with the intrapersonal scale (-.52, i.e. self-regard (-.66), independence (-.56), Assertiveness (-.58)) and with adaptability (-.55), stress tolerance (-.54) and general mood (-.60 i.e optimism (-.62)). Furthermore, people who are obsessive (scale 7Pt and Obs) and experience anxiety (Anx), show a low total EQ (-.49, -.68 and -.59), have a low self-regard (-.51, -.54 and -.54), are not able to deal with stress (Stress management, -.55 and -.58 and stress tolerance, -.59 and -.56) and don't feel overall happy with their life (general mood: -.55, -.55 and -.56). Finally, people exhibiting behaviours or attitudes that contribute to bad work performance (Wrk) also have a low total EQ score (-.74), low intrapersonal skills (-.66, i.e. self-regard: (-.62), Assertiveness

(-.50), independence (-.50)), are pessimistic (-.53) and unhappy (-.59), and have less stress tolerance (-.53). Overall, we can conclude that there is a good concurrent validity between the two tests. However, only a few of the scales presented a large effect size, while most others only showed small or at best medium effect sizes. This indicates that although there is a link between the two tests, the EQ-i is measuring something different than the behavioural and personality characteristics measured by the MMPI-2, supporting its construct validity.

3.6 Regression analysis

In order to investigate which of the MMPI-2 variables best predicts EQ-i, a regression analysis was performed. Our previous analysis and results determined which variables (namely those with medium (z=.30) and large (z=.50) effect sizes) were put into the regression analysis. After controlling for gender, education and employment the MMPI-2 scales accounted for a large proportion of the variance in the different EQ-i scales (range from 7% to 47%). Results are summarized in table 9. All mentioned predictors correlated negatively with the EQ-i scales unless otherwise specified.

The MMPI-2 scales L, scale 0(Si), Work Interference, Depression, Obsessiveness, Low Self-Esteem and Cynicism explained 47% of the variance in the Total EQ-i score. The Intrapersonal scale was best predicted by 7(Pt), 0(Si) and content scales Low Self-Esteem, Depression, and Obsessiveness. Both F and Anxiety scales had a positive β coefficient. Clinical scale 0(Si) and content scale Negative Treatment Indicators were found to be the only two predictors for Emotional Self-Awareness. Assertiveness was negatively predicted by scale 0(Si) and Low self esteem. Scale 0(Si), 7(Pt), Depression and Low Self-Esteem explained 44% of the variance for Self-Regard. Self-Actualisation was best predicted by scale 0(Si), 2(D), Depression and Low Self-Esteem and positively by Anxiety. The Independence scale was best predicted scale 7(Pt), 0(Si), Low Self-Esteem, Obsessiveness, Work Interference and positively by both Anxiety and Negative Treatment Indicators. The validity scale F, clinical scale 0(Si) and content scales Antisocial Practices and Social Discomfort were the predictors for the Interpersonal scale. Interpersonal Relationships were best predicted by a combination of F scale, scale 0(Si), Depression and Social Discomfort. Low Self-Esteem and Work Interference were observed to be predictors for the Problem Solving scale. The MMPI-2 validity scales L and K both had a positive relationship with Reality Testing while scale 8(Sc), Obsessiveness, Low Self-Esteem and Bizarre Mentation were negatively correlated. A combination of scale 0(Si), Anxiety, Obsessiveness and Social Discomfort proved to be good predictors for Flexibility. The best predictors for Stress Management, were scales Anxiety, Obsessivenss and Anger. For Stress Tolerance the content scale Cynicism had a positive β coefficient while scale 7(Pt), 0(Si), Anxiety, Fears, Obsessiveness and Work Interference were negative predictors. Both Anger and Type A content scales proved to be good predictors for the Impulse Control scale and explained 30% of the total variance. A combination of Scale 0(Si), 2(D), 7(Pt), Depression, Obsessiveness and Health Concerns (positively) accounted for 47% of the variance in General Mood. Happiness was predicted by scale 2(D), 4(Pd), Depression, Social Discomfort and Work Interference (positively). Finally significant predictors for the Optimism scale were validity scale F (positive β coefficient), clinical scale 7(Pt) and 0(Si) and content scales Low Self-Esteem, Depression and Work Interference.

EQ-i scales		Δ adj. R^2	Significant predictors
Total EQ-Score	Education*	.04	
	MMPI-2 scales	.51	L (+), Si, WRK, DEP, OBS, LSE, CYN (+)
Intrapersonal	Education *	.03	
	MMPI-2 scales	.49	F(+), Pt, Si, LSE, DEP, OBS, ANX (+)
ES	Gender*	.03	
	MMPI-2 scales	.21	Si, TRT
AS	Education*	.02	
	MMPI-2 scales	.34	Si, LSE
SR	Gender & education*	.01	
	MMPI-2 scales	.45	Si, Pt, DEP, LSE
SA	Education & employment*	.04	
	MMPI-2 scales	.27	Si, D, ANX, DEP, LSE
IN	Gender*	.03	
	MMPI-2 scales	.32	Pt, Si, ANX (+), LSE, OBS, WRK, TRT(+)
Interpersonal	Gender & Education*	.10	
	MMPI-2 scales	.24	F, Si, ASP, SOD
IR	Gender & education *	.02	
	MMPI-2 scales	.36	F, Si, DEP, SOD
Adaptability	Education & employment*	.04	
	MMPI-2 scales	.33	K, Pt, OBS, SOD, WRK,
PS	Gender & education*	.03	
	MMPI-2 scales	.10	LSE, WRK
RT	Gender, education & employment	.02	
	MMPI-2 scales	.40	L (+), K (+), Sc, OBS, LSE, BIZ
FL	Education*	.05	
	MMPI-2 scales	.24	Si, ANX, OBS, SOD
Stress Management	Gender & education*	.04	
	MMPI-2 scales	.35	ANX, OBS, ANG
ST	Gender, education & employment	.09	
	MMPI-2 scales	.36	Si, Pt, ANX, FRS, OBS, CYN (+), WRK
IC	Education*	.01	
	MMPI-2 scales	.31	ANG, TPA
General Mood	Education &	.02	

	employment*		
	MMPI-2 scales	.49	Si, D, Pt, DEP, HEA (+), OBS
HA	Education *	.02	
	MMPI-2 scales	.45	D, Pd, DEP, SOD, WRK (+)
OP	Education & employment*	.02	
	MMPI-2 scales	.37	F (+), Pt, Si, LSE, DEP, WRK,

Note: ES = Emotional Self-Awareness, AS = Assertiveness, SR = Self-Regard, SA = Self-Actualisation, IN = Independence, EM = Empathy, IR = Interpersonal Relationship, RE = Social Responsibility, PS = Problem Solving, RT = Reality Testing, FL = Flexibility, ST = Stress Tolerance, IC = Impulse Control, HA = Happiness, OP = Optimism, F = Infrequency, L = Lie, K = Correction, D = Depression, Pd = Psychopathic Deviate, Pt = Psychastenia, Sc = Schizophrenia, Si = Social Introversion, ANX= Anxiety, FRS= Fears, OBS= Obsessiveness, DEP= Depression, HEA= Health Concerns, BIZ= Bizarre Mentation, ANG= Anger, CYN= Cynicism, ASP= Antisocial Practices, TPA= Type A, LSE= Low Self-Esteem, SOD= Social Discomfort, FAM= Family Problems, WRK= Work Interference, TRT= Negative Treatment Indicators.

* The variables: Gender, Education and Employment were only mentioned in the table when they were retained in and thus contributed to the model.

All significant predictor had negative β coefficients except the ones marked (+)

Table 9. Stepwise regression

4. Conclusions and directions for future research

Overall, the present study provided support for the reliability and validity of the Bar-On Emotional Quotient Inventory (Bar-On, 1997b), as a measure of emotional intelligence, in a Flemish sample.

The internal consistency proved to be satisfactory. Results of the exploratory factor analysis did not confirm Bar-On's (1997) findings claiming a 13 factor structure of the EQ-i, but partially supported the alternative findings of Palmer et al.(2003) who found six factors. The current study found evidence for a seven factor structure using parallel analysis, which is known to be a more accurate method when determining the correct number of components (Zwick, & Velicer, 1986). Another main difference with the Bar-On study is that we used a principal axis factor analysis (Direct Oblimin with Kaiser Normalisation) instead of an orthogonal (Varimax) rotation procedure which could also explain why our results are more similar to these of Palmer et al. (2003). Our first factor was very similar to the first factor found by Bar-On and Palmer et al. and was labelled Emotional disposition with items from Self-Regard, Optimism, Happiness and Stress Tolerance and only moderate loadings of items from Self-Actualisation. The second factor called Interpersonal EQ had high loadings from items of Interpersonal Relationship, Empathy and Emotional Self-Awareness. Factor 3 was named: Impulse control and our fourth factor to emerge was Problem Solving. Both factors were very similar to the third and fourth factor found by Palmer et al. Palmer et al. (2003) found a sixth factor which consisted of items loading from Flexibility and Independence, we on the other hand found two separate factors for that. Our 5th factor consisted of items loading from Independence and Assertiveness which was similar to one of the 13 factors found by Bar-On and our sixth factor Flexibility/Stress Tolerance had items loading from those two scales. Our last factor Interpersonal Adaptation/Self-Actualisation included loadings from Self-Actualisation, Interpersonal Relationships, Happiness and Flexibility. It would probably be useful replicate this study in larger, and independent samples.

With regards to gender effects, our results were consistent with the findings of Bar-On (1997), revealing no difference in overall emotional intelligence between males and females. However, consistent gender differences were found with respect to some components (i.e. interpersonal and intrapersonal skills, Problem Solving, Flexibility and Stress Tolerance) although differences were small.

When looking at educational level as a measure for academic success, results showed that overall EQ-scores increase with level of education. The least educated group showed significantly lower scores than the highest educated group with regards to many aspects of emotional intelligence. These results confirmed recent studies which stated that emotional intelligence is linked to academic success (Khajehpour 2011, Parker et al., 2004, Parker et al., 2004, Parker et al., 2006, Qualter et al., 2011, Van der Zee et al., 2002). Based on our study, we don't have enough evidence to come to any conclusions about the predictive value of emotional intelligence, but it seems clear that there is some connection to educational level. We obtained similar results regarding employment status: the unemployed group scored significantly lower on Total EQ and on several subscales than the employed group. Again these findings correspond with those reported by Bar-On (1997), indicating a link between emotional intelligence and occupational success. Interesting to note is that lower levels of education or unemployment, seemed to result in significantly lower scores on the same scales. This could simply be a reflection of the fact that the unemployment rate might be higher within the lower education group and that in the current study both groups largely contained the same individuals, and thus as a logical consequence had comparable EQ-scores. Another possible explanation however is that the same aspects of EI, that are associated with a higher risk of academic failure, also pose an increased risk for later unemployment.

Regarding the concurrent validity between the EQ-i and the MMPI-2 we found that people high on emotional intelligence experience fewer psychological problems and pathology than people low on emotional intelligence. This is in line with previous research of Schutte et al., (2007); Martins et al., (2010) etc… claiming a strong association between emotional intelligence and mental health. Our observations were made based on a non-clinical population, it would also be interesting to investigate emotional intelligence in clinical settings, for example the link between emotional intelligence and different clinical syndromes or personality disorders. Furthermore it would be useful to study the impact of emotional intelligence in relation to treatment and prediction of treatment outcome.

We also explored the incremental validity of MMPI-2 scales to predict emotional intelligence beyond the control variables (gender, employment, education). In general the MMPI-2 scales appeared to be good predictors for the EQ-i scales with large proportions of the variance explained. Especially clinical scales 2(D), 7(Pt) and 0(Si) proved to be significant negative predictors. Furthermore results showed that content scales Obsessiveness, Low Self-Esteem, Depression and Social Discomfort were strong negative predictors for some of the EQ-i scales. For a few EQ-i scales, Anxiety was a good negative predictor, while for other scales Anxiety was a positive predictor.

Finally some attention should be given to the fact that we did not include the Restructured Clinical (RC - Tellegen, Ben-Porath, McNulty, Arbisi, Graham & Kaemmer, 2003) scales in our research, this will be an important follow up study, also taking other scales of the Restructured MMPI-2 (Ben-Porath & Tellegen, 2008; Tellegen & Ben-Porath, 2008) into account, once the Dutch manual is published. The RC scales were originally developed to correct the high intercorrelations and extensive covariance problem of the clinical scales and were added to the MMPI-2 in 2003. Studies showed an improved convergent and discriminant validity. In 2008 a new version of the MMPI-2, the MMPI-2-RF (Restructured Form) was developed. This much shorter version with 338 items selected from the MMPI-2 item pool has the RC scales at its core.

To summarise, the present study provided support for the validity of a measure of emotional intelligence, the Bar-on Emotional Quotient Inventory (Bar-on, 1997) in a Flemish sample and supported its relation to academic success, professional success and psychological wellbeing.

5. References

Armstrong, A.R., Galligan, R.F., & Critchley, C.R. (2011). Emotional Intelligence and psychological resilience to negative life events. *Personality and Individual Differences,* 51, 331 - 336.

Austin, E.J., Saklofske, D.H., & Egan, V. (2005). Personality, well-being and health correlates of trait emotional intelligence. *Personality of Individual Differences,* 38, 547 - 558.

Bar-On, R. (1997a). Development of the Bar-On EQ-I: A Measure of Emotional Intelligence. Paper presented at the 105th Annual Convention of the American Psychological Association, Chicago, August.

Bar-On, R. (1997). *The Emotional Intelligence Inventory (EQ-i): technical manual.* Toronto, Canada : Multi-Health Systems.

Bar-On, R. (2000). Emotional and Social Intelligence: Insights from the Emotional Quotient Inventory. In R. Bar-On, and J.D.A. Parker, (Eds.), *The Handbook of Emotional Intelligence (17, 363-388).* Jossey-Bass, San Francisco.

Ben-Porath, Y.S., & Tellegen, A. (2008). *MMPI-2-RF. Manual for Administration, Scoring, and Interpretation.* Minneapolis: University of Minnesota Press.

Butcher, J.N., Derksen, J., Sloore, H., & Sirigatti, S. (2003). Objective Personality assessment of people in diverse cultures: European adaptations of the MMPI-2. *Behaviour Research and Therapy, 41,* 819-840.

Ciarrochi, J.V., Chan, A.Y.C. & Caputi, P. (2000). A critical evaluation of the emotional intelligence construct. *Personality and Individual Differences,* 28, 539-561.

Ciarrochi, J., Deane, F.P., & Anderson, S. (2002). Emotional intelligence moderates the relationship between stress and mental health. *Personality and Individual Differences,* 32, 197- 209.

Cattell, R.B. (1966). The scree test for the number of factors. *Multivariate Behavioural Research, 1,* 141 - 161.

Cohen, J. (1988). *Statistical Power Analysis for the Behavioral Sciences*. Hillsdale, New Jersey: Lawrence Erlbaum Associates.

Davies, M., Stankov., L. & Roberts R.D. (1998). Emotional intelligence : in search of an elusive construct. *Journal of Personality and Social Psychology*, 75, 989-1015.

Davis, S.K., & Humphrey, N. (2012). Emotional intelligence predicts adolescent mental health beyond personality and cognitive ability. *Personality and Individual Differences*, 52, 144 - 149.

Dawda, D. & Hart, S.D. (2000). Assessing emotional intelligence : reliability and validity of the Bar-On Emotional Quotient Inventory (EQ-i) in university students. *Personality and Individual Differences*, 28, 797-812.

Derksen, J.J.L., de Mey, H.R.A., Sloore, H., & Hellenbosch, G. (2006). *MMPI-2: handleiding bij afname, scoring en interpretatie*. Nijmegen, The Netherlands: PEN Test Publisher.

Derksen, J.J.L., Jeuken, J., & Klein-Herenbrink, A.J.M. (1998). Bar-On Emotional Quotient vragenlijst. Nijmegen: PEN Psychodiagnostics Dutch translation and adaption.

Derksen, J., Kramer, I., & Katzko, M. (2002). Does a self-report measure for emotional intelligence assess something different than general intelligence ? *Personality and Individual Differences*, 32, 37 – 48.

Dulewicz, V. & Higgs, M. (2000). Emotional intelligence. A review and evaluation study. *Journal of Managerial Psychology*, 15, 341-372.

Emmons, R.A., & Kaiser, H.A. (1996). Goal orientation and emotional well-being linking goals and affect though the self. In L.L. Martin & A. Tesser (Eds.), *Striving and feeling. Interactions among goals, affect and self-regulation* (4, 79 - 98). Lawrence Erlbaum Associates, Mahwah: New Jersey.

Friedman, A.F., Lewak, R., Nichols, D.S. & Webb, J.T. (2001). Psychological assessment with the MMPI-2. Lawrence Erlbaum Associates, Publishers. Mahwah, NJ & London.

Gallagher, E.N., & Vella-Brodrick, D.A. (2008). Social support and emotional intelligence as predictors of subjective well-being. *Personality and Individual Differences*, 44, 1551 - 1561.

Goleman, D. (1995). *Emotional Intelligence: why it can matter more than IQ*. New York: Bantam Books.

Goleman, D. (1998). *Working with emotional intelligence*. New York: Bantam Books.

Hedlund, J. & Sternberg, R.J. (2000). Too Many Intelligences? Integrating Social, Emotional, and Practical Intelligence. In R. Bar-On, and J.D.A. Parker (Eds.), *The Handbook of Emotional Intelligence* (7, 136-167). Jossey-Bass, San Francisco.

Horn,J.L. (1965). A rationale and test for the number of factors in factor analysis. *Psychometrika*, 30, 179 - 185.

Jacobs, M., Snow, J., Geraci, M., Vythilingam, M., Blair, R.J.R., Charney, D.S., Pine, D.S., & Blair, K.S. (2008). Association between level of emotional intelligence and severity of anxiety in generalized social phobia. *Journal of Anxiety Disorders*, 22, 1487 - 1495.

Karimi, M., & Besharat, M.A. (2010). Comparison of alexithymia and emotional intelligence in gifted and non-gifted high school students. *Procedia Social and Behavioral Sciences*, 5, 753 - 756.

Khajehpour, M. (2011). Relationship between emotional intelligence, parental involvement and academic performance of high school students. *Procedia. Social and Behavioral Science*, 15, 1081 - 1086.

Martins, A., Ramalho, N., & Morin, E. (2010). A comprehensive meta-analysis of the relationship between emotional intelligence and health. *Personality and Individual Differences*, 49, 554 - 564.

Mayer, J.D., Caruso, D.R. & Salovey, P. (1999). Emotional intelligence meets traditional standards for an intelligence. *Intelligence*, 27, 267-298.

Mayer, J.D., Caruso, D.R. & Salovey P. (2000). Selecting a Measure of Emotional Intelligence: The Case for Ability Scales. In R. Bar-On, and J.D.A. Parker (Eds.), *The Handbook of Emotional Intelligence* (15, 320-342). Jossey-Bass, San Francisco.

Mayer, J.D., Salovey, P., & Caruso, D.R., (2002). *Mayer-Salovey-Caruso Emotional Intelligence Test (MSCEIT) user's manual*. Toronto: Multi-Health Systems.

McClelland, D.C. (1973). Testing for competence rather than for "intelligence". *American Psychologist*, January, 1-14.

Nemiah, J.C., & Sifneos, P.E. (1970). Affect and fantasy in patients with psychosomatic disorders. In O.W. Hill, *Modern trends in psychosomatic medicine*. Vol 2 (26-34). London: Butterworth.

Newsome, S., Day, A.L. & Catano, V.M. (2000). Assessing the predictive validity of emotional intelligence. *Personality and Individual Differences*, 29, 1005-1016.

O'Connor, B..P. (2000). SPSS and SAS Programs for determining the number of components using parallel analysis and Velicer's MAP test. *Behavior Research Methods, Instruments, & Computers*, 32, 396 - 402.

O'Connor, R.M., Jr., & Little, I.S. (2003). Revisiting the predictive validity of emotional intelligence: self-report versus ability-based measures. *Personality and Individual Differences*, 35, 1893 - 1902.

Palmer, B.R., Manocha, R., Gignac, G., & Stough, C. (2001). Examining the factor structure of the Bar-On Emotional Quotient Inventory with an Australian general population sample. *Personality and Individual Differences*, 35, 1191 - 1210.

Parker, J.D.A., Creque, R.E., Barnhart, D.L., Irons Harris, J., Majeski, S.A., Wood, L.M., Bond, B.J., & Hogan, M.J. (2004). Academic achievement in high school: does emotional intelligence matter ? *Personality and Individual Differences*, 37, 1321 - 1330.

Parker,J.D.A., Hogan, M.J., Eastabrook, J.M., Oke, A., & Wood, L.M. (2006). Emotional intelligence and student retention: Predicting the successful transition from high school to university. *Personality and Individual Differences*, 41, 1329 - 1336.

Parker, J.D.A., Summerfeldt, L.J., Hogan, M.J., & Majeski, S.A. (2004). Emotional differences and academic success: examining the transition from high school to university. *Personality and Individual Differences*, 36, 163 - 172.

Parker, J.D.A., Taylor, G.J. & Bagby, R.M. (2001). The relationship between emotional intelligence and alexithymia. *Personality and Individual Differences*, 30, 107-115.

Petrides, K.V., & Furham, A. (2001). Trait Emotional Intelligence: psychometric investigation with reference to established trait taxonomies. *European Journal of Personality*, 15, 425 - 448.

Qualter, P., Gardner, K.J., Pope, D.J., Hutchinson, J.M., & Whiteley, H.E. (2011). Ability emotional intelligence, trait emotional intelligence, and academic success in British secondary schools: A 5 year longitudinal study. *Learning and Individual Differences* doi:10.1016/j.lindif.2011.11.007.

Reiff, H.B., Hatzes, N.M., Bramel, M.H., & Gibbon, T. (2001). The relationship of LD and gender with emotional intelligence in college students. *Journal of Learning Disabilities*, 34, 66 - 78.

Schutte, N.S., & Malouff, J.M. (2011). Emotional intelligence mediates the relationship between mindfulness and subjective well-being. *Personality and Individual Differences*, 50, 1116 - 1119.

Schutte, N.S., Malouff, J., Hall, L., Haggerty, D., Cooper, J., Golden, C., & Dornheim, L. (1998). Development and validation of a measure of emotional intelligence. *Personality and Individual Differences*, 25, 167-177.

Schutte, N..S., Malouff, J.M., Simunek, M., McKenley, J., & Hollander, S. (2002). Characteristic emotional intelligence and emotional well-being. *Cognition and Emotion*, 16, 769 - 786.

Schutte, N.S., Malouff, J.M., Thorsteinsson, E.B., Bhullar, N., & Rooke, S.E. (2007). A meta-analytic investigation of the relationship between emotional intelligence and health. *Personality and Individual Differences*, 25, 167-177.

Sjöberg, L. (2001). Emotional Intelligence and Life Adjustment: A validation study. SSE/EFI Working Paper Series in Business Administration, No 2001:8.

Salovey, P. & Mayer, J.D. (1990). Emotional Intelligence. *Imagination, Cognition and Personality*, 9, 185-211.

Swart, A. (1996). The relationship between well-being and academic performance. Unpublished master's thesis, University of Pretoria, South-Africa. In *Bar-On, R. (1997). The Emotional Intelligence Inventory (EQ-i) : technical manual*. Toronto, Canada : Multi-Health Systems.

Tellegen, A., & Ben-Porath, Y.S. (2008). *MMPI-2-RF Technical Manual*. Minneapolis, MN: University of Minnesota Press.

Tellegen, A., Ben-Porath, Y.S., McNulty, J.L., Arbisi, P.A., Graham, J.R., & Kaemmer, B. (2003). *The MMPI-2 Restructured Clinical (RC) scales: Development, validation and interpretation*. Minneapolis: University of Minnesota Press.

Van Der Zee, K., Thijs, M., & Schakel, L. (2002). The relationship of emotional intelligence with academic intelligence and the Big Five. *European Journal of Personality*, 16, 103 - 125.

Zeidner, M., Matthews, G., & Roberts, R.D. (2009). *What we know about emotional intelligence. How it affects learning, work, relationships, and our mental health*. Cambridge: MIT Press.

Zeidner, M., Shani-Zinovich, I., Matthews, G., & Roberts, R.D. (2005). Assessing emotional intelligence in gifted and non-gifted high school students: Outcomes depend on the measure. *Intelligence*, 33, 369 - 391.

Zwick, W.R., & Velicer, W.F. (1986). Comparison of five rules for determining the number of components to retain. *Psychological Bulletin*, 17, 253 – 269.

Section 5

Qualitative Psychology

10

Qualitative Research Methods in Psychology

Deborah Biggerstaff
Warwick Medical School
University of Warwick, Coventry
UK

1. Introduction

In the scientific community, and particularly in psychology and health, there has been an active and ongoing debate on the relative merits of adopting either quantitative or qualitative methods, especially when researching into human behaviour (Bowling, 2009; Oakley, 2000; Smith, 1995a, 1995b; Smith, 1998). In part, this debate formed a component of the development in the 1970s of our thinking about science. Andrew Pickering has described this movement as the "sociology of scientific knowledge" (SSK), where our scientific understanding, developing scientific 'products' and 'know-how', became identified as forming components in a wider engagement with society's environmental and social context (Pickering, 1992, pp. 1). Since that time, the debate has continued so that today there is an increasing acceptance of the use of qualitative methods in the social sciences (Denzin & Lincoln, 2000; Morse, 1994; Punch, 2011; Robson, 2011) and health sciences (Bowling, 2009; Greenhalgh & Hurwitz, 1998; Murphy & Dingwall, 1998). The utility of qualitative methods has also been recognised in psychology. As Nollaig Frost (2011) observes, authors such as Carla Willig and Wendy Stainton Rogers consider qualitative psychology is much more accepted today and that it has moved from "the margins to the mainstream in psychology in the UK." (Willig & Stainton Rogers, 2008, pp. 8). Nevertheless, in psychology, qualitative methodologies are still considered to be relatively 'new' (Banister, Bunn, Burman, et al., 2011; Hayes, 1998; Richardson, 1996) despite clear evidence to the contrary (see, for example, the discussion on this point by Rapport et al., 2005). Nicki Hayes observes, scanning the content of some early journals from the 1920s – 1930s that many of these more historical papers "discuss personal experiences as freely as statistical data" (Hayes, 1998, 1). This can be viewed as an early development of the case-study approach, now an accepted methodological approach in psychological, health care and medical research, where our knowledge about people is enhanced by our understanding of the individual 'case' (May & Perry, 2011; Radley & Chamberlain, 2001; Ragin, 2011; Smith, 1998).

The discipline of psychology, originating as it did during the late 19th century, in parallel with developments in modern medicine, tended, from the outset, to emphasise the 'scientific method' as the way forward for psychological inquiry. This point of view arose out of the previous century's Enlightenment period which underlay the founding of what is generally agreed to be the first empirical experimental psychology laboratory, established by Wilhelm Wundt, University of Leipzig, in 1879. During this same period, other early psychology researchers, such as the group of scientific thinkers interested in perception (the Gestaltists: see, for example, Lamiell, 1995) were developing their work. Later, in the 20th century, the introduction of Behaviourism became the predominant school of psychology in America and Britain. Behaviourism emphasised a reductionist approach, and this movement, until its displacement in the 1970-80s by the 'cognitive revolution', dominated the discipline of psychology (Hayes, 1998, pp. 2-3). These approaches have served the scientific community well, and have been considerably enhanced by increasingly sophisticated statistical computer programmes for data analysis.

A recent feature of the debate in the future direction for psychology has been a concern for the philosophical underpinnings of the discipline and an appreciation of their importance. In part, this is an intrinsic part of theoretical developments in psychology and the related social sciences, in particular sociological research, such as Grounded Theory, developed by the sociologists Glazer and Strauss during the 1960s and 1970s (e.g. Charmaz, 1983; Glaser & Strauss, 1967; Searle, 2012); modes of social inquiry such as interviewing and content analysis (Gillham, 2000; King & Horrocks, 2010); action research (Hart & Bond, 1999; Sixsmith & Daniels, 2011); discourse and discourse analysis (Tonkiss, 2012; Potter & Wetherell, 1995); narrative (Polkinghorne, 1988; Reissman, 2008); biographical research methods (Roberts, 2002); phenomenological methods (Giorgi,1995; Langdridge, 2007; Lawthom &Tindall, 2011; Smith et al., 2009); focus groups (Carey, 1994; Vazquez-Lago et al., 2011); visual research methods (Mitchell, 2011); ethnographic methods (Boyles, 1994; Punch, 2011); photo-biographic-elicitation methods (Rapport et al., 2008); and, finally, the combining or integrating of methods, the approach often known as 'mixed methods' (Frost, 2011; Pope et al., 2007; Thomas et al., 2004; Todd et al., 2004).

Qualitative methods have much to offer when we need to explore people's feelings or ask participants to reflect on their experiences. As was noted above, some of the earliest psychological thinkers of the late 19th century and early 20th century may be regarded as proto-qualitative researchers. Examples include the 'founding father' of psycho-analysis, Sigmund Freud, who worked in Vienna (late 19th century - to mid 20th century), recorded and published numerous case-studies and then engaged in analysis, postulation and theorising on the basis of his observations, and the pioneering Swiss developmental psychologist, Jean Piaget (1896 - 1980) who meticulously observed and recorded his children's developing awareness and engagement with their social world. They were succeeded by many other authors from the 1940s onwards who adopted qualitative methods and may be regarded as contributors to the development of qualitative methodologies through their emphasis of the importance of the idiographic and use of case studies (Allport,1946; Nicholson, 1997)[1] . This locates the roots of qualitative thinking in the long-standing debate between empiricist and rationalistic schools of thought, and also in social constructionism (Gergen, 1985; King & Horrock, pp. 6 – 24)[2].

---

[1] Allport states "[…] among the methods having idiographic intent, and emphasised by me, are the case study, the personal document, interviewing methods,matching, personal structure analysis, and other procedures that contrive to keep together what nature itself has fashioned as an integrated unit – the single personality." (Allport, 1946, pp. 133).

[2] A notable milestone in the development of qualitative methodologies in the UK for example, was the publication, in 1992, of a paper proposing a role for qualitative methods for psychology, by Karen Henwood and Nick Pigeon in the *British Journal of Psychology*.

More recently, in the UK, the British Psychological Society now has a members' section for Qualitative Methods in Psychology (QMiP) which held a successful inaugural conference, in 2008, at the University of Leeds. The Section now boasts a membership of more than 1000 members, making it one of the largest BPS Sections. The undergraduate psychology curriculum, which confers BPS graduate basis for registration (GBR), now includes qualitative research methods teaching in the core programme for UK universities degrees. Elsewhere, qualitative psychology has taken a little longer to be accepted e.g. by the American Psychological Association (APA). This is somewhat surprising given the large volume of qualitative research papers which originate from the American research community. However, US researchers, alongside their international colleagues, have finally managed to petition successfully for the inclusion of qualitative methodologies to be admitted to Section 5, the methodology section, of the APA, during 2011.

These developments can be tracked by a search for qualitative research across the main electronic databases and exploring the 'hits' recovered. A quick scan using the umbrella terms 'qualitative' and / or 'qualitative research' for example, provides the researcher with a result for a relatively low number of papers from the earlier years of last century. However there is a noticeably sharp increase in the number of papers published from 1990 onwards. A search of the main databases, using the term "qualitative" as a key word (January, 1990 - December, 2011) produced a retrieval rate for qualitative papers of over 51744 hits (CINAHL); 122012 hits (PsycInfo); 12108 for Medline (OVID); and 18431 for Applied Social Sciences Index and Abstracts (ASSIA). Prior to 1990 the number of papers recorded in these databases is noticeably lower: searching in ASSIA for papers published between 1985 - 1990, for example, results in 13 papers, while a Medline search for the years 1985 - 1990 returns 6 papers. Searching in CINAHL for the same period (1985 - 1990) results in no papers (zero result).

2. What is qualitative psychology?

So, what exactly is qualitative research? A practical definition points to methods that use language, rather than numbers, and an interpretative, naturalistic approach. Qualitative research embraces the concept of *intersubjectivity* usually understood to refer to how people may agree or construct meaning: perhaps to a shared understanding, emotion, feeling, or perception of a situation , in order to interpret the social world they inhabit (Nerlich, 2004, pp. 18). Norman Denzin and Yvonna Lincoln define qualitative researchers as people who usually work in the 'real' world of lived experience, often in a natural setting, rather than a laboratory based experimental approach. The qualitative researcher tries to make sense of social phenomena and the meanings people bring to them (Denzin & Lincoln, 2000)[3].

In qualitative research, it is acknowledged that the researcher is an integral part of the process and who may reflect on her/his own influence and experience in the research

(See Henwood, K. & Pidgeon, N. (1992) Qualitative research and psychological theorising. *British Journal of Psychology*, **83**: 97 - 111).

[3] For readers interested in more on the history of the philosophy of science and its relationship to developments in psychology, I recommend the following authors: Andrew Pickering (1992); John Richardson (1996); Mark Smith (1998); Clive Seale (2012); and especially Jonathan Smith and colleagues with the publication of *Rethinking Methods in Psychology* (Smith et al., 1995b).

process.[4] The qualitative researcher accepts that s/he is not 'neutral'. Instead s/he puts herself in the position of the participant or 'subject' and attempts to understand how the world is from that person's perspective. As this process is re-iterated, hypotheses begin to emerge, which are 'tested' against the data of further experiences e.g. people's narratives. One of the key differences between quantitative and qualitative approaches is apparent here: the quantitative approach states the hypothesis from the outset, (i.e. a 'top down' approach), whereas in qualitative research the hypothesis or research question, is refined and developed during the process. This may be thought of as a 'bottom-up' or emergent approach, as, for example, in Grounded Theory (Charmaz, 1995).This contrast is part of the epistemological positions that shape our assumptions about the world. King and Horrocks summarise some of these main differences in position as being either realist, contextual or constructionist. They compare these to assumptions about the world, the knowledge produced and the role of the researcher (King & Horrocks, 2010). These authors, along with others, such as Colin Robson, advocate adopting a pragmatic approach to qualitative research. As Robson observes, "Pragmatism is almost an 'anti-philosophical' philosophy which advocates getting on with the research rather than philosophizing – hence providing a welcome antidote to a stultifuying over-concern with matters such as ontology and epistemology." (Robson, 2011, pp.30)[5].

It may be helpful to think of qualitative research as situated at one end of a continuum with its data from in-depth interviews, and with quantitative 'measurable' data at the other end (see **Figure 1**). At the centre-point of this continuum may rest such data as content analysis and questionnaire responses transformed from the written or spoken word into numerical 'codes' for statistical analysis. Examples include standardised questionnaires, e.g. for depression and anxiety such as Hospital Anxiety and Depression Scale (HADS), or Beck's Depression Inventory. With limited space given on questionnaires, respondents can only give the briefest answers to pre-formulated questions from the researchers. Respondents' replies are coded and 'scored', but does that mean that we can measure feelings or emotion? How do we 'calculate' levels of depression or anxiety? How does the experience of depression affect people's lives? Have we, as researchers, asked appropriate questions in the first place? Qualitative research methodology looks to answer these types of questions – the *exploratory* approach. An example of this exploratory approach is Jonathan Smith's work examining young mothers' lived-world experiences of the psychological transition to motherhood (see, for example, Smith, 1999; 1998; 1994).

[4] This is in contrast to the positivist, *hypothetico-deductive* methodology, associated with the philosopher Karl Popper, and enthusiastically adopted by the psychology discipline, of 'refuting the null hypothesis', commonly taken to be the 'gold standard' of quantitative scientific research methodology i.e. where hypotheses are defined at the start of the research (see, for example, Popper,1935/2002). One of the challenges however of attempting to fit the 'scientific' approach into researching human behaviour, is that sometimes this scientific experimental methodology, the design of which originates in the laboratory, may not quite provide what is needed when attempting to investigate psychological and human behaviours. The Medical Research Council (MRC) in the UK also acknowledges this. In 2008 they provided new guidance to their 2000 *MRC Framework for the development and evaluation of RCTs for complex interventions to improve health* to include non-experimental methods, and complex interventions outside healthcare. See
http://www.mrc.ac.uk/Utilities/Documentrecord/index.htm?d=MRC004871

[5] See also Robson, 2011, pp. 30 – 35 for further discussion on this topic.

Epistemological position	Realist	Contextual	Constructionist
Assumptions about the world	There exists unmediated access to a 'real' world where process and relationships can be revealed	Contrast is integral to understanding how people experience their lives	Social reality is constructed through language which produces particular versions of events
Knowledge produced	Seeks to produce objective data which is reliable and likely to be representative of the wider population from which the interview sample is drawn	Data are inclusive of context aiming to add to the 'completeness' of the analysis by making visible cultural and historical meaning systems	Does not adhere to traditional conventions. Knowledge brought into being through dialogue
Role of researcher	Researcher aims to avoid bias. Remains objective and detached	Subjectivity of researcher is integral to process. Researcher active in data generation and analysis	Researcher 'co-producer' of knowledge. Therefore needs to be reflexive and critically aware (e.g. of language)

Source: adapted from King & Horrocks, 2010, pp. 20

Table 1. Epistemological positions that shape our world

Today, a growing number of psychologists are re-examining and re-exploring qualitative methods for psychological research, challenging the more traditional 'scientific' experimental approach (see, for example, Gergen, 1991; 1985; Smith et al., 1995a, 1995b). There is a move towards a consideration of what these other methods can offer to psychology (Bruner, 1986; Smith et al.,1995a). What we are now seeing is a renewed interest in qualitative methods which has led to many researchers becoming interested in how qualitative methods in psychology can stand alongside, and complement, quantitative methods. This is important, since both qualitative and quantitative methods have value to the researcher and each can complement the other albeit with a different focus[6] (Crossley, 2000; Dixon-Wood & Fitzpatrick, 2001; Elwyn, 1997; Gantley et al., 1999; Rapport et al., 2005). Seminal qualitative-focused works from authors such as Jerome Bruner, Donald Polkinghorne and Jonathan Smith and colleagues' in the early 1990s highlight the importance of 're-discovering' qualitative methods in the field (Bruner, 1990, 1991, 2000; Polkinghorne, 1988; Smith et al., 1995a; 1995b).

[6] I thank the book's editor, Gina Rossi for this helpful comment.

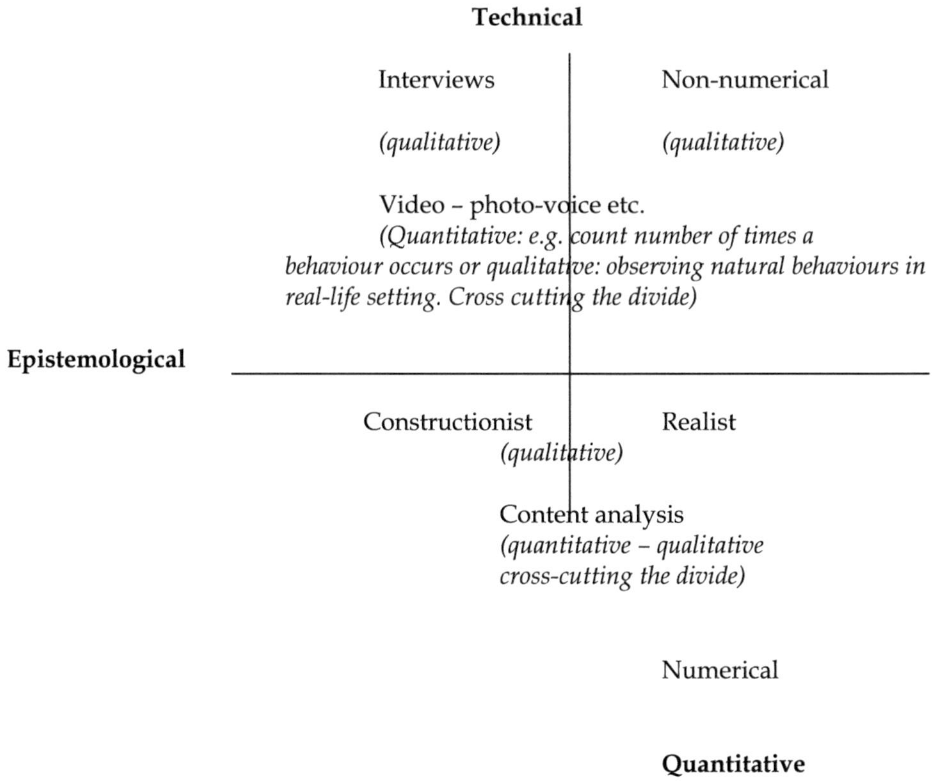

Source: adapted from Henwood, 1996.

Fig. 1. The quantitative – qualitative continuum

Jonathan Smith and his colleagues, for example, announce at the beginning of their *Rethinking psychology,* that "Psychology is in a state of flux" with an "unprecedented degree of questioning about the nature of the subject, the boundaries of the discipline and what new ways of conducting psychological research are available." (Smith et al., 1995a, pp. 1). Rom Harré, heralded these new ways of thinking as marking the 'discursive turn' (Harré, 1995a, pp. 146), while Ken Gergen, writes about there being a 'revolution in qualitative research' (Gergen, 2001, pp. 3).

Additionally, as Karen Henwood suggests, integrating qualitative with quantitative methods in psychology also provides researchers with a tool for the potential "democratisation of the research process". She observes how among clinical psychologists working in the United Kingdom's National Health Service (NHS) for instance, the research process can be "opened to include the views of service users"with an increasing emphasis on exploring "people's personal and cultural understandings and stocks of knowledge" (Henwood, 2004, pp. 43). Henwood suggests that integrating methods may thus also help establish and embed research validity by communicating responsibly and honestly when exploring multiple perspectives.

In a parallel movement, qualitative methods have also come to be increasingly acknowledged across the social sciences more generally (Banister, et al. 2011; Oakley, 2000;

Potter, 1996; Radley & Chamberlain, 200; Richardson, 1996; Strauss & Corbin, 1990; Willig, 2008). Meanwhile, as already noted above, the use of narrative and meaning in psychology and the human sciences also re-emerged (Bruner, 1990, 1991; Crossley, 2000; Polkinghorne, 1988; Reissman, 2008). Interestingly, Polkinghorne observes that, in contrast to other related disciplines in the social sciences, psychology very largely ignored the use of narrative until the end of the 1980s - early 1990s with a shift towards a "renewed interest in narrative as a cognitive structure" (Polkinghorne, 1988, pp. 101) as an element in the field of cognitive psychology. Polkinghorne suggests that the re-emergence of narrative thinking in psychology took place during this period due to the increased attention being given by psychologists to the utility of exploring life histories, self-narrative (for example in establishing one's personal identity) and a renewal of interest in the case study and biographical research (Roberts, 2002). Polkinghorne, along with other authors, such as Jerome Bruner (1990, 1991, 2002) and Ricoeur (1981/1995) proposes that our use of narrative is linked to the perception of time and our place in the lived-world where

> "[...] people use self-stories to interpret and account for their lives. The basic dimension of human existence is temporality, and narrative transforms the mere passing away of time into a meaningful unity, the self. The study of a person's own experience of her or his life-span requires attending to the operations of the narrative form and how this life story is related to the stories of others."
>
> (Polkinghorne, 1988, pp. 119).

During the same period, (i.e. over the past ten - fifteen years), psychology and social science journals, such as the *British Journal of Psychology, Journal of Health Psychology, Social Science and Medicine* etc., as, indeed, did the *British Medical Journal,* began to include qualitative research papers, indicating that a qualitative approach, in parallel with the quantitative scientific paradigm, can illuminate important areas in the behavioural sciences and psychology. In the early days there was some debate about academic 'rigour' and validity suggesting some unease about using qualitative methods, both in psychology and related areas. This is now much improved as researchers address these issues (Bloor, 1997; Henwood, 2004; Yardley, 2008). However, this is less of a challenge today, with increasing acceptance of these methods and the introduction of appraisal checklists. Nevertheless, as with any research, poor understanding of the methodology and what it can offer, or the inappropriate selection of a method, is likely to lead to poor quality results and the resultant lack of any real insight into the area being explored. Today, the introduction of evidence-based tools such as the Critical Appraisal Skills Programme (CASP) based at the Centre for Evidence Based Medicine, University of Oxford, include a qualitative paper checklist on their website providing evidence of a much greater acceptance of these methods (CEBMhttp://www.sph.nhs.uk/what-we-do/public-health-workforce/resources/critical-appraisals-skills-programme).

Additionally, the British Psychological Society has now developed guidelines for the appraisal of qualitative papers indicating the wider academic acceptance of qualitative psychology today. As Peter Banister and his colleagues note, writing in the preface to their *Qualitative methods in psychology,* in benchmarking UK psychology degrees, The Quality Assurance Agency of 2007, include a section on the need for students to cover both quantitative and qualitative research methods. This includes being able to analyse both types of data. This ability is now (2010) also highlighted as being a requirement for conferring of BPS Chartership status (Banister et al., 2011: vii - viii)

Thus, in order to best gain insight into the field of qualitative psychology some of this background knowledge of the specific theoretical and philosophical underpinnings outlined earlier is needed by researchers today who decide to explore their chosen research topic using qualitative methods. These theoretical and philosophical concerns inform the discipline and it is important that the researcher understands this.

2.1 Pluralism in qualitative research: Synthesizing or combining methods

The importance of researching and studying people in as natural a way as possible is emphasised i.e. the 'real world' approach (Robson, 2011). This is contrasted with the positivist approach of refuting the null hypothesis. The need for the researcher to put herself in the position of the 'subject' in her attempt to understand how the world is from that person's perspective is emphasised. King and Horrocks, for instance, discuss these different, sometimes competing 'quant - qual' approaches to research. These authors suggest that, while often presented as the challenge of two 'paradigms,' it may be an unhelpful way to approach the quantitative - qualitative continuum (King & Horrocks, 2010, pp. 7). This is because some researchers today are beginning to think further about how we might optimise results by synthesizing qualitative and quantitative data to interpret our research evidence. Thus, we may further understand (*verstehen*), our findings, by drawing on social theory, from Max Weber's work (Whimster, 2001, pp. 59-64). This interpretive approach, originating, as it does, from the field of social sciences, aims to develop new conceptual understandings and explanations in social theory (Pope, et al., 2007, pp. 72 onward).

Cresswell and Clark (2007) recognise that, in order to avoid losing potential value of some data, it may be preferable to adopt 'mixed methods'. This is often of value in, for example, health research where health evidence is needed from both quantitative and qualitative perspectives. This helps bring together diverse types of evidence needed to inform healthcare delivery and practice (Pope et al., 2007). I offer some suggestions and guidance for when either a qualitative or quantitative approach might be most useful, or alternatively, when it might be helpful to consider using combined methods i.e. a 'mixed methods' approach. The research focus can then be viewed from a number of vantage points, the approach known as *triangulation* (Banister et al., 2011; Huberman & Miles, 1998, pp. 199). Since triangulation is an approach which may be adopted across different qualitative methods, this is discussed next.

3. Triangulation

The term 'triangulation', according to Huberman and Miles, is thought to originate from Campbell and Fiske's 1959 work on "multiple operationalism" developed from geometry and trigonometry (Huberman & Miles, 1998). Huberman and Miles caution that the term 'triangulation' may have more than one interpretation. However, it is usually used to describe data verification of data, and considered as a method for

> "...checking for the most common or the most insidious biases that can steal into the process of drawing conclusions."
>
> (Huberman & Miles, 1998, pp. 198)

When researchers employ triangulation, multiple measures are used to ensure that any data variance is not due to the way in which the data were collected or measured. By linking different methods, the researcher intends that each method enhances the other, since all the information that is collected potentially offers to be contextually richer than if it were seen from only one vantage point. Each area provides a commentary on the other areas of the research (Frost, 2009). Triangulation can be a useful tool to examine data overload, where researchers analysing data may miss some important information due to an over-reliance on one portion of the data which could then skew the analysis. Another use is to provide checks and balances on the salience of first impressions. Triangulation is also a useful tool to help avoid data selectivity, such as being over-confident about a particular section of the data analysis such as when trying to confirm a key finding, or without taking into account the potential for sources of data unreliability (Huberman & Miles, 1998, pp.198-9).

It should be noted however, that, although triangulation is generally considered helpful when using qualitative methods, it can just as equally be applied to quantitative or mixed-methods research. It is a pragmatic and strategic approach, whether applied to qualitative or qualitative research (Denzin & Lincoln, 1998). It may be viewed as providing a way of expanding the research perspective and becomes another means of strengthening research findings (Krahn et al.,1995).

Banister et al. (2011) point out that any method of enquiry, whether quantitative or qualitative, can be open to bias and/or value laden, a fact that should be acknowledged,

> "[...] a researcher and research cannot be value-free, and that a general 'objectivist' notion that science can be value-free is impossible, given that we are all rooted in a social world that is socially constructed. Psychology (at least in the West) has general values (even if these are often left implicit) of communicating broadening knowledge and understanding about people, with a commitment to both freedom of enquiry and freedom of expression."
>
> (Banister et al., 2011, pp. 204)

Triangulation can help balance out, if not overcome, some of the challenges inherent in research, of whatever methodological persuasion (Todd et al., 2004). Triangulation can be separated into four broad categories: data triangulation, investigator triangulation, triangulation of method and triangulation of theory.

3.1 Data triangulation

Using one data origin may sometimes not be ideal. Collecting information from more than one source can extend and enhance the research process. Banister and colleagues suggest that more than one viewpoint, site, or source, increases diversity, thus leading to increased understanding of the research topic (Banister et al., 2011; Cowman, 1993). The authors propose it can be helpful to look at data collected at different times, or stages, of fieldwork, in order to re-evaluate ("*re*search") the material. This might mean checking if anything has been overlooked or given too much emphasis, during the research process. The use of triangulation can be very helpful when verification of data is needed, such as when doing action research or an ethnography (Walsh, 2012, pp. 257 onward).

The approach supports research being a reflexive, organic process, enriched by researchers' increasing depth of knowledge as they investigate the area (Finlay, 2003). This is linked to the role of *reflexivity* in qualitative research, considered by many to be an essential component in qualitative inquiry (Banister et al., 2011, pp. 200-201; Frost, 2011, pp. 11-12). The researcher is expected to be able to stand back from the completed research and consider, in retrospect, the selected methodology, whether the approach adopted suited the analysis undertaken what the experience may have been like for both the researcher and the participants etc. Other factors which may be considered include whether flaws were found in the research design, how the research study might be improved or refined, what further research might be needed etc. Some researchers advocate keeping a journal or diary recording these reflexions during the actual research process (Robson, 2011, pp. 270).

3.2 Investigator triangulation

Investigator triangulation is a multi-vantage point method which, as the name suggests, uses different approaches to research into the one area, thus exploring a number of aspects of the topic being examined. In health psychology, for example, it can be a useful way to study certain types of patient groups such as children and their lives (Greig et al., 2008, pp. 88-89). Eiser and Twamley (1995), writing about children and illness, consider that triangulation provides a useful approach for researching children. They discuss research areas such as children's understanding of illness and issues arising from a child's consent to treatment. They point out that children have a different, more limited, vocabulary from adults. The authors state that, when researching illness and children, "...the greater involvement of the family all necessitate a distinctive approach" (Eiser & Twamley,1995, pp. 133). These authors conclude that combining methods involved in using triangulation helps improve investigators' understanding of the issues being researched. They observe that,

> "Quantitative and qualitative research methods can be complementary. While quantitative work provides us with focused and highly generalizable information, qualitative work is particularly useful for new or sensitive areas where little may be known, or where the aim is to obtain understanding of more subjective and cultural aspects of illness."
>
> (Eiser & Twamley,1999, pp. 145)

They conclude by citing Roche, stating,

> "...each type of approach while distinctly different in orientation, focus and application is able to contribute to the understanding of health problems and the development of solutions. The strengths of one approach do not diminish the other. Qualitative and quantitative techniques are complementary and both are powerful tools in their own right."
>
> (Roche,1991, pp. 136, cited by Eiser & Twamley, *ibid.*)

Judith Sixsmith and John Daniels, for instance, consider investigator triangulation has the potential to enrich the research process. The authors, however, also flag up the possibility of difficulties in using this method. This can be further complicated when representing a range of perspectives, such as when incorporating stakeholders' views. The authors suggest that "it cannot be assumed that that those around the table will have an equally shared degree of responsibility and contribution. If not, then once again fairness is challenged and ultimately more problems are created than solved."

(Sixsmith & Daniels, 2011, pp. 32-32)

3.3 Method triangulation

Triangulation by method uses several approaches to collect data and information about the topic being explored. Here the researcher chooses the method of inquiry according to the question being researched e.g. by observing behaviours (an observational approach) or exploring how participants feel e.g. using interviews. Multiple methods help avoid any problems of the research findings being an artefact of the particular method used (Banister et al., 2011). This can help resolve issues around any questions of validity or distortion (Flick, 1992; 2007, pp. 37 - 53). Triangulation of method can, therefore, give different information about the research area, where, drawing on the early gestalists work on field and ground, the whole becomes 'more than the sum of the parts' (Helson, 1933; Perls et al., 1951). It is possible to combine qualitative and quantitative methods using data synthesis and triangulation, such as in 'mixed-methods' (Cresswell & Clark, 2007; Pope et al., 2007). This methodological approach might encompass either combining different types of data within a research project, perhaps by surveying a large number of participants , thus obtaining quantitative data, before moving on to an in-depth interview element by using a smaller, purposeful sample, to provide further illumination or explanation of the survey findings (qualitative data). Alternatively, researchers might synthesize the evidence from the research data across several qualitative and / or quantitative studies in order to elaborate further on the research context concerned (Pope et al., 2007; Thomas et al., 2004). This can be viewed as a pragmatic approach in order to obtain the best information from the evidence available.

3.4 Theoretical triangulation

In contrast, theoretical triangulation explores, and is informed by, more than one theory or theoretical framework. This approach aims to explore the diversity and complexity that is frequently the reality of research particularly when examining human behaviours. This is especially likely where large, multidisciplinary research teams come together to work on a project such as in health research, economics, organisational behaviour and psychology. Theoretical triangulation acknowledges, and allows for, the broad range of theories, complexity and diversity of the real world and how different theories may be accounted for in research (Kok et al., 2004). This is linked to the concept of *levels of triangulation* where an attempt is made to investigate the topic at differing levels, where connections are made to both the explanations at the individual level and at a society level (Banister et al., 2011). This can lead to *'contextualization'* of the picture to gain a greater understanding of the research 'fit' with the environment.

4. Qualitative methods and the implications for psychological research

The emphasis on interpretation and meaning has several implications for the qualitative psychology researcher and for service delivery areas such as health psychology and health services research. Gantley et al. (1999) in their text *An Introduction to Qualitative Methods for Health Professionals*, provide a useful summary:

1. Interpretative analysis concentrates on understanding the views of research participants; it makes explicit the distinction between respondents' views and researcher's interpretation
2. Interpretative analysis accepts that there are different coexisting interpretations of any phenomenon, e.g. a sore throat, and may attach equal importance to each interpretation.
3. The recognition of multiple meanings challenges one of the basic tenets of western biomedicine and evidence-based medicine, that of **positivism**.

(Source: adapted from Gantley et al., 1999)

Positivism is a philosophical approach dating from the nineteenth century. It underlies scientific and other approaches that privilege measurement and counting. This approach inevitably informs our view of the world -but it is not the only way of seeing. Thus, the qualitative - quantitative methodology debate on research may be seen as a reflection on the different emphasis between *values versus facts*.

In psychological and health research, qualitative methods may stand alone, or be used as part of the research process. When used in conjunction with quantitative methodologies (as, for example, in a mixed methods approach), or when using data from several sources, the use of qualitative methodology can help explore more thoroughly complex beliefs, attitudes and experiences. This approach, as we have seen earlier, uses triangulation, since the research focus is viewed through different research 'lenses', or examined by the researcher from a number of angles or vantage points (Huberman & Miles, 1998, pp. 199).

Some of the most frequent uses for qualitative research especially, for example, in health psychology and health services research, addresses issues in research processes and beliefs. These might include process: how an outcome is reached or why people follow a certain course of action, or behaviour e.g. in service delivery. An example might be exploring reasons for parents bringing their children to an 'out-of-hours' clinic rather than booking an appointment at their general practitioner's surgery. A recent example, with a European perspective, is a qualitative study exploring primary care physicians' attitudes to prescribing antibiotics to their patients and the challenges of antimicrobial resistance in Spain (Vazquez-Lago et al., 2011).

Other uses for qualitative research are:

Examining research questions to inform and guide questionnaire development e.g. as a preliminary exploratory stage of design, or to gain greater understanding of research questionnaire data e.g. after questionnaires have been returned - using qualitative in-depth interviews to explore further some of the issues mentioned by respondents.

Hypothesis generation (e.g. in a Grounded Theory approach) where categories or outcomes cannot be determined before data collection. This would involve the progressive identification and integration of categories of meaning from the data obtained. In turn, this data can then be used either to inform the research process and method or, alternatively in the generation of theory.

4.1 Different uses for four approaches commonly encountered in research

Silverman (1993) summarises some of these different approaches commonly adopted in research. These are set out below (**Table 2**) with the differences contrasted between quantitative compared to qualitative.

Methodology		
Approach	*Quantitative research*	*Qualitative research*
Observation	Preliminary work e.g. prior to designing questionnaire	Fundamental to understanding another culture
Textual analysis	Content analysis - counting in terms of researchers' categories	Understanding participants' categories
Interviews	'Survey': mainly fixed choice questions to random samples	'Open ended' questions to small numbers of participants (in-depth interviews)
Transcripts	Used infrequently to check accuracy of records	Used to understand how participants organise their talk / think about their experiences

Source: adapted from Silverman, 1993.

Table 2. Different uses for four research approaches

5. Some of main qualitative methods used in psychology

5.1 Introduction

Rigorous research methodologies form a necessary foundation in evidence-based research. Until recently such a statement has been read as referring solely to quantitative methodologies such as in the double blind randomised controlled trial (RCT) encountered in healthcare research. Quantitative methods were designed for specific purposes and were never intended to take researchers to the heart of patients' lived experiences. The experimental, quantitative research methods, such as the RCT, focus on matters involved in the development of clinical drug trials and assessing treatment outcomes, survival rates, improvements in healthcare and clinical governance and audit.

Qualitative paradigms, on the other hand, offer the researcher an opportunity to develop an idiographic understanding of participants' experiences and what it means to them, within their social reality, to be in a particular situation (Bryman, 1992). Qualitative research has a role in facilitating our understanding of some of the complexity of bio-psycho-social phenomena and thus offers exciting possibilities for psychology in the future. Qualitative research is developing therefore new ways of thinking and revisions to the more established methods are constantly being introduced and debated by researchers across the world. These methods include: Content / thematic analysis (CA/ TA); Grounded Theory in psychology (GT); Discursive psychology / Discourse analysis (DA); Narrative psychology (NA); Phenomenological psychology methods such as interpretative phenomenological analysis (IPA).

5.2 Content Analysis and Thematic Analysis

Content Analysis, or Thematic Analysis (the terms are frequently used interchangeably and generally mean much the same), is particularly useful for conceptual, or thematic, analysis or relational analysis. It can quantify the occurrences of concepts selected for examination (Wilkinson & Birmingham, 2003). CA or TA, has become rather a 'catch-all term' (Boyle, 1994), but this approach is useful when the researcher wishes to summarise and categorise themes encountered in data collection. These can include: summaries of people's comments from questionnaires, documents such as diaries, historical journals, video and film footage, or other material: the list is not exhaustive. The approach is also useful in guiding the development of an interview schedule. However, this method provides - *summaries* of frequency of the content. The method may therefore be considered too limited where an in-depth approach is required.

Interview data need methods of analysis capable of providing the researcher with greater insight into participants' views, the psychological and phenomenological background to participants' stories and their narrated experiences and feelings. Other qualitative methods are explored for utility of purpose here. One such method, originally developed from sociological research is Grounded Theory (GT).

5.3 Grounded Theory

Grounded Theory (GT) is frequently considered to offer researchers a suitable qualitative method for in-depth exploratory investigations (Charmaz, 1995; Strauss & Corbin, 1990; Willig, 2008). It is a rigorous approach which provides the researcher with a set of systematic strategies (Charmaz, 1995). While this method shares some features with phenomenology, (see below), GT assumes that the analysis will generate one over-arching and encompassing theory. GT was, in its original version, designed to investigate social processes from the bottom up, or the "*emergence* of theory from data" (Willig, 2008, pp. 44). GT methods developed from the collaboration of sociologists Glazer and Strauss during the 1960s and 1970s (e.g. Glaser & Strauss, 1967). It is a set of strategies that has been of immense use in sociological research as an aid to developing wider social theory (hence its name). As Willig observes, GT can be an attractive method for psychologists who have trained in quantitative methods since the building blocks, identified using the GT approach, aim to generate categories from the data collected, thus moving from data to theory (Willig, 2008, pp. 34 onward). Its originators, Glaser and Strauss (1967), considered the separation of theory from research as being a rather arbitrary division. They set about devising an approach whereby the data collection stage may be blurred or merged with the development of theory in an attempt to break down the more rigid boundaries between the usual data collection and data analysis stages. GT approaches data by blurring these different stages and levels of abstraction. A GT analysis may proceed by checking and refining the data analysis by collecting more data until 'data saturation' can be achieved (Charmaz, 1996). However, for many psychological investigations, it may be obvious at an early stage that, due to the complexity of people's lived experiences, participants' narratives about their lives, feelings and/ or emotions, may not always be best served by adopting GT as a method (i.e. generation of one main theory).

Carla Willig (2008), for example, observes that GT, as a methodology for psychological research, may not offer psychologists a particularly reflexive approach. She considers it sometimes has a limited applicability, proposing that, "It could be argued that research questions about the nature of experience are more suitably addressed using phenomenological research methods." (Willig, 2008, pp. 47). In all fairness, GT was originally developed for researching from a sociological perspective and, while there is some commonality between sociology and social psychology, the use of GT to analyse data might not always provide a sufficiently robust and flexible way of capturing psychological nuances and complexities contained in participants' narratives about lived experiences. GT, as a methodology, was therefore adopted and adapted by some qualitative psychologists (Pidgeon & Henwood, 1997). Willig concludes that GT can be "reserved for the study of social psychological processes" as a descriptive method (Willig, 2008, pp. 47).A further challenge, when considering using GT, is the challenge provided by the different types of GT that have developed within the field such as the debate on the two main 'schools' of GT: Straussian and Glaserian (see Stern, 1994, pp. 213 on for discussion).

5.4 Discursive psychology and Discourse Analysis

As its name suggests, Discourse Analysis (DA) is primarily concerned with the nuances of conversation (Potter, 1996). The term 'discourse' can cover anything related to our use of language whether a single utterance or moment of speech (speech fragment) through to a conversation between two people, or the delivery of a political speech. It may refer to how language may be systematically ordered as in language 'rules' or different conventions such as medical jargon or legal terminology (Tonkiss, 2012, pp. 406). The 'turn to language' in researching society and in the discursive psychology field has been inspired by theories emerging from other disciplines and consideration of speech use as both communication and performance (Seale, 2012). As Willig observes (2008, pp. 95) DA is more than a methodology, since social scientists have become interested both in how we use language in communication and also how we 'socially construct' our environment and lived experience by the use of language (see, for example, Bruner, 1986, 1991; Gergen, 2001). It has become more of a critique of how we describe the world and the nuances of the discourse and language we use. Discursive psychology highlights how 'knowledge' is socially constructed and reported for example in "existing institutional practices that may be considered unjust." (Holt, 2011, pp. 66). Where some psychologists may wish to explore conversation by exploring the finer nuances of conversation such as the length of a pause, the terms of speech people use, or other variations of discourse, then DA can be a very useful method (Potter & Wetherell, 1987; Willig, 2008, pp. 96-106).

The discursive approach looks to verbal behaviour as a more direct means of uncovering underlying cognitions (Harré,1995) rather than assigning a numerical value 'score' or scale to a behaviour. This approach takes the view that interpretation and empathy are involved in attempting to understand human behaviour. Self-report, from people being studied, can then become a valuable resource in its own right:

> "Thus the experimenter or observer has to enter into a discourse with the people being studied and try to appreciate the shape of the subject's cognitive world. But at this point it no longer makes sense to talk of observers and subjects at all. They are only coparticipants in the project of making sense of the world and our experience of it."
>
> (Harré & Gillett, 1994, pp. 21)

This approach to studying human behaviour uses words, contained in language, as symbols with meaning, where the 'subject' i.e. the person, is seen as discursive in order that they may make sense of their environment by signifying "the order of things" (Foucault, quoted by Harré & Gillett, 1994, pp. 26).

The discursive view sees people as active agents within their own lives and, as such, cannot, "be defined in isolation from a context and whose mental processes can be unravelled by objective measurement and description." (Harré & Gillett, 1994, pp. 26).

However, when considering the selection of a qualitative method, and thinking about using discourse analysis, we need to be clear about what our research aims and objectives are. Participants' narratives frequently include elements relating to feelings and emotions rather than how reality is manufactured and portrayed in conversation. Willig suggests that discourse analysis can be used to explore "the internal organisation of the discourse itself and ask 'what is this discourse doing?'" (Willig, 2008, pp. 99). Here is a prime distinction between DA and other psychological qualitative methods such as IPA, in that DA explores the *role* of language in participants' descriptions of events and conversations while the phenomenological approach examines how people *ascribe meaning* to their experiences in their interactions with their environment (Biggerstaff & Thompson, 2008; Pringle et al., 2011; Shinebourne, 2011; Smith et al., 2009; Smith et al., 1999).

5.5 Narrative analysis

Linked to discourse, we now turn to consider briefly narrative in psychology and the rise of narrative analysis. Narrative in both psychology and medicine has much in common with studying narrative as a more general linguistic form (Bruner, 2002; Greenhalgh& Hurwitz, 1999; Polkinghorne, 1988; Webster, 1996). Indeed, some of the earliest thinkers in the field of psychology used methods we more usually associate with narrative to describe our experiences of encountering and engaging with the world. One of the foremost psychological thinkers of the late nineteenth century, Brentano, in his foreword to his 1874 text, *Psychology from an empirical standpoint,* states, "My psychological standpoint is empirical: experience alone is my teacher." (Brentano, cited in Moran & Mooney, 2002, pp. 32).

A narrative approach entails examining people's use of stories, accounts of events etc. and also of listening to these stories (Sarbin, 1986). The related discipline of 'narratology' has developed from the disciplines of linguistics and literary criticism where narratives are treated as a search for meaning in the lived experience of people (Bruner, 2002; Holloway & Freshwater, 2007). This search for meaning has much in common with phenomenological methods of enquiry and the search for meaning or significance as we strive to make sense of our lives and our 'being in the world' (Brockmeier, 2009). He observes,

> "[…]the *quest* for meaning: the meaning, or significance, that we give to our lives, to our being in the world. This question arises again and again in the life of each individual in a particular, in fact, unique, way, and it hence requires a patient and ongoing examination of the multifarious forms and practices in which individuals make sense of their lives. One might think of the river in which you never step twice."
>
> (Brockmeier, 2009, pp. 217).

Using psychology of narrative, for example, the researcher may examine people's life stories or their accounts of such experiences (Esin, 2011). It explores the biographical lives of participants' lives or social and cultural stories (Goodley, 2011). Psychology of narrative can be helpful to explore and interpret findings from such research, since this type of enquiry helps the researcher to enter more fully into understanding people's lives and their experiences (Crossley, 2000; Greenhalgh & Hurwitz, 1999 & 1998; Murray, 2008 & 1995). Esin defines essential features of narrative as connections between events that help make these events meaningful for the audience, stating that "Sequence is necessary for narrative. A narrative always responds to the question 'And then what happened?'" (Esin, 2011, pp. 93).

Narrative in psychology can provide an important method for exploring psychological development, self-understanding and people's inter-relationship with their world (Gergen, 2001b). Examining human experiences and 'making sense' of our environment offers a core method of enquiry across many disciplines and cultures (Brockmeier, 2009; Brown et al., 1996; Bruner, 1999; Bruner, 2002; Charon, 2005; Harré, 2003; Murray, 2008; Riessman, 2008).

The use of narrative methods in both psychology and medicine, assumes a narrator and a listener. Narrative is an interactive transaction with the potential for narrator and listener to assign their own meanings to their experiences as the topic under discussion unfolds (Bruner, 1991; 1990). Bruner for example, proposes that the interpretation of people's actions and their narratives about what happens to them provides us with explanations of those experiences. Such interpretation "is concerned with 'reasons' for things happening, rather than strictly with their 'causes' " (Bruner, 1991).

5.6 Phenomenological psychology

When we want to learn how we can best explore participants' lived experiences, a different approach can be helpful, that of phenomenology. The aim of the phenomenological psychologist is to help make implicit 'taken-for-granted' elements of our lives explicit (Giorgi, 1995, pp. 33). Phenomenological research has developed from the philosophy of the European phenomenological 'school' of philosophy, the most prominent proponents of which are Edmund Husserl, Martin Heidegger and Maurice Merleau-Ponty. More recently, some phenomenological researchers have been influenced by what has become known as the Duquesne school, which includes Giorgi, Van Kaam and others. The group acquired this title because some of the founders to this approach either worked in, or had links with, Duquesne University in the United States. The Dutch school of phenomenology, which includes authors such as Langeveld, is known as the 'Utrecht school' (see Cohen & Omery, 1994, pp.138 onward, for further discussion regarding different phenomenological schools). This is by no means a complete list: there are many other phenomenological researchers in psychology such as Scott Churchill (USA), Karin Dahlberg (Sweden), and Les Todres (UK). Over the past decade in the UK, Jonathan Smith has led the development of a phenomenological method specific to psychology, that of interpretative phenomenological analysis (IPA). Smith developed this method from his work exploring people's lived experiences based on European phenomenological philosophers such as Husserl. His original development of the IPA method was based on the detailed interpretive analysis of in-depth interviews (Smith & Osborn, 2008; Smith et al., 1999)[7]. When we wish to explore the 'being-in-the-world' psychology of

[7] The IPA website and research forum may be found at: www.ipa.bbk.ac.uk

experience, the idiographic case-study approach proposed by methods such as IPA can be especially helpful (Smith et al., 2009). IPA was specifically developed by Jonathan Smith (Smith et al., 1995) to rigorously explore idiographic, subjective experiences and, specifically, social cognitions. It is now widely used within British psychology (e.g. Clare, 2003; Duncan et al., 2001; French et al., 2005; Smith, 2011; Thompson et al. 2002).

Phenomenology in psychology places the experience of the self at the centre of the current psychological dialogue about people's lived experiences and their meanings (Cohen & Omery, 1994; Giorgi, 1995; Giorgi & Giorgi, 2008; Langdridge, 2007; Smith et al., 1995; Spinelli, 2005). The qualitative psychologist is aiming to see and understand what surrounds us (Cohen & Omery, 1994). When exploring the 'taken for granted' - the everyday lives of participants, especially those aspects relating to the psychology of how people feel about an issue, event, or experience for example - the use of a phenomenological approach highlights such issues and brings them to the fore. This might be useful for example, when considering the background of health service delivery (Oakley, 1993, pp. 235).

IPA's theoretical basis stems from the phenomenology originating with Husserl's attempts to construct a philosophical science of consciousness, with hermeneutics (the theory of interpretation), and symbolic interactionism. This last proposes that meanings an individual may ascribe to an event are of central concern, but that access to such meaning can only be obtained through an interpretative process. IPA acknowledges that the researcher's engagement with the participant's 'text' has an interpretative element, in contrast to some other methods (e.g., discourse analysis, DA; see Potter, 1996). IPA assumes an epistemological stance whereby, through its careful and explicit interpretative methodology, it becomes possible to access the meanings an individual gives to their feelings and their cognitive inner world. IPA also draws on Gadamer's philosophy of hermeneutics and the study of the understanding of the text (Smith, 2007).

Attention is drawn however to one of the main differences between IPA and Discourse Analysis (DA): DA aims to examine the *role* of language in describing a person's experience, whereas IPA intends to explore how people may ascribe *meaning* to their experiences when interacting with their environment (Smith et al., 1999). It is thus especially suited to behavioural and psychological studies that relate findings to the bio-psycho-social theories informing discourse among healthcare professions (Smith, 1996; Smith, 2004; Willig, 2008). IPA is a qualitative methodology with a clearly set out methodology that is both rigorous and yet sufficiently flexible fit for a wide range of types of study (Biggerstaff & Thompson, 2008; Brocki & Wearden, 2006; Smith & Osborn, 2008; Willig, 2008). It is important to note that IPA is only one version of phenomenological research methodologies (Willig, 2008) and other phenomenological approaches are also useful to the qualitative researcher (Giorgi, 1995). As van Manen observes

> "the simple phenomenological precept (is) to always try to understand someone from his or her situation. [....]
>
> The phenomenological approach asks of us that we constantly measure our understandings and insights against the lived reality of our concrete experiences, which, of course, are always more complex than any particular interpretation can portray"
>
> (van Manen, 1998, pp. 8,pp. 10)

Phenomenological methods have some elements in common with Grounded Theory, discussed above, in that the theoretical framework may be uncovered during the research analysis - i.e. theory emerges and informs the data analysis in a cyclical, or iterative, fashion (Strauss & Corbin, 1990). As with GT, the aim of the IPA researcher is to uncover, develop and verify data as it emerges. This is achieved by a careful and systematic process which uncovers themes and connections in an orderly sequence. The overall aim of adopting a phenomenological approach is to explore the world of 'lived experience.'[8] The difference in IPA and Grounded Theory may be summarised by suggesting that IPA reflects the diversity of experience rather than a more condensed single theoretical viewpoint, or core category, an approach usually arrived at through the use of Grounded Theory (Chamberlain, 1999).

IPA is still evolving as researchers use and debate the method. It does, however, have the advantage of being especially developed by practising psychologists and is therefore an obvious candidate in current psychological qualitative analytical methodology. It is increasingly found to be an accessible approach and a method which is idiographic, inductive and interrogative (Smith, 2004) and aims to provide insight into the heart of participants' lived experiences (Biggerstaff &Thompson, 2008; Pringle et al., 2010).

6. Emergent qualitative methods

The rise of technology and digital photography and use of the internet and video editing tools, have enabled researchers to consider the potential of these newer, and potentially rich, resources of data from film, video and DVD. Newer, emergent, qualitative methodologies especially in technology and visual research methods, can prove attractive and useful to researchers. Accessing information resources online can provide today's psychology researcher with rich data and fruitful new areas to explore. Examining resources such as diaries or personal eye-witness accounts can also provide the researcher with data. Again, these become easier to access if they have been uploaded as a research resource online, although with any such repository it is advisable to seek permission to use before beginning a research project since such data may raise copyright issues.

Using qualitative data analysis of video interviews recording people's experiences of health and illness, in the UK, for example, has led to a unique website resource for health research 'DIPex' (Ziebland & McPherson, 2006). Increasingly, psychologists are looking to use the internet and online platforms for their research. The internet offers the possibilities of online interviews, discussion forum analysis, or what people may have written online e.g. in blogs. The *Healthtalk online* project (www.healthtalkonline.org) arising from the DIPex project, is a rich resource for people who can view video clips and transcript excerpts from patients discussing their experiences and feelings about their illnesses, how they cope with their condition, their fears and anxieties, how they fought back and similar narratives. Commentaries from clinicians providing information about the illnesses being discussed are also available on the website. Additional sources of advice and resources are offered providing a solid platform supporting patients, their families and loved ones during their illnesses.

---

[8] From the concept of the Life-world or *Lebenswelt*, from Husserl's unpublished works after his death (see for example Ashworth, 2008: 10 - 12; Philipse, 1995: 277; Cohen and Omery, 1994: 139, for further discussion).

7. Ethics of researching online

When researching into online discussion forums and chat rooms etc., the researcher needs to remain mindful of possible ethical issues. The majority of comments posted by people online, for instance, may originally have been written and uploaded to a website for a different purpose. Contributors may have intended their internet 'posts' to be private, or at least their personal views and opinions were written to share with like-minded people, perhaps going through similar experiences or coping with similar situations. People may not be happy to agree to their original postings on a website being analysed by researchers and used for a different purpose. Such concerns should be considered on a case by case basis.

New ways of researching are being developed as research teams debate these issues and explore these resources (Willig, 2008). Standard ethical practices may need adapting to account for the internet age. However, where material is in the open domain, it may be easier for researchers to make a case justifying its use as source material. This would still need to be checked out with your university or health services research ethics committee (e.g. NHS National Research Ethics Service NRES in UK) and appropriate professional codes of practice. For UK psychologist researchers and students, for example, this would be research governance codes of the relevant university or institution and the British Psychological Society, possibly in conjunction with the NHS , if patients were involved. This is especially pertinent since it is not usually possible to contact patients to obtain informed consent from such resources later (and any such consent would be retrospective and difficult to obtain). Such ethical issues are being addressed today by research bodies. The Association of Internet Researchers, for example, has developed ethics guidelines for researchers[9]. The British Psychological Society provides an ethical code of conduct and research guidance to working online[10]. This emphasises the need for qualitative psychology researchers to be able to assess both the context and aims of their proposed research when selecting their methodology and to be aware of the need for vigilance in keeping abreast for new guidance on these issues as it is released.

Similar criteria may be used for both selecting an appropriate qualitative method and in the critical appraisal of published qualitative research in order to establish a systematic and thorough approach to appraising the evidence from qualitative research papers.

8. Evaluating qualitative psychology research: Some suggested criteria

In this final section of the chapter I set out some suggestions to help readers evaluate qualitative research. I have drawn from several sources but particularly acknowledge the contribution of Mays and Pope (2000), Mays et al., (2007), who have written extensively on this issue in health research and Uwe Flick, Lucy Yardley and Jonathan Smith who consider the importance of quality and validity when evaluating qualitative research in psychology (Flick, 2007; Smith, 2011; Yardley, 2008) .

8.1 General features

In general, as with reviewing a quantitative research paper, we need to ask what the paper contributes to knowledge of the research area. Does the study have something new to say

[9] Association of Internet Researchers http://aoir.org/documents/ethics-guide /

[10] See British Psychological Society www.bps.org.uk/webethic

about the topic for instance? Alternatively, perhaps the researchers have explored the chosen topic from a different angle, or incorporated different viewpoints from their participant sample. As identified earlier in this chapter, people are seen as an important resource for collaboration, thus highlighting the need for qualitative research to acknowledge reflexivity and subjectivity (Sixsmith & Daniels, 2011, pp. 26 - 7). An example of this type of approach might be where the research examines the views of a minority whose opinions have not previously been sought. In turn, such a paper would then pave the way for further research.

Next we need to think about the method(s) the researchers have used for their study. Does it seem appropriate? Does the study design lend itself to using a qualitative approach? In examining the reasons for conducting any such study, we need to bear in mind questions such as: does the research team situate their reasons for carrying out their work within an appropriate body of research literature?

Alternatively, the approach used may incorporate theoretical interest. Perhaps the research topic is approached in a different way, or from a different and newer theoretical context? Again, this needs to be clear to the reader with appropriate support from the theoretical literature. Does the research reported contribute to the development of knowledge in the direction of theory?

8.2 Outline of methods used

As with quantitative research appraisal, we need to evaluate researchers' sampling methods. A clear rationale for how participants were approached and selected for inclusion in the study should be clearly set out and a clear rationale should be stated for this sample. Do the researchers use a purposive sample? Have they used 'snowballing', that is following up introductions to potential other participants from volunteers in the study? This is a useful approach for accessing 'hard-to-reach' groups of people in society. Have the researchers continued interviewing participants until data saturation is reached (i.e. when no new themes emerge from their analysis)? What do they decide to do about *disconformatory cases*, (i.e. where a participant's viewpoint and emergent themes may differ from other participants)? This is acceptable in qualitative research, indeed understandable, since sample sizes are usually smaller than in a quantitative study.

Whatever the research team have done, their approach needs to be set out clearly. As in quantitative research, the research method and approach must be capable of replication by other researchers so detail is important. Demographics such as numbers of participants, gender, age group, descriptive vignettes with pseudonyms, if used, etc. should also be clearly stated.

The ethical principles of informed consent should be set out clearly. For example, how was consent obtained and was it recorded on paper? A clear explanation for the choice of data collection and method used is needed. It is important that the research team provide reflexive discussion about how they handled the researcher - situation interface: for example, issues encountered during data collection, what they decided to do about any group dynamics, such as may occur during focus group research for example (Ali & Kelly, 2012; Burman & Whelan, 2011).

The paper should clearly state how data were collected and managed. This includes information about areas such as data collection and storage: how was the transcription of recorded interviews handled, how are data stored, and for how long does the research team plan to store their data? Exact details are usually governed by local or national research data governance but these details must be considered. Research governance details are particularly important in qualitative research since a person's audio interview is more likely to be unique to that individual compared to a briefer set of responses contained from a questionnaire for example. While researchers generally are able to offer anonymity, such as using pseudonyms, it can be harder for the qualitative researcher to offer total confidentiality since a person's narrative about an experience may be unique to them, thus offering more likelihood for possible identification. If this is the case, then the researcher must inform the reader what steps they have taken to protect their participants – perhaps by changing identifying features or details of that particular participant's situation (Frith, 2007, pp. 126).

How data are recorded is also important. The use of field notes is recommended, and can prove invaluable as an *aide-memoire,* they also provide 'back-up' insurance should there be recording failure. However, data verification is also very important. I strongly recommend all interview and focus group data be recorded, whether using audio or video, in order to obtain the highest quality 'raw data' prior to analysis.

8.3 Data analysis

When undertaking critical appraisal, the researchers need to provide a clear description of the framework they used for data analysis. Whatever method is used for analysis, and, as we have seen, a wide choice of possible qualitative research methods are available, the method adopted should be stated with clarity and be capable of replication by another researcher. Whatever research method is selected, this must be clearly stated and set out in a way that is capable of replication. Research methods should be referenced by the authors in the literature. However, if no pre-existing framework exists, then the authors should be very explicit about the approach they have adopted. Their reasons for this development must be justified by providing appropriate support from relevant literature (this may happen if a researcher is developing a new methodology for instance). For a clear audit trail, these processes and procedures should be clearly described.

What categories were used for analysis? How did the researchers decide on these categories? These areas need adequate discussion. For instance, if there are references to raw data sources, did the researchers use more than one data source? How did the researchers identify their themes and data categories? Are issues of data verification, such as asking an expert colleague to check thematic categories, considered? Do the researchers report how they decided on the categories? Adequate discussion is necessary since such themes provide the main results from which conclusions are drawn. This point leads on to findings and discussion.

8.4 Findings and discussion

When reading findings and conclusions it is important to consider carefully how the confirmation of findings was handled: were any *reliability checks* used by researchers? If there are excerpts from data transcripts (usual in qualitative papers) then what do these excerpts tell us about the research results (Frith, 2007, pp. 124-5). Are any quotations used to highlight findings? It is helpful if the paper states whether the excerpts are illustrative, or provide contrasting viewpoints by participants. It is also helpful to ask oneself whether the researchers comment if they consider their findings are transferable from one context to another and, should that be the case, what particular elements do they highlight as being most important or relevant?

When we consider these results and themes as a whole, do we find the researchers' conclusions useful and applicable? Do the conclusions drawn seem reasonable and appropriate, given what we know about the background and stated aims for the study? Does the paper state if excerpts provided are illustrative or, have the researchers provided the reader with contrasting viewpoints?

Another area to examine is that of 'credibility checks'. Sometimes researchers may feedback their proposed analysis to individual participants and ask for comments. Not all methods adopt this approach. However, if this has been carried out by the research team, is the process clear to the reader?

Sometimes there may be an alternative explanation or thematic summary to a particular perspective. This needs to be considered and discussed by the research team. Do the researchers adopt a reflexive approach? If so, do they state how they handled these reflections and how these relate to their reported findings? As discussed earlier (section 3.1). reflexivity is important in qualitative research since researchers need "to be aware of their own positions and interests and to explicitly situate themselves within the research."(Finlay, 2003, pp. 5). From the perspective of the critical reader, it is helpful to stand back from the results and ask oneself if the researchers' results and conclusions drawn are credible and appropriate in relation to the original research question. Other areas which need to be considered include whether these results relate back to the research literature and theoretical background reported in the authors' original literature review and research aims.

Finally, the reviewer needs to consider whether the researchers discuss whether their findings are transferable from one context to another. Are the results and conclusions useful and applicable?

9. Balancing the strengths and weaknesses of qualitative research in psychology

One of the main strengths of the qualitative approach, and thus its attractiveness to psychologists, is that it allows the researcher to explore the meanings people give to their experiences. These approaches can help provide us with more insightful information and quality data on how people think about their world, their lived-world experiences. It provides the researcher with an open-ended approach and one where the participant takes the lead in data collection (the researcher usually remains responsible for data analysis and interpretation). The usual use of a smaller sample size also enables that this detailed, richness of data, can be finely nuanced and in-depth.

Furthermore, the researcher is able to utilise complementary data sources. There are opportunities for the researcher to incorporate multiple methods in order to obtain richer data, or what is sometimes known as thick description (for instance in ethnographic methods). As David Walsh observes, the researcher, "then finds a whole web of cultural structures, knowledge and meanings which are knotted and superimposed on one another and which constitute a densely layered **cultural script**"

(Walsh, 2012, pp. 247, original author's emphasis)

Data sources in qualitative research include interviews, focus groups, observation techniques, analysis of text, such as historic diaries and journals, film, video or art work. Validity can be confirmed with research participants. Finally, qualitative research does not pretend to be other than it is: it is situation specific

Of course, some of these features also have their counterpart. For example the issue of data being context specific means that it is not always generalisable to a different context. This should be borne in mind when considering qualitative approaches. The researcher is not separate from the research process but instead can be seen as part of the process. This may have an impact on the research and the data collected and the researcher usually acknowledges her role in the research process (Willig, 2008).

Although the smaller size of qualitative data sets and the eventual findings may limit generalisable applicability, nevertheless such findings may reflect and inform what is happening within a larger population. This can then be examined further. The idiographic approach that forms a major trend in qualitative research does however take account of individuals, their values, and their experiences in a way that places people at the centre of the field of study.

To summarise, **Table 3** provides a brief check-list for the appraisal of qualitative psychology research papers. When assessing a paper for quality the reader may wish to consider the following points adapted from the British Psychological Society guidelines for authors and reviewers. These guidelines are available online:http://www.bps.org.uk

Checklist for evaluating qualitative psychology research
How does this work contribute to our knowledge of this area? Does it enhance or develop knowledge? Do the researchers provide the reader with a different perspective on research findings in the field?
Are the research findings of worth or relevance?
Is there evidence of a clear research question to the reader?
Have the researchers used an appropriate design for the research question and theoretical approach?
Are we provided with sufficient information to relate the findings reported here to another setting? (Context)
Are there a good range of possible cases or settings used for this study? (Sampling)
Considering data collection and analysis. Have the researchers used a systematic approach?
Does the paper specifically address issues relating to sound audit processes? Are such processes reported clearly. Is informed consent reported?
Is the reported account sufficiently reflexive? How do the authors incorporate this in their research?

Source: acknowledgement to The British Psychological Society. See www.bps.org.uk

Table 3. Checklist for evaluating qualitative research in psychology

10. Use of the internet and computer software in qualitative analysis

Computer software (e.g. NUD*ST, NVIVO, Atlas-ti, and information technology such as the behavioural coding and analysis software programmes provided by Noldus) has been available for qualitative analysis, in one form or another, for some time now. Programmes are now very sophisticated. Today software programmes can store transcripts of interviews, upload video files and act as thematic notebooks for researchers to store and share work with colleagues. As with any statistical software, it takes time for researchers to learn the programme in addition to learning how to conduct a qualitative analysis. Where a computer programme has been used, look for evidence that shows how the researchers conducted the analysis and how they used the computer programme to arrive at their results (but remember the adage GIGO : garbage in, garbage out). Computer programmes can be useful to help researchers store, share and sort their data.While they may not yet be a substitute for rigorous analysis, they can be a helpful tool for the qualitative researcher to think about, categorise, and sift through the large volume of data generated by qualitative research methods.

Additionally, today there are many rich e-resources available to qualitative researchers via the internet such as the Vision 2 Lead (V2L) website for "e-learning, e-community and e-leadership" with its "12 questions for qualitative e-researchers for 2012" (see http://blog.vision2lead.com/e-interviews-2/12-e-research-ideas-for-2012/) and international e-journals for qualitative research such as *The Weekly Qualitative Report* and *The Qualitative Report,* a peer-reviewed open access journal for qualitative researchers originating from Nova South eastern University, Florida, US.[11] E-communities such as these and the Sage publishing house's online community *Methodspace* across the UK, US and Europe, help develop a truly international research community of qualitative researchers, thus enhancing debate and encouraging new research networks for developing qualitative methods.

11. Summary and conclusions

Qualitative research methods have much to offer psychological research. As with any research approach, there are strengths and weaknesses. These should be carefully and systematically weighed up and assessed by the researcher before any firm decision is made. The methodology selected needs to be fitted to the aims and objectives of the research proposed.

The exploration, interpretation and our understanding of data is a skill that the qualitative researcher can develop to uncover new ways of viewing the world. A qualitative approach can provide arich source of data. It is frequently an in-depth process, therefore sample sizes tend to be smaller than numbers usually seen in quantitative research. As Carla Willig observes, the exploration of qualitative research methods is an exciting 'adventure' of discovery (Willig, 2008). It is an approach I recommend to any reader thinking about embarking on their own research voyage. Qualitative psychology research helps uncover aspects of life which may not have been explored in much detail. This in-depth approach can help us understand experiences of the lived-world, and participants' behaviours, feelings and emotions.

[11] The Qualitative Report and Weekly Qualitative Report http://www.nova.edu/ssss/QR/index.html

In conclusion, therefore, rigorous methodologies in qualitative psychology are now recognised as being an essential component for evidence-based research whether for quantitative or qualitative research (Biggerstaff & Thompson, 2008). This is especially important when exploring people's behaviours, their experiences of their interactions with, and engagement in, their world and organisations. Many areas of psychology, in particular social, organisational, and health psychology have embraced qualitative psychology methods in order to gain a better understanding of how behaviours relate to people's experiences, e.g. their response to treatment (see, for example, Mays & Pope, 2000, 1995; Murphy & Dingwall, 2001; Murphy et al., 1998).

In the past, there has been a great deal of debate in the discipline of psychology, as in other areas of social sciences, surrounding the relative merits of qualitative and quantitative approaches with much discussion on issues such as 'quality' and ensuring 'rigour' in qualitative research. However, there is now a growing acceptance and recognition that we gain greater understanding of participants' psychological experiences of their lived-experiences by including qualitative methods, and the issue of validity has become recognised (Yardley, 2008). These have challenged quantitative exclusivity in the field of psychology. Qualitative psychology has established itself in research methods for psychology postgraduate training and UK undergraduate psychology degree courses now include it as a core element in the curriculum. Today, to ignore qualitative research in examining psychological experiences would be akin to 'throwing the baby out with the bath water'. As we have seen in this chapter, searching the main research databases produced a large volume of qualitative research literature and qualitative methodologies can help provide rich answers to our questions. As ever, the skill lies in asking the right questions and selecting the most appropriate methods to answer our inquiry.

12. References

Allport, G. W. (1946. Personalistic psychology as science: a reply. *Psychological Review*, 53: 132-135,

Ali, S. & Kelly, M. (2012). Ethics and social research. In C. Searle (Ed.) *Researching society and culture 3rd edition*. London: Sage.

Ashworth, P. (2008). Conceptual foundations of qualitative psychology. In J. A. Smith (Ed.). *Qualitative psychology: A practical guide to research methods.* London. Sage Publications.

Banister, P., Dunn, G., Burman, E., Daniels, J., Duckett, P., Goodley, D., Lawthom, R., Parker, I., Runswick-Cole, K., Sixsmith, J., Smailes, S., Tindall, C. & Whelan, P. (2011). *Qualitative methods in psychology: A research guide. 2nd edition.* Maidenhead: Open University Press/ McGraw Hill.

Biggerstaff, D. L. & Thompson, A. R. (2008). Interpretative phenomenological analysis (IPA): A qualitative methodology of choice in healthcare research. *Qualitative Research in Psychology*, 5: 214 - 224.

Bloor, M. (1997). Techniques of Validation in Qualitative Research: a Critical Commentary. In G. Miller & R. Dingwall (Eds.) *Context and Method in Qualitative Research.* London: Sage Publications.

Bowling, A. (2009) *Research methods in health: investigating health and health services* (3rded.) Maidenhead: Open University Press.

Boyle, J. S. (1994). Styles of ethnography.In J. M. Morse (Ed.).*Critical issues in qualitative research methods.* Thousand Oaks: Sage.

Bryman, A. (1992) Quantitative and qualitative research: further reflections on their integration. In J. Brannen, (Ed.) *Mixing Methods: qualitative and quantitative research.* Aldershot: Ashgate.

Brentano, F., C., von (2002/ 1874) Psychology from an Empirical Standpoint: Foreword from the 1874 edition and The Distinction between Mental and Physical Phenomena. In D. Moran & T. Mooney (Eds.) *The phenomenology reader.* London: Routledge.

British Psychological Society. (2010). *Accrediation through partnership handbook: guidance for undergraduate and conversion psychology* programmes. Leicester: British Psychological Society.

Brocki, J. M., & Wearden, A. J. (2004). A critical evaluation of the use of interpretative phenomenological analysis (IPA) in health psychology. *Psychology and Health,* 21 (1): 87- 108.

Bruner, J. (1986). *Actual minds, possible worlds.* Cambridge, MA: Harvard University Press.

Bruner, J. (1990). *Acts of Meaning.* Cambridge, MA: Harvard University Press.

Bruner, J. (1991). The narrative construction of reality.*Critical Inquiry,*18: 1- 21.

Bruner, J. (1999). Narratives of ageing.*Journal of Ageing Studies,* 13 (1): 7 – 9.

Bruner, J. (2002). *Making Stories: Law, Literature, Life.* New York: Farrar, Strauss & Giroux.

Burman, E. & Whelan, P. (2011). Problems in / of qualitative research. In P. Banister, G. Dunn, E. Burman, et al.(Eds.) *Qualitative methods in psychology: A research guide. 2nd edition.* Maidenhead: Open University Press/ McGraw Hill.

Carey, M. A. (1994). The group effect in focus groups: planning, implementing, and interpreting focus group research. In J. M. Morse (Ed.) *Critical issues in qualitative research methods.* Thousand Oaks: Sage

Centre for Evidence-Based Medicine (2012). Solutions for Public Health, National Health Services. In collaboration with University of Oxford. CEBM http://www.sph.nhs.uk/what-we-do/public-health-workforce/resources/critical-appraisals-skills-programme (Accessed 26th March, 2012)

Charmaz, K. (1983). Loss of self: a fundamental form of suffering in the chronically ill. *Sociology of Health and Illness,* 5 (2): 168 – 195.

Charmaz, K. (1995). Grounded theory. In J. A. Smith, R. Harré, & L. Van Langenhove, (Eds.) *Rethinking methods in psychology.* London: Sage

Clare, L. (2003). Managing threats to self: awareness in early stage Alzheimer's disease. *Social Science and Medicine,* 57: 1017 – 1029.

Cohen, M. Z. & Omery, A. (1994) Schools of phenomenology: implications for research. In J. M. Morse (Ed.) *Critical issues in qualitative research methods.* Thousand Oaks: Sage.

Cowman, S. (1993). Triangulation: a means of reconciliation in nursing research. *Journal of Advanced Nursing,* 18: 788-792.

Creswell, J. W. & Clark, P. V., L. (2007).*Designing and conducting mixed methods research.* Thousand Oaks: Sage.

Critical Appraisal Skills Programme (CASP). (2012). http://www.casp-uk.net/ (Accessed 26th March, 2012)

Crossley. M. L. (2000). *Introducing Narrative Psychology: Self, trauma and the construction of meaning.* Buckingham: Open University Press.

Denzin, N.K. & Lincoln, Y.S. (Eds.) (1994 / 2000).*Handbook of qualitative research.* London: Sage Publications.

Denzin, N., K. & Lincoln, Y. S. (Eds.) (2008). *The landscape of qualitative research.* London: Sage

Dixon-Wood, M., & Fitzpatrick, R. (2001) Qualitative research in systematic reviews: has established a place for itself. *British Medical Journal,* 323: 765- 766.

Duncan, B., Hart, G., Scoular, A. & Brigg, A. (2001). Qualitative analysis of psychosocial impact of diagnosis of Chlamydia trachomatis: implications for screening. *British Medical Journal,* 315: 1659 – 1663.

Elwyn, G. J. (1997). So many precious stories: a reflective narrative of patient based medicine in general practice, Christmas, 1996. *British Medical Journal,* 315, 1659 - 1663.

Esin, C. (2011). Narrative analysis approaches. In N. Frost (Ed.). *Qualitative research methods in psychology: combining core approaches.* Maidenhead: McGrawHill/Open University Press.

Finlay, L. (2003). The reflexive journey; mapping multiple routes. In L. Finlay & B. Gough (Eds.) *Reflexivity: A Practical Guide for Researchers in Health and Social Sciences.* Oxford: Blackwell.

Fitzpatrick, R. (1997). The assessment of patient satisfaction. In C. Jenkinson (Ed.) *Assessment and evaluation of health and medical care* Buckingham: Open University Press.

Flick, U. (2007). *Managing quality in qualitative research.* London: Sage

Flick, U. (1992). Triangulation revisited: strategy of or an alternative to validation of qualitative data. *Journal of Theory of Social Behavior,* 22: 175 – 197.

French, D. P., Maissi, E. & Marteau, T. M. (2005). The purpose of attributing cause: beliefs about the causes of myocardial infarction. *Social Science and Medicine,* 60: 1411 – 1421.

Frost, N. (2011). *Qualitative research methods in psychology: combining core approaches.* Maidenhead: McGrawHill/Open University Press.

Frost, N. (2009). 'Do you know what I mean?': the use of a pluralistic narrative analysis approach in the interpretation of an interview. *Qualitative Research,* 9 (1): 9 – 29.

Gantley, M., Harding, G., Kumar, S., Tissier, J. (1999). *An Introduction to Qualitative Methods for Health Professionals.*London: Royal College of General Practitioners.

Gergen, K. J. (2001) *Social Construction in Context.* London: Sage Publications.

Gergen, K. J. (1985).The social constructionist movement in modern psychology.*American Psychologist,* 40: 266 – 275.

Gillham, B. (2000). *The research interview.* London: Continuum

Giorgi, A. (1995). Phenomenological Psychology.In J. A. Smith, R. Harré & K. Van Langenhove (Eds.) *Rethinking Psychology.* London: Sage Publications

Glaser, B. G. & Strauss, A. L. (1967).*The discovery of grounded theory.* Chicago: Aldine.

Goodley, D. (2011). Narrative inquiry. In P. Banister, G. Dunn, E. Burman, et al.(Eds.) *Qualitative methods in psychology: A research guide. 2nd edition.* Maidenhead: Open University Press/ McGraw Hill.

Greenhalgh, T. & Hurwitz, B. (Eds.) (1998).*Narrative Based Medicine: Dialogue and discourse in clinical practice.* London: BMJ Books.

Greig, A., Taylor, J., & MacKay, T. (2008). *Doing research with children.*2nd edition. London: Sage.

Harré, H. (1995a). Discursive psychology. In J. A. Smith, R. Harré, & L. Van Langenhove, (Eds.) *Rethinking psychology.* London: Sage.

Hart, E., & Bond, M. (1999). *Action research for health and social care.* Buckingham: Open University Press.

Hayes, N. (Ed.) (1998). *Doing qualitative analysis in psychology.*Hove: Psychology Press.

Helson, H. (1933). The fundamental propositions of Gestalt psychology.*Psychological Review,* 40 (1): 13 -32.

Henwood, K.L. (1996). Qualitative inquiry: perspectives, methods and psychology. In J .T.E.Richardson (Ed.) *Handbook of Qualitative Research Methods for Psychology and the Social Sciences.* Leicester: The British Psychological Society.

Henwood, K. (2004). Reinventing validity: reflections on principles and practices from beyond the quality-quantity divide. In Z. Todd, B. Nerlich, S. McKeown, D. D. Clarke. (Eds.) *Mixing methods in psychology: the integration of qualitative and quantitative methods in theory and practice.*Hove: Psychology Press.

Henwood, K. & Pidgeon, N. (1992) Qualitative research and psychological theorising.*British Journal of Psychology,* 83: 97 - 111.

Holt, A. (2011). Discourse analysis approaches. In N. Frost (Ed.) (2011). *Qualitative research methods in psychology: combining core approaches.* Maidenhead: McGrawHill/Open University Press.

Huberman, A.M. & Miles, M.B. (1998).Data Management and Analysis Methods.In N.K.Denzin & Y.S. Lincoln.*Collecting and Interpreting Qualitative Materials:Handbook of qualitative research.Volume 3.* London: Sage Publications.

King, N., &Horrocks, C. (2010).*Interviews in qualitative research.* London: Sage.

Kok, G., Schaalma, H., Ruiter, R. A. C., Van Empelen, R. (2004). Intervention mapping: a protocol for applying health psychology theory to prevention programmes. *Journal of Health Psychology,* 9 (1): 85 – 98.

Langdridge, D. (2007). *Phenomenological psychology: Theory, research and method.* Harlow: Pearson Prentice Hall.

Lamiell, J. T. (1995). Rethinking the role of quantitative methods in psychology. In Smith,J. A., Harré, R. & Van Langenhove, L. (Eds.) (1995b). *Rethinking methods in psychology.* London: Sage

Lawthom, R. & Tindall, C. (2011). Phenomenology. In P. Banister, G. Dunn, E. Burman, et al. (Eds.) *Qualitative methods in psychology: A research guide. 2nd edition.* Maidenhead: Open University Press/ McGraw Hill.

May, T. (Ed.) *Social research: issues, methods and process.* 4th ed. Maidenhead: McGrawHill/ Open University Press.

May, T., & Perry, B. (2011).Case study research. In T. May (Ed.) *Social research: issues, methods and process.* 4th ed. Maidenhead: McGrawHill/ Open University Press.

Mays, N., & Pope, C. (2000).Assessing quality in qualitative research.*British Medical Journal,*320 : 50 – 52.

Mays, N., & Pope, C. (2000). Qualitative research: rigour and qualitative research. *British Medical Journal,* 320: 50 - 52.

Mitchell, C. (2011). *Doing visual research.* London: Sage.

Morse, J.M. (Ed.) (1994) *Critical Issues in Qualitative Research Methods.* Thousand Oaks: Sage Publications.

Murphy, E. & Dingwall, R. (1998).Qualitative methods in health services research. In N. Black, J. Brazier, R. Fitzpatrick, B. Reeves (Eds.). *Health Services Research Methods: A guide to best practice.* London: BMJ Books.

Murphy, E. &Dingwall, R. (2001).Qualitative Methods in Health Technology Assessment. In A. Stevens, K. Abrams, J. Brazier, R. Fitzpatrick & R. Lilford (Eds.) *The Advanced Handbook of Methods in Evidence Based Healthcare.* London: Sage Publications.

Murphy, E., Dingwall, R., Greatbatch, D., Parker, S., Watson, P. (1998). Qualitative research methods in health technology assessment: a review of the literature. *Health Technology Assessment,*2 (16). Wessex: NCCHTA.

Nerlich, B. (2004). Coming full (hermeneutic) circle. In Z. Todd, B. Nerlich, McKeown, & D. D. Clarke (Eds.) *Mixing methods in psychology: the integration of qualitative and quantitative methods in theory and practice.* Hove: Psychology Press.

Nicholson, I. (1997). Humanistic psychology and intellectual identity: The "Open" system of Gordon Allport. *Journal of Humanistic Psychology,* 37: 61 – 76.

Oakley, A. (1993). *Essays on women, medicine and health.* Edinburgh: Edinburgh University Press.

Oakley, A. (2000). *Experiments in Knowing: Gender and Method in the Social Sciences.* Cambridge: Polity Press

Perls, F., Hefferline, R. & Goodman, P. (1951).*Gestalt therapy.* New York: Dell.

Piaget, J. & Inhelder, B. (2000/1969).*The psychology of the child.*Basic Books.

Pickering, A. (Ed.) (1992). *Science as Practice and Culture.* Chicago: University of Chicago Press.

Pidgeon, N. & Henwood, K. (1997). Using grounded theory in psychological research. In N. Hayes (Ed.). *Doing qualitative analysis in psychology.* Hove: Psychology Press.

Polkinghorne, D. E. (1988).*Narrative knowing and the human sciences.* New York: State University of New York Press.

Pope, C., Mays, N., Popay, J. (2007). *Synthesizing qualitative and quantitative health evidence: a guide to methods.* Maidenhead: McGrawHill/ Open University Press.

Popper, K. (1935/2002). *The Logic of Scientific Discovery.* London: Routledge

Potter, J. (1996). Discourse analysis and constructionist approaches: theoretical background. In J. T. E. Richardson (Ed.).*Handbook of Qualitative Research Methods for Psychology and the Social Sciences.* Leicester: B.P.S. Books

Potter, J., & Wetherell, M. (1995). Discourse analysis. In J. A. Smith, R. Harré, & L. Van Langenhove (Eds.).*Rethinking methods in psychology.* London: Sage

Pringle, J., Drummond, J., McLafferty, E., Hendry, C. (2010). Interpretative phenomenological analysis: a discussion and critique. *Nurse Researcher,* 18 (3): 20 – 24.

Punch, K. F. (2011). *Introduction to research methods in education.* London: Sage.

Punch, K. J. (2011). *Introduction to social research: quantitative and qualitative approaches.* London: Sage. *2nd edition.*

Quality Assurance Agency. (2007). *Subject benchmark statement psychology.* London: Quality Assurance Agency for Higher Education.

Radley, A. & Chamberlain, K. (2001). Health psychology and the study of the case: from method to analytic concern. *Social Science and Medicine,* 53: 321 - 332.

Ragin, D. F. (2011). *Health psychology: an interdisciplinary approach to health.* Boston: MA: Pearson.

Rapport, F., Doel, M. A., Wainwright, P. (2008). The doctor's tale: enacted workspace and the general practitioner. Forum: Qualitative Social Research, 9 (2): Art. 2, http://nbn-resolving.de/urn:nbn:de:0114-fqs080227 (accessed, 9th December, 2011)

Rapport, F., Wainwright, P., Elwyn, G. (2005). "Of the edgelands": broadening the score of qualitative methodology. *Medical Humanities*, 31: 37 -42.

Reissman, C. K. (2008). *Narrative methods for the human sciences*. Thousand Oaks: Sage.

Richardson, J. T. E. (Ed.). (1996). *Handbook of Qualitative Research Methods for Psychology and the Social Sciences*. Leicester: B.P.S. Books

Ricoeur, P. (1981 / 1995). *Hermeneutics and the Human Sciences*.Trans. & Ed. J. B. Thompson. Cambridge: Cambridge University Press.

Roberts, B. (2002). *Biographical Research*. Buckingham: Open University Press.

Robson, C. (2011). *Real world research: A resource for social-scientists and practitioner- researchers.* 3rd edition. Oxford: Blackwell Publishing.

Shinebourne, P. (2011). Interpretative phenomenological analysis. In N. Frost (Ed.). *Qualitative research methods in psychology: combining core approaches.* Maidenhead: McGrawHill/Open University Press.

Silverman, D. (1993). Theory and Method in Qualitative Research. Ch.1, in *Interpreting Qualitative Data: Methods for Analysing Talk, Text and Interaction.* London: Sage Publications.

Sixsmith, J., & Daniels, J. (2011). Action Research. In P. Banister, G. Dunn, E. Burman, et al.(Eds.) *Qualitative methods in psychology: A research guide. 2nd edition.* Maidenhead: Open University Press/ McGraw Hill.

Smith, J. A. (1994). Reconstructing selves: a case study of changing identities during the transition to motherhood.*Journal of Language and Social Psychology*, 10: 225 - 243.

Smith, J. A. (1998). Developing theory from case studies: self-reconstruction and the transition to motherhood.In N. Hayes (Ed.).*Doing qualitative analysis in psychology*.Hove: Psychology Press.

Smith, J. A. (1999). Towards a relational self: social engagement during pregnancy and psychological preparation for motherhood. *British Journal of Social Psychology,*38: 409 - 426.

Smith, J. A. (2007). Hermeneutics, human sciences and health: linking theory and practice. *International Journal of Qualitative Studies on health and Well-being*.2: 3 - 11.

Smith, J. A. (Ed.) (2008). *Qualitative psychology: a practical guide to research methods.* London: Sage.

Smith, J. A. (2011). Evaluating the contribution of interpretative phenomenological analysis. *Health Psychology Review*, 5 (1)): 9 - 27.

Smith, J. A. & Osborn, M. (2008).Interpretative Phenomenological Analysis. In J. A. Smith (Ed.), *Qualitative Psychology: A practical guide to research methods* (2nded.) (pp. 53 - 80). London: Sage.

Smith, J. A., Flowers, P., & Larkin, M. (2009).*Interpretative phenomenological analysis: Theory, method and research.* London: Sage.

Smith,J. A., Harré, R. & Van Langenhove, L. (Eds.) (1995a). *Rethinking psychology*. London: Sage.

Smith,J. A., Harré, R. & Van Langenhove, L. (Eds.) (1995b). *Rethinking methods in psychology.* London: Sage

Smith, J. A., Jarman, M., Osborn, M. (1999).Doing Interpretative Phenomenological Analysis. In M. Murray & K. Chamberlain (Eds.), *Qualitative Health Psychology: Theories and Methods* (pp. 218 - 240). London: Sage.

Smith, M.J. (1998). *Social Science in question*. London: Sage Publications

Spinelli, E. (2005). *The interpreted world: An introduction to phenomenological psychology* (2nd ed.) London: Sage.

Strauss, A. & Corbin, J. (1990).*Basics of Qualitative Research: Grounded Theory procedures and techniques.* London: Sage Publications.

Thomas, J., Harden, A., Oakley, A., et al. (2004) Integrating qualitative research with trials in systematic reviews. *British Medical Journal*, 328: 1010 - 1012

Thompson, A. R., Kent, G. & Smith, J. A. (2002). Living with vitiligo: dealing with difference. *British Journal of Health Psychology*, 7: 213 - 223.

Todd, Z., Nerlich, B., McKeown,S, Clarke, D. D. (Eds.) (2004). *Mixing methods in psychology: the intergration of qualitative and quantitative methods in theory and practice.* Hove: Psychology Press.

Tonkiss, F. (2012). Discourse analysis. In C. Searle (Ed.). *Researching society and culture. 3rd edition.* London: Sage.

Van Manen, M. (1998). Modalities of body experience in illness and health. *Qualitative Health Research*, 8, (1): 7 - 24.

Vasquez-Lago, J. M., Lopez-Vazquez, P., López-Durán, A., Taracido-Trunk, M., & Figueiras, A. (2011). Attitudes of primary care physicians to the prescribing of antibiotics and antimicrobial resistance: a qualitative study from Spain. *Family Practice*, doi:10.1093/fampra/cmr084

Walsh, D. (2012). Doing ethnography. In C. Searle (Ed.) *Researching society and culture*, 3rd edition. London: Sage.

Whimster, S. (2001). Max Weber: work and interpretation. In G. Ritzer & B. Smart (Eds.). *Handbook of social theory*. London: Sage.

Willig, C. (2008) *Introducing qualitative research methods in psychology: Adventures in theory and method. 2nd ed.* Maidenhead: McGrawHill/ Open University Press.

Willig, C. & W. Stainton Rogers (eds) (2008) *Handbook of Qualitative Research in Psychology.* London: Sage.

Yardley, L. (2008). Demonstrating validity in qualitative research. In J. A. Smith (Ed.) *Qualitative psychology: a practical guide to research methods* (pp. 235 - 251). London: Sage.

Ziebland, S., &McPherson, A. (2006).Making sense of qualitative data analysis: an introduction with illustrations from DIPex (personal experiences of health and illness).*Medical Education*, 40: 405 - 414.

Ziebland S., & Wright, L (1997). Qualitative research methods In C. Jenkinson (Ed.) *Assessment and evaluation of health and medical care* Buckingham: Open University Press.

11

Issues of Information Exchange Efficiency in Long-Term Space Flights

V. Gushin and A. Yusupova
Institute for Biomedical Problems, Moscow, Russia

1. Introduction

A human being can live in outer space only in the artificially created environment of a spacecraft. Space vacuum, galactic space radiation, meteorite currents, super-low temperatures outboard give rise in space crew members to a natural feeling of threat to their health and survival. In this connection a high level of psychic tension persists even in a trouble-free space flight due to a natural worry about one's safety which is not relieved even during sleep.

As the time of a space flight increases, a cosmonaut's emotional sphere comes to be affected predominantly by uniformity (monotony) of the closed environment and by limitation of social contacts. The impact of these factors enhanced by zero gravity leads on to the appearance of dysfunctional changes. Their incrementing intensity manifests itself in cumulative weariness and central nervous system asthenisation due to an inadequate reaction of the nervous system to stimuli. Asthenisation, a condition experienced following space flights (as well as after serious illnesses, traumas, and mental overstrain), manifests itself after 1-2 months of long-term space flights due to sensory deprivation existing in space flight condition (Myasnikov, Zamaletdinov, 1997). In asthenisation, strong extrinsic stimuli may evoke a poor response, while on the other hand slight stimuli may produce a positive reaction (Myasnikov, Stepanova et al., 2000). A sign of deterioration in cosmonauts' psychic condition is a frequent appearance of frankly negative emotional responses especially if they leave a lasting negative track behind themselves in the form of low mood. Normally emotional responses (defined as the emotional component of responses to various external and internal stimuli) are transitory, clearly oriented and extremely diverse, and, most important, are not very strong. If however negative emotions predominate and become stagnant, establishing a steadily negative mood background together with irritability, aggressiveness, constant complaints of feeling unwell, of fatigue, headache etc., and if at the same time we observe paradoxical forms of emotional reactions with inadequate outbursts of irritation in response to insignificant stimuli, then this should be regarded as evidence of intense psychological trouble. In such condition a person often manifests speech peculiarities which are not normally characteristic of him or her, such as swearwords, expletives, sounds and words filling pauses, unusually loud or, on the contrary, unusually low speech with increased/decreased tonality and speed (Myasnikov et al., 1982). So individual speech style changes. It should also be pointed out that asthenisation of cosmonauts' nervous and psychic sphere which mostly affects controlling systems, may have a negative impact on the interpersonal relationships in a space crew and on the crew-ground interaction, as well as affect performance of each crew member.

The influence of the social isolation factor in sealed cabin is displayed in the form of compulsory socializing of cosmonauts (obligatory contacts during communication with a limited circle of people in Mission Control). These limited social contacts are at the same time excessive because one has to socialize too closely with a limited circle of people. This specific situation makes it a necessity to reconsider many conventional rules and role orientations and results in an impossibility to satisfy a number of social and mental needs. (Novikov, 1981). Limitation of social contacts can induce negative emotional reactions, which have an influence on professional activities, and can for instance hamper communication of crew members with the ground services and become a source of conflict.

The analysis of space crew's communication with the Mission Control Center (MCC) is a standard operational procedure of the psychological support group in the Institute for Biomedical problems, Russia. For more than 20 years it has been used for monitoring the behavioral health of Russian crewmembers in space and long-term space simulations. Since 1992, we apply speech content analysis to reveal relationship dynamics within the group and between crew and MC. Since 2000, we apply the content analysis method to study communication of International Space Station (ISS) crews with MC.

The main reason for using content analysis for space crews communication is the necessity of non-invasive methods in crews' routine. ISS audiocommunication channels include those which are private and those which are open and automatically recorded. Crewmembers sign an informed consent thus agreeing with publicity of information surpassing this channel.

Daily work on ISS includes a considerable number of work tasks. An additional intervention in crew's schedule with one more methods concerning relationship dynamics, may lead to collection of biased data.

2. Space crew communication as a type of professional activity

The object of psychology in studying any type of professional activity is always psychological factors and processes which induce, program and regulate a person's professional activity as well as expression of personality traits through which this activity is implemented (Shadrikov, 1983). As the experience of psychological analysis of cosmonauts professional activity confirms, such processes manifest it selves in large-scale communication of a crew with various ground services (launching plant, technical and landing complexes, Mission Control etc.) and with other space objects included in the circuit of the automated system of the space flight control. First of all, part of this communication is the verbal communication of space crew members with Mission Control transferred through an open communication channel accessible for everybody of the Mission Control personnel (as distinguished from private communication channels used for special tasks of flight support, and among other things for medico-psychological purposes). In the course of such communication, cosmonauts provide Mission Control with a detailed and regular information about technological operations performed onboard, about space vehicle status, their health state, and appearing problems. In response an operators group of Mission

Control which usually includes experienced cosmonauts who have flown in space provide the crew with recommendations, instructions, directing and controlling the crew's work. Earlier such communication was limited to communication sessions, but now a space crew can communicate with Mission Control at any time during a space flight.

From the psychological point of view such cooperation ensures for a space crew information which is important for the crew members both professionally and for their personal relationships. It allows them to know better their way in the current situation, to make timely and appropriate decisions on the space ship control and its technical systems maintenance, to stay informed about life on Earth (Myasnikov et al, 2001). On their part, Mission Control operators need communication with the crew in order to get current information about the mission plan performance by the crew, which is used for the strategic and the short-time planning of the cosmonauts' activity, technical and medical support of the crew, timely consultation on various issues etc.

Therefore, information exchange is an intrinsic part of the professional activity of cosmonauts and Mission Control, and the communication efficiency directly determines the appropriateness of flight control decisions taken by the communication parties. A good personal and intergroup contact, a mutual understanding and cooperation in decision making ensures the mission plan realization and satisfies the crew's need for new informational challenges and socialization in a wider circle of persons. Adequate, open and friendly contact between the ground and the space professional groups determines, on the one hand, emotional tonus and performance of the cosmonauts and, on the other hand, precludes the development of so called deprivation effects caused by the impact of factors of a prolonged space flight. Combining engineering and technological and medical and psychological aspects of this professional activity makes communication of the crew and Mission Control an important source of unbiased current information from the engineering and technological and medical and psychological points of view. Due to this, a record and a later detailed analysis of communication of a space crew and Mission Control have been an intrinsic part of the Russian mission support system starting from the years 70 of the past century.

3. Methodology of space crew psychological status control

Psycho-diagnostics in the medical support system of manned space missions aim at the identification of various forms of adaptive behavior of people in special working conditions. In other words, psycho-diagnostics of cosmonauts' health status is are a synthesis of clinical, psychological and professional evaluations made conjointly by an expert-doctor and an expert-psychologist using accepted procedures, evaluation scales and terminology. In a space flight unlike clinical conditions, expert evaluation and diagnostics are performed on the basis of a remote observation (no direct contact with a 'patient'), with a scarcity of diagnostic data and impossibility in certain cases to make some necessary additional studies (Orbitalnaya stanciya Mir, 2002).

Psychological control and support of cosmonauts and astronauts at 'Mir" Space Station performed by Moscow Medico-Biological Problems Institute led the Institute's specialists to the development of a method which allows to remotely control and evaluate the personnel's psycho-emotional status basing on the expert evaluation of the content of their communication with external parties and on the device-aided analysis of the time spans of such communication. The principal sources of psychological data derived from a monitoring of interpersonal interaction in a space crew are the crew's communication with Mission Control, video communication sessions, and also direct communication of the psychological support group with the cosmonauts (Gazenko et al, 1976; Kelly, Kanas, 1993; Gushin, 1995; Caldwell, 2000). The main advantage of the usage of the crew's wireless communication for the evaluation of the cosmonauts' psycho-physiological status is its psychological 'noninvasiveness', since the board-ground wireless communication is a regular procedure in a space flight. Diagnostic criteria developed by psychologists of Russian Public Scientific Center of Moscow Medico-Biological Problems Institute allow to objectively and quantitatively evaluate the psychological climate in a space crew without compelling the cosmonauts to undergo additional test procedures which would demand extra time and without installing additional equipment at the space station (Myasnikov, Stepanova, 2000). On the basis of these criteria Mission Control psycho-neurologists can provide flight directors with their professional opinions on the psycho-physiological status of space crew members for the purpose of correcting the work-and-sleep schedule.

How expert diagnostic assesment is organized during a space flight is represented on Figure 1. As we can see, information is transmitted from the board of a space vehicle through wireless and video telecommunication channels, biotelemetry channels to the experts (doctors and psychologists) being part of the medical support group. The experts analyzing the incoming information make partial expert judgments on the crew members behavior and group interaction. The chief psycho-neurologist summarizes these data and makes a diagnosis of the state of health within a day, within a week or other time periods, and also before the cosmonauts should perform especially difficult types of work, for instance, extravehicular activity. At the same time the experts decide whether the flight should continue along the regular plan or some required preventive (curative) measures should be taken.

We have to hardly mention that the efficiency of preventive care is determined for a great deal by the experts' general medical and clinical psychology knowledge of the phenomenology of a certain psycho-neurological state, of the underlying psycho-physiological mechanisms, as well as of the influencing factors. The basic premise for the analysis of information coming from onboard is that space flight conditions induce a certain psychological or neurological effect indirectly, which means that the same flight condition effect (e.g., constant noise on the ISS) does not result to the same psychological disturbances. The psychological effect depends on the initial and the current functional status of a crew member and his or her adaptive capabilities.

Until recently such analysis was a descriptive qualitative analysis. In order to make it more illustrative, a scale of expert evaluations has been developed which helps to render the work-rest distribution in quantitative characteristics ranged by number of points. After many years of making expert opinions (Orbitalnaya stanciya Mir, 2002), the specialists drew up a list of individual and group-related indicators of the psycho-neurological status of crew members (Myasnikov at al., 2002) which up till now have been monitored in the study of information coming from onboard (Chart 1). Myasnikov and Zamaletdinov who have been practicing this approach distinguished 14 individual and 5 group-related indicators used in the dynamic evaluation of the cosmonauts' mental state. These indicators were formulated on the ground of expert assessments. The individual indicators are: dominant interests, proposals (complaints), deprivation phenomena, emotional response, mood, volitional actions, general behavior, health, sensorial sphere, motor performance, speech, sleep, psycho-physiological tension and professional activity. A special cluster of scales describes efficiency of group interaction thus allowing to judge about the small group's structure (formal and informal leaders, outcastes) and about the presence or absence of frictions in the space crew. An indicator of leadership is in the first place the fact of dominating in communication and the issues raised during it. Signs of a wrapped conflict in crew members are: the narrowing of the contacts circle and the exclusion of the unwelcome partner from it, or limiting the verbal interaction with such partner down to the minimum determined by the need to participate in a common activity, that is the formalization of the relationships with such partner.

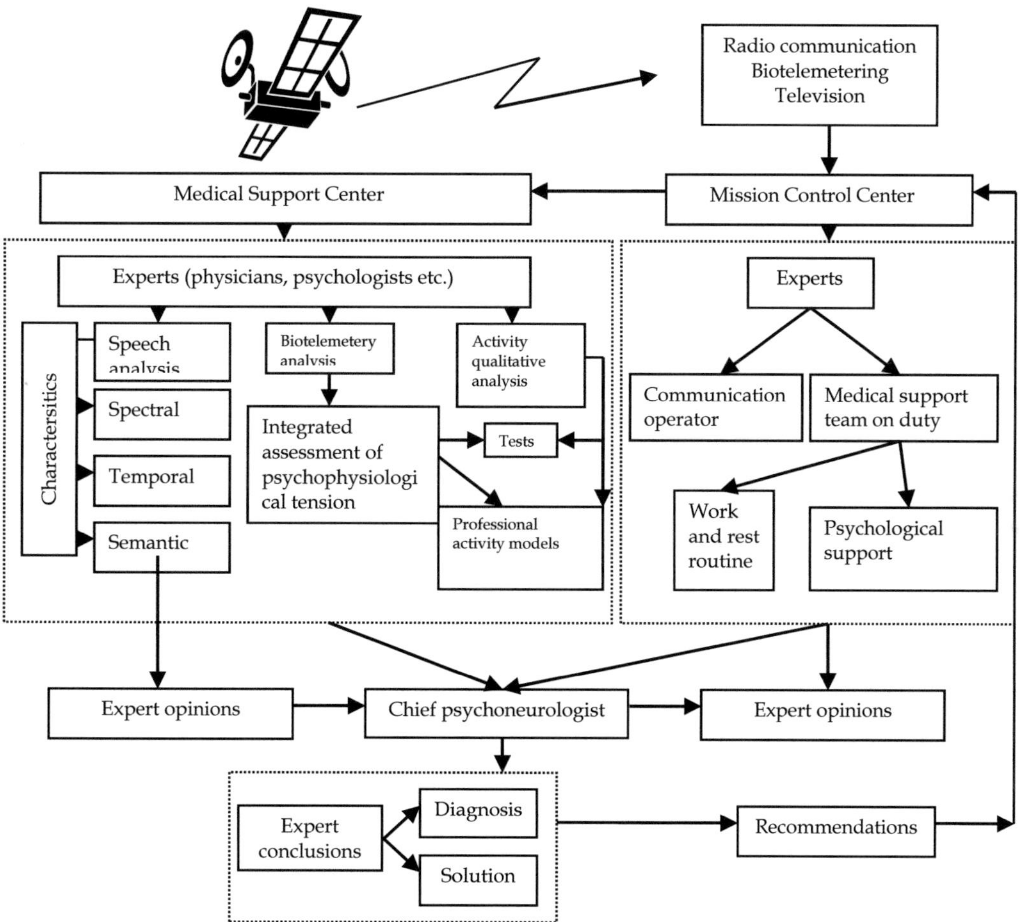

Fig. 1. Expert diagnostics organization during a space flight (Myasnikov, Zamaletdinov, 1997).

In their daily psycho-neurological opinions (which is a regular standard procedure in prolonged space flights) the experts describe unfavorable group dynamics phenomena registered in the course of observation (conflicts, formation of coalitions, mutual estrangement etc.). Besides, the degree of the mental ill-being in the group is assessed quantitatively through the method of expert evaluation on the basis of scales (such scales as "difficulties of group dynamics" in the space crew, "conflicts within the space crew and between the crew and the ground control").

As a novelty, the approach by Myasnikov and Zamaletdinov introduced 7 degrees of intensity for each diagnostic indicator. The diagnostic zones were subdivided into relative zones: optimal (from the 1st to the 3rd degree of the qualitative evaluation), transitional (from the 4th to the 5th degree) and unfavorable (from the 6th to the 7th degree). Once again, these intensity degrees were formulated by experts on the ground of their experience. A precondition for a correct assessment of an indicator is the fact that this indicator has appeared in at least two successive communication sessions. So, quantitative values representing qualitative changes along all or the majority of indicators make up quite an informative system of a dynamical remote evaluation. Research conducted during space flights (Gazenko et al, 1976; Grigorev, 1986) revealed that various parameters of verbal activity (length of communication session, content of voice messages (speech semantics), thematic variety of speech, emotional expressiveness of voice messages, character related properties of voice and speech etc.) are relatively stable indicators of the individual verbal behavior of a cosmonaut.

Individual indicators	Complaints Deprivation phenomena Emotional response Mood State of motivation and volition sphere Various aspect of general behavior Health State of sensorial sphere Motor performance Speech Sleep Psycho-physiological tension Dominant and associate interests Performance Operator activity Initiative Professional proposals and actions
Group-related indicators	Mutual understanding Group cohesion In-group control Group operation Nature of contacts with ground services

Chart 1. Basic Indicators Used in the Study of Information Coming from Onboard of a Spacecraft for Making Expert Opinions (according to "Mir" Space Station, 2002).

Until very recently, the remote psychological monitoring system was quite efficient in monitoring and progress forecast of the space crew activity. However, the experience of expert and diagnostic tasks solutions accumulated by space psychology and medicine revealed certain methodological difficulties. They are determined by the absence of a reliable conceptual model and objectively established criteria of the work of an expert dealing with remote control and information scarcity. As a result, such work of an expert has more to do with art than science, demands years of preparation, and such expert evaluations are to a certain degree subjective, determined by the expert's personal style and experience. Besides that, a problem was the ethic aspect of the method and a disfavor with which cosmonauts treated the studies of their psychological compatibility and mental health set against the background of the social acknowledgement of their achievements as those of national heroes. The fact of having assessment results which were not quite perfect could influence the possibility of cosmonaut's future flights. These factors hindered to a certain degree the development of psychological aspects of expert and diagnostic work.

4. Methods

Commencing our research of communication in actual long-duration space flights we have developed our analysis method based on the data of the space analogue experiment called SFINCSS-99 involving long-term isolation (Yusupova et al, 2006). The system of categories we developed worked sufficiently in the situation of long term isolation; however, when continuing our research in actual space flights, we had to face the fact that our analysis categories were not universal. The categories which we had used in the space analogue turned out to be too general for the analysis of the speech of space crews in long-duration space flights, that is they did not possess sufficient resolution capability and, in our view, differentiated the utterances inadequately. This inadequacy was quite expectable. According to T.G. Vinokur (Vinokur, 2007), variants of communicative verbal behavior, that is communicative styles absorb a practically 'open range' of individual interplays between the speaker and the listener, and the types of communicative styles can be defined in the terms *adequate to the components of the given heterogeneous segment of verbal behavior*. Therefore, the terms (categories) should be modified each time when the situation in which communication changes takes place.

The communication structure in space flights on ISS differed both from the communication in the above simulation experiments and from the communication of the Mir Space Station as well. At the stage of ISS development, the major share of communication was devoted to solving specific operational issues, and non-operational issues were seldom discussed. A special factor was that communication was effected simultaneously by two national Mission Control Centers (the Russian and the US MCC) and according to the regulations, the astronauts and cosmonauts could address each of them.

In order to upgrade our content analysis categories, we repeatedly listened to the records a space crew's communication for one week evaluated by the Mission Control specialists as 'normal': during this week there had been no contingency events and no large-scale innovations which would have changed the work schedule of the crew established on ISS. We registered standard phrases and dialogues trying to find textual differences related to changes in the ways of information conveyance, interpersonal interaction regulation and feelings expression (in accordance with the three communicative functions which we were looking for in the text). We also took note of terms and phrases which occurred rarely but were typical of the communicators.

The result of this preliminary research was a modified categories chart (see Chart 2). The categories were arranged in three groups according to the Bales' (1950) communication analysis scheme and communicative functions established by B.F. Lomov (Lomov, 1981).

Modified Categories as Adapted to Space Analogue	**Modified Categories as Adapted to Real Space Flight**	**Category Functions**
Demands for information	Primary demands for information	Informative function of communication
	Clarifying (secondary) demands for information	
Information sharing (orientation) / Opinion	Informing after a demand	
	Informing without a demand	
	Ignoring a demand	
	Professional jargon, use of acronyms	
Demands for action	Requests	
Compliments, gratitude, approval, consent	Emotional consent	Emotional function of communication
Disapproval, discontent, discord	Emotional discord	
Warm-hearted humor, jokes, phatic expressions	Humor and jokes (tension release)	
Satire, acidity	Satire, acidity	
Complaints, laments/ antagonism	Operational complaint	
	Socially directed complaint	
Compliments, gratitude, approval, consent	Rational consent	Socio-regulatory function of communication
Disapproval, discontent, discord	Rational discord	
Request / intention of joint activity, solidarity, offers	Encouragement, sympathy, gratitude	
	Calls by name	
Justification, defense	Self-justification	
Refusal of joint activity, refusal of help, refusal of offers	Refusal to cooperate	

Chart 2. Bales' method categories modified to capture special features of communication on ISS.

We paid special attention to drawing up the codebook which should have reflected the basic provisions of our research method. A codebook is a manual used by an expert-encoder who collects empirical data and encodes the predetermined units of analysis (Neuendorf, 2002). Therefore, the codebook together with the coding form (chart of categories used to record the number of these categories in speech) are the principal documents of content analysis. Since we used the quantitative content analysis (Krippendorf, 1980), once the codebook and the coding form had been adopted, they did not change in the course of the four missions data collection in order to ensure the research data consistency.

One more relevant feature of the space flight communication analysis is how often such communication can be listened to. In our case, the choice of the days of the week was determined by the access to the encrypted communication channel which we gained. It was Tuesdays in case of the crews I, III, IV and Tuesdays plus Thursdays in case of the crew II.

5. Certain results and discussion

Certain issues we faced were connected to communicative styles of the two MCs, and their efficiency. It is ordinary that every nation has its specific style of communication that lay down implicit communication rules. However, in a situation where people work in extreme environments, the communication procedure should be built to be as effective as possible, if we think about communication efficiency as of its level of information transmission. Comparing styles of communication typical for American and Russian MCs, we found a significant difference between them. Certain sorts of utterances used by MC may raise or reduce the effectiveness of communication between MC and space crew.

5.1 Separation of communication channels

The analysis of the national MCCs' communication with ISS shows that the most striking feature of this communication is the division of communication channels between the Russian MCC and the USA MCC (Yusupova, Gushin, 2006). The Russian cosmonauts communicated with the Russian Mission Control, and the US astronauts communicated with the US Mission Control (see Figure 2). Each of the national MCCs preferred to communicate with their own crewmembers in terms of giving and receiving information. On average, the national MCCs spoke with their own crewmembers 98% of the communication time and with the other nationality crewmembers 2% of the communication time. There was very little international communication, and this was true of all communication components: informative, socio-regulatory and emotional.

The phenomena of what we called the contours of informational exchange was recognized during our ISS communication studies. It was clear that there were steady preferences in choosing the interlocutor between crewmembers and MC operators. The design of communication connections became more complex since ISS crews include members of two countries as a minimum, and are being controlled by two MCs - an American and a Russian one. The interlocutor is chosen not only by his psychological features that would go well with the crewmember, but also by preferred (native) language. This creates a certain disproportion in information receipt, which may lead to various misunderstandings between the two MCs.

Therefore, the onboard - Earth communication had two communicative channels: one channel was the Russians to Russians communication and the other channel was the Americans to Americans communication. In connection with this, a danger emerges that the Mission Control Centers may have two independent opinions each of which conditioned by insufficient information. Thus, we can speak about three visions of the situation onboard of ISS:

1. The vision achieved by the Russian MCC.
2. The vision achieved by the US MCC.
3. The vision achieved by the crewmembers.

Certainly, not all informational exchange of ISS and Earth goes through the audio communication. For instance, there is also an exchange of electronic messages and of control charts and work results. In our opinion, the separation of communication channels may lead to a loss of some information and affect the joint performance of the MCCs and the crews.

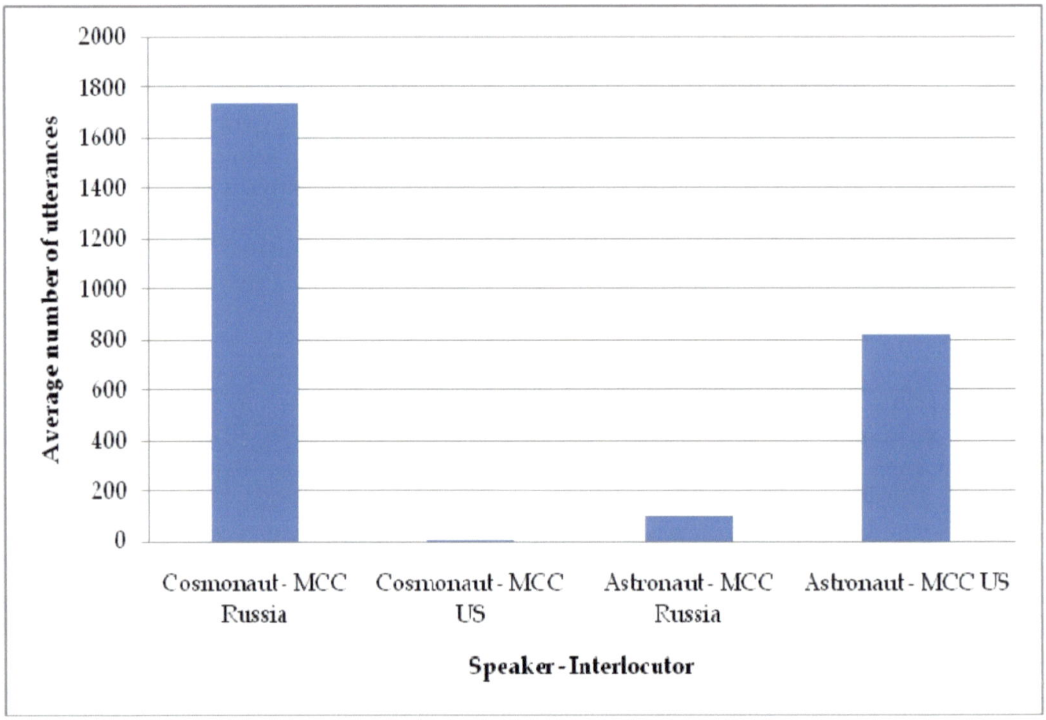

Fig. 2. Average numbers of utterances in space crewmembers - MCC communication.

5.2 Informing without a demand or after a demand

Clarifying the issue why the Russian cosmonauts were the communicative leaders in the majority of cases cannot go without an analysis of the distribution of informative function utterances. The existence of two almost completely independent communication channels as shown above allows to make such analysis.

Analyzing the special features of the usage of primary demands for information, we can see the following characteristics of the cosmonauts' communication with Mission Control. For instance, we see one and a half times more questions made by the Russian MCC than by the cosmonaut in the first mission. In an audio communication session this sounds like that: *"ISS, answer MCC! – In contact? – What is the pressure onboard? What are the oxygen values? Have you done the full work today? Have you done sports?"* or like that: *"Have you turned off the taps? What is the pressure? What about oxygen? Have you cleaned out the sacks or are they still lying there in a heap? Have you moved the fire extinguisher? Is cryogen on? Have you ridden the exercise bike? Is that lamp burning?"*. In case of the US astronauts' communication with the national Mission Control, such things are almost always reported by the astronauts without questions having been asked by Mission Control.

When we analyzed the first crew's data, we presumed that such predominance of questions on the part of the Russian Mission Control compared to the US Mission Control was due to the fact that the Russian cosmonaut was the crew commander, as the most of information is usually expected from crew commanders. Our analysis of the second and the fourth crews confirmed this idea, for the US Mission Control indeed addressed more questions to the astronauts - crew commanders than the astronauts to Mission Control. However, the correlation of the questions in the Russian communication channel remained the same.

Unfortunately, this "questions shower" phenomenon can hardly encourage cosmonauts' performance. The Russian cosmonauts often had to spend their time looking for the information being requested in that particular moment, which distracted them from working and increased the communication time. To support this view, we can cite some more of the audio communication (of the second crew):

MCC: *Have you ridden the exercise bike?*
Cosmonaut: *No, I haven't. We are going to ride it in the night.*
MCC *(calmly): Are you joking.*
Cosmonaut: *I am quite serious, I've given you an example of this fussing – an hour for this, an hour for that, forty minutes for this, forty minutes for that. That's why nothing is done. Yes, I've finished with the cargo ship [the logistics module] – but the other things – just in snatches. This is like, you know, in your garage – you fetched potatoes, then onions, then you ran somewhere else, sorted out your things, then fetched water, then gas – and here you've been running all day and what have you done? Nothing. And here it is like that.*

This feature of communication of the Russian MCC with the cosmonauts manifested itself also in the requests distribution. So, the Russian Mission Control addressed to the first crew's cosmonaut 3,3-times more requests than the cosmonaut to Mission Control (so the correlation was 3,3:1); in the second crew this correlation was 7:1; in the third crew - 18:1; in the fourth crew - 11:1. In our opinion, this feature is especially characteristic of the Russian MCC's communicative style which aims at extracting information from cosmonauts, at constantly controlling cosmonauts' actions. *"I am answering all your questions like a schoolboy at the blackboard"* - said the Russian crew commander when he was once again poured with questions for which he had no time to answer. The Mission Control's strategy of 'extracting information' was also from time to time opposed by the Russian cosmonaut of the second crew.

MCC: *Let's sum up today's results. Have you done your sports in full?*
Cosmonaut: *In full.*
MCC: *Say a few words about the plants which are growing. [Referring to the experiment of growing vegetables on ISS]*
Cosmonaut: *They are growing.*
MCC: *Growing? ... Fine.*

The US MCC and the astronauts communication, though seemingly relaxed, turns out to be more efficient: information is reported by the astronauts without questions being asked, when they have collected and prepared all the data which need to be reported to Mission Control. The astronauts begin their information sharing like: *"I want to report that..."* Therefore, the informational exchange takes much less time (see Figure 3).

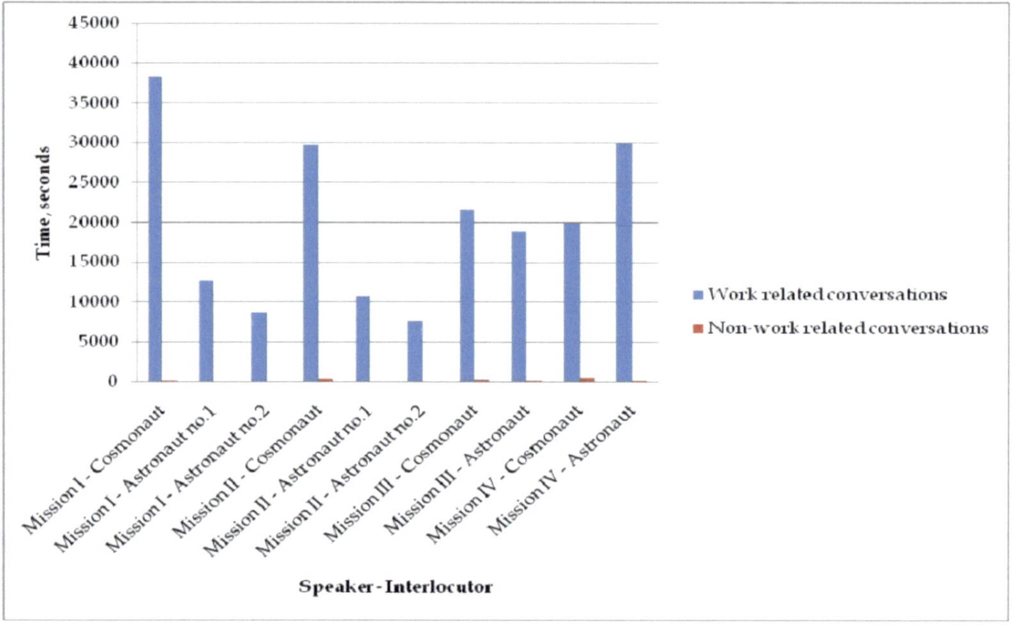

Fig. 3. Time spent by the crewmembers on work related and non work related communication with the Mission Control Centers at similar mission stages.

5.3 Informing and phatic component

We have to point at the high figures of the 'Informing after a demand' category in the Russian cosmonauts' speech which, however, is quite natural due to the fact that they are often asked questions. On the contrary, it was typical for the MCCs to inform the cosmonauts without a demand; the figure of this category was 1,8-times bigger than the figure of the 'Informing after a demand' category. Mainly the Russian communicators ask repeated questions, and the Russian Mission Control staff ask repeated questions more often than the Russian cosmonauts do. Most probably, this is related to the factors of the communication irregularity and of the pouring the cosmonaut with questions. These differences may be conditioned by the communicative style developed in a certain culture, and so may be the differences in the phatic component of communication described below.

Despite the smaller total volume of communication, the number of utterances in the 'Encouragements, sympathy, gratitude' category in the first three crews was the same in case of the US and the Russian crewmembers, while in the fourth crew, the US astronaut used more utterances of this category than the Russian cosmonaut. Positive phatic (small talk) utterances were used in the speech of the astronauts and the US MCC as a natural thing in the course of communication, between this and then: *"I appreciate you folks for letting us know!", "Thanks for the heads up!"*. On the contrary, in the majority of cases, the Russian MCC provides phatic elements as a separate communication block, clearly separating the phatic and the informative components:

MCC *(wearily): Congratulations with the first of April, dear [crewmembers]. Today is the first of April and you should laugh well.*
Cosmonaut *(wearily): I began laughing already yesterday when I got your radiogram.*

Space crewmembers, being excellent specialists but also different personalities, form their own communication styles with MCs as well. These styles may include highly effective examples as well as neglecting styles leading to poor effectiveness level. As the communication between MCs and space crews is under control of psychological services, certain changes in training of the both communication sides should lead to enhancement of informational exchange efficiency.

5.4 Consents and discords

In the first mission, we noticed a predominance of utterances which contained the cosmonaut's consents with the interlocutor's position. The number of utterances of this type clearly prevailed over disapprovals, arguments, expressions of negative emotions, self-justifications, refusals to cooperate. At the same time, we noticed the tendency of the communicative leader - the Russian crew commander to avoid discussing sensitive issues. On the contrary, in the second mission, the number of discords, self-justifications and refusals to cooperate was 1,7-times bigger than the number of rational and emotional consents. We should point out that this ratio emerged owing to the cosmonaut - flight engineer who was the communicative leader. In the third and the fourth missions, the Russian cosmonauts were less dominating in communication with Mission Control and expressed what they thought of information which they received more seldom compared to the first two missions.

In the second mission, encouragements were a reaction of the Russian Mission Control Center to the increasing number of emotional discords of the cosmonaut and might be regarded as a kind of coping strategy (see Figure 4).

A considerable quantity of emotional discords and satire of the Russian cosmonaut in the second mission can be accounted for by several external stress generating reasons known in the mass media. But it is sure that the cosmonaut's negative utterances were often a reaction to the Mission Control actions. For example, *"We have written to Earth in what way we dispose of waste, and if Earth don't know this, then it's their problem"*. After another series of repeated questions: *"Do you at least take notes when I report?"* or *"Well again, you write with your one hand and strike out with your other hand, do you?"*.

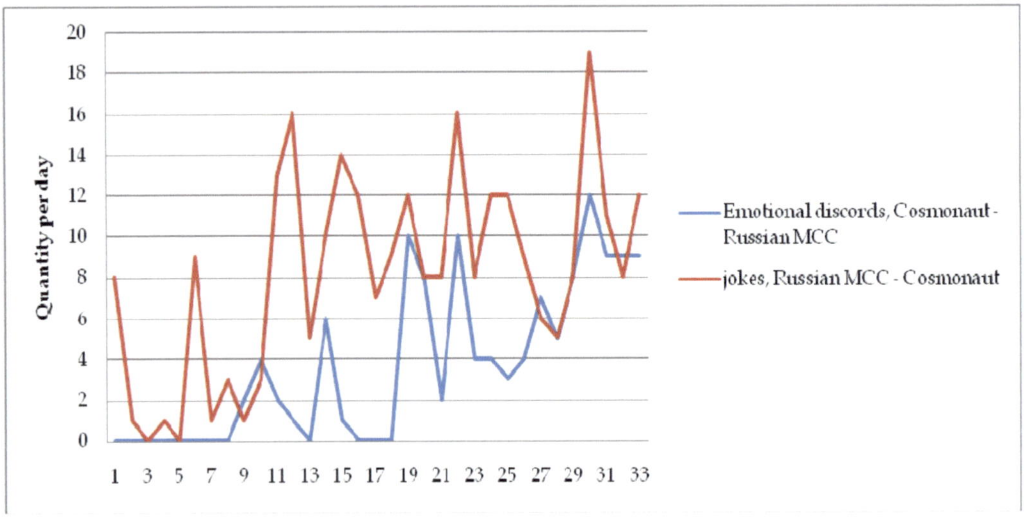

Fig. 4. Emotional discords addressed by the cosmonaut to the Russian MCC and jokes addressed by MCC to the cosmonaut.

6. Phenomena identified by the analysis of isolated small groups communication

The results of the previous part of the present chapter show the existing communication difficulties we detected in several space missions. These difficulties are to overcome with help of communication trainings of crews as well as ground personnel. During 20 years that we were collecting data in different isolated crews, we found out that there is a number of repeating communication phenomena that is typical for isolated small groups.

The phenomenon of isolated small group remote communication with the outside world takes place when due to their professional activity, a group of people are isolated from the usual socio-psychological contacts, have a restricted freedom of movement, no usual comfort, experience sensorial deprivation (there is no usual informational flow coming from the environment), and constantly face danger. Categories of personnel which communicate remotely in extreme environments are ocean-going ship crews, polar winterers, staff on oil platforms and distant mineral deposits, weather stations staff, prolonged expeditions personnel, cosmonauts and astronauts etc.

We should pay attention to the fact that isolated crewmembers experience difficulty in satisfying their need to reduce the ambiguity of how their behavior is perceived in a given situation. Firstly, the range of available standards of behavior is considerably restricted due to a small number of communication partners and a decreased informational flow, since communication in isolation is restricted. Describing communication of isolated subjects with the external world, specialists emphasized several times the involuntary nature of such communication because a person may not speak as much as he or she would want to and when and with whom he or she would want to.

We should bear in mind that isolated people communicate in an environment extremely poor in information, distinguished by monotony and sensorial deprivation. Undoubtedly, on certain adaptation stages, this gives rise to an increased need, on the one hand, to compensate for the usual informational flows (in particular, the yearning of speaking with family and friends, the social inclusion in the life of people far away) and, on the other hand, to receive diverse new information.

However, special research has demonstrated that a mere increase of informational flows is not a fully adequate compensatory mean of psychological support in isolation. Adapting to sensorial deprivation and monotony in isolation, a person starts to communicate both with the crewmates and the distant society at a lower level of informational exchange (Gushin, 1997). So, the general volume of communication decreases, the range of topics and the circle of interlocutors narrow down - the 'psychological closing' phenomenon emerges. That is why the external group's attempts to communicate with the isolated crew with the same intensity as before isolation are often opposed by the crew. The isolated crew claims that contacts distract them from work and attempt to avoid communication.

Secondly, in space flight, the reflecting process itself is distorted when a group of people larger than the one the subject is accustomed to, pay their attention to him or her and consequently the subject may reassess his or her personal value and conceive himself or herself as a 'star'. An important aspect of communication in such conditions is that contacts take place against the 'public privacy' background (Leonov, Lebedev, 1975) when the isolated person feels to be carefully observed. Due to an almost total absence of communication privacy, cosmonauts' communication with Earth loses its freedom and confidence, becomes more formal and at the same time self-presenting, dramatic, since a cosmonaut has to constantly comply with a certain social role associated with a high social status. The feeling that one is being constantly evaluated leads on to the appearing signs of social facilitation as it is currently understood - that is, an increased social agitation occurring in the presence of other people and aggravated by the lack of personal space (crowding). So, the general increase of psycho-physiological agitation complicates the crew's performance in the new and little-studied conditions.

People are naturally attracted to the ones they like and want to speak to and they prefer to keep distance from the ones they dislike and have no wish to communicate with. We can suggest that the opposite is also true - an increasing distance between communication parties makes the interlocutor less attractive and reduces the person's wish to communicate. Consequently, it is no wonder that the isolated person, being at a significant distance from the support group, being highly motivated to perform and worrying about how he or she is evaluated by strangers whom he or she hardly can influence, wants to avoid such strangers by hiding from video monitoring and by reducing audio contacts.

So, remote communication of isolated small groups is restricted, involuntary andpublic. The functions of the isolated small group's communication are not only informational exchange, but also a compensation for sensorial deprivation, monotony, for a lack of openness and confidence in contacts. Finally, when speaking with the outside world, each communicator reflects not only his or her opinion but that of their group.

6.1 Influence of isolated small group's evolution on communication

At the initial stages of its formation, a small group, in particular, a space crew, is quite open towards the influence of society. In a real or simulated social isolation, a crew which has participated in a full-fledged group training grows gradually cohesive and becomes a 'cooperation group' having a well developed internal structure and a high degree of member interaction (Umansky, 1980).

However, together with cohesion, the isolated small group experiences a sharp decrease of the influence of society due to the limited contacts. In fact, for the isolated crew, society means support group and group of confidants (family and friends), and they communicate with these groups by different information channels - mainly, audio communication channels in case of the support group and computer messages in case of the confidants. Consequently, the small group's communication turns from the full-fledged single-circuit communication into the limited two-circuit communication (Chart 3).

Further on (according to our information, in 4 to 6 weeks), the crew evolves as 'autonomy group' which is distinguished (according to Umansky, 1980) by the development of group identity, the construction of group rules, the rise of group cohesion and at the same time of separation. Potentialities of the group as a holistic entity increase, new tasks and goals appear which have evolved inside the group and might contradict those set up by society. In particular, Tuckman's research (Tuckman, 1965) points to such group evolution stages when group behavior which was originally generated by the need to resolve the problems of society generates a new type of behavior which is not induced directly by environment and is oriented to the group's own problems. This stage is certainly a higher stage of group evolution which enables the group to cope with emerging problems by themselves and it is a very important condition helping to cope with unfavorable environment in an expedition, space flight etc. On the other hand, owning to isolation and a decreased social control, there is a danger that the autonomy group may evolve into an unfavorable group form - 'corporation group' (Novikov, 1981, Umansky, 1980) which is distinguished by group egoism and aggressive behavior.

The problem is that specific living conditions in isolation, sensorial deprivation, monotony, involuntary communication, decrease of social control, public privacy speed up the coming of this stage of group evolution and aggravate its course. Describing communication of a group which have been acting autonomously for a long time, with an external group (a visiting crew), Novikov says that the autonomous group members experienced the feeling of being invaded and intruded on. No doubt, communication with the support group is experienced by the isolated small group less acutely, but sometimes the support group's attempts to make a closer contact might be regarded by the isolated group as intrusion.

The isolated crew perceives communication with the support group as imposed and tries to minimize it along with the general decrease of informational flows. On the other hand, they need to compensate for sensorial deprivation and monotony which they achieve through making informal contacts with the confidants more active. So, the need for socialization gradually specializes: the isolated group emphasizes not the quantity of communication, which gets smaller in connection with the general decrease of informational exchange in an environment poor in information, but the quality. In this sense, we can compare a group which has reached a high level of internal development to how a mature person who is getting older limits his or her interpersonal contacts and simultaneously makes models of his or her contacts more complex. At the group level, this is manifested in the emergence of the 'divided communication' phenomenon that we discovered: which means a decrease of communication with the support group, clear preferences with respect to communicator choice, filtration of information which the isolated group communicates outwards and at the same time intensification of contacts with the confidants.

	Stages of Group Evolution (according to L.I. Umansky, 1984)	*Communication Type*	*Kind of Interaction with Society*
Ground Group Training	1) Conglomerate Group	single-circuit communication 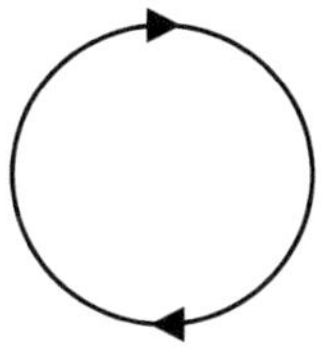	Open interaction with society
	2) Nominal Group		
	3) Association Group		
Orbital Flight	4) Cooperation Group (a well developed structure, a high level of cooperation – emerging in 4 to 6 weeks)	two-circuit communication 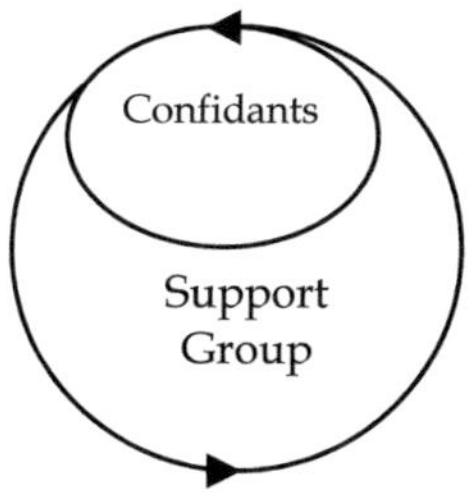	1. Isolation from the larger community. 2. The larger community disintegrates into the support group and the group of confidants. 3. Communication decreases.
	5) Autonomy Group (group identification, separation, joint effort)	two-circuit, divided communication 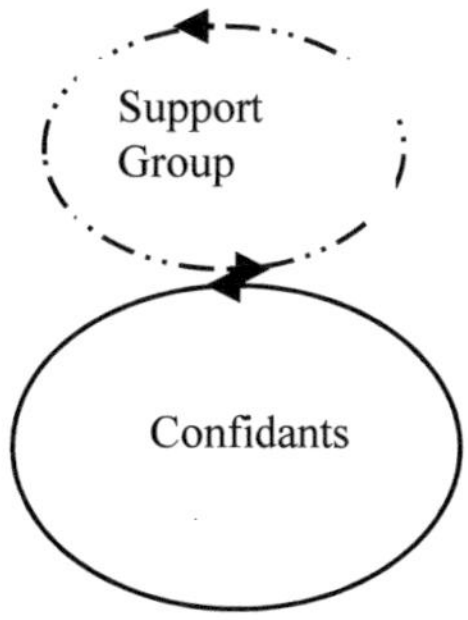	1. Decrease of social control. 2. Involuntary nature of communication.
Mission to Mars (a possible variant)	6) Corporation Group (group egoism, opposition, aggressivity)	No-circuit, monoreferential communication 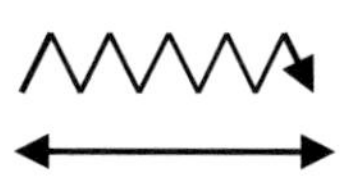	1. Delays in communication with Earth. 2. Absence of direct help of Earth.

Chart 3. Communication of isolated small group: ground training, flight on orbital space station, mission to Mars.

6.2 Remote communication as intergroup interaction

According to Tajfel (1978), the identification of oneself as a group member leads to the comparison of one's group and its members with other groups - and a further discrimination of other groups by the way of in-group favoritism and out-group hostility. This phenomenon emerges even if there are no objective contradictions or conflicting interests among the groups. In Ageev's view, this is related to the fact that the structure itself of intergroup activity contains factors reducing the adequacy of intergroup perception, which is the basis for in-group favoritism and out-group hostility. Adequacy of intergroup perception depends on the goals and values of joint intergroup activity, on criteria of evaluation of groups' achievements in such joint activity and, finally, on a group's success in an intergroup situations (Ageev, 1990).

The isolated group's interaction with the group of confidants is much simpler because this group is nominal or associated, that is to say that it is not so rigid, which facilitates communication. Moreover, in this communication circuit, a cosmonaut behaves as a group member to a much lesser degree and acts more like an individual. In communication with the confidants, a cosmonaut not only compensates for monotony, involuntary nature of contacts in space flight but also resolves the conflict between the growing aspiration to self-realization and self-assertion and the intensifying tendencies towards a person's involvement into the group structure and his or her integration into the group.

Extreme manifestations of intergroup problems may lead on to the development of group egoism, the aggravation of the small group's isolation from society, accompanied by a complete loss of mutual trust by the relevant groups against the background of the small group's monoreference, that is the isolated crew's orientation only to their own egocentric and eccentric (sometimes even delusive) ideas (Tuckman, 1965). A vicious circle occurs: autonomisation means that the isolated group orients itself not to the external but to the internal rules and ideas and try to get their own way in their communication with the outside world. They often do not find consent or understanding and therefore limit their external contacts, stop giving to the external communication parties information about what happens in isolation. Furthermore, the isolated group's contacts with the support group (and the correcting feedback) are limited by that the isolated group do not want to and have no need to speak with strangers which have different rules and ideas, while communication with the confidants is restricted due to rigorous operational limits.

In their turn, the support group which represent society do not have complete information about what happens onboard and have no possibility to give the crew really efficient recommendations to purposefully correct the crew's behavior. Therefore at the stage of the isolated group's autonomisation, due to the general decrease of the group's informational exchange with society, the limitedness of society's representation in communication circuit and the emergence of 'allotted communication', society forms an extreme difficulty in correcting the group's directedness so as this happens in usual conditions when social environment can constantly and efficiently optimize the functioning of a group which is open to the influence of society.

In this case, from an open exchange of relevant interpretations (Tuckman, 1965) which allows to gain an insight into the groups' intentions and to propose an alternative, communication turns into no-circuit, monoreferent when having no feedback, and each party communicates to the other some information which the other party cannot completely understand and therefore cannot respectively correct its behavior. In such situation, each group overtly demonstrates that their intentions and requirements do not meet the tasks set up by the other group in front of them, and an inevitable an intergroup conflict emerges.

6.3 Influence of adaptation to isolation and conformism

In case of the normal course of isolation (no accidents, illnesses etc.), the level of the crew's adaptation to difficult conditions rises. In this case, changes in communication, such as the increasing autonomisation should in our opinion be interpreted from the point of view of that the isolated group's judgments are influenced by judgments of the social majority (in this case represented by the Mission Control group). This is reflected by the socio-psychological phenomenon of conformity to group norms as defined by Homans and Asch (Homans, 1961, Asch, 1955). Social psychologists regard conformity not simply as a negative phenomenon, for it is often an expedient form of behavior facilitating the interaction process by providing an individual with behavioral standards acceptable to the group. Moreover, we think that the abidance by the group's behavioral standards is especially important for performing in extreme environment and is a condition for the conservation and survival of the isolated small group (Jetten, Postmes, McAuliffe, 2002).

In the period of acute adaptation to new extreme environment of isolation or space flight, there increases an uncertainty in evaluation of the actual situation. The objective criteria of such evaluation are vague due to an inadequately formed flight model. There emerges the state of internal uncertainty which makes a person more amenable to influences from outside. Experiencing a need to reduce this uncertainty, the crew actively communicates with Mission Control. Simultaneously, a person's amenability to opinions of the support group which help him or her to cope with hard conditions rises steeply.

However, the isolated group's competence grows in the course of flight, and with the lapse of time, they start to consider themselves to be not less and even more competent than the external majority with respect to a large part of situations onboard. They accumulated judgments stemming from their own experience and not learnt from other people. Such judgments are more stable and less exposed to change in case of being attacked. In the course of mastering the unfavorable environment, a person's self-esteem grows, and, as it is known that people with a high self-esteem prefer to keep to their opinions and do not easily yield to persuasion. Due to this, the need for recommendations from outside decreases as well as the original amenability to Mission Control opinions. Thus, the opposition to opinions from outside (the inconformity with respect to the external group) grows parallel to the growth of the small group's capabilities during group cohesion and adaptation to difficult conditions.

The degree of the small group's conformity depends on the size of the majority group (Asch, 1955). However, as we already mentioned, for the isolated group, society 'shrinks' to two rather small groups: the Mission Control group and the confidants group. With the decrease of the degree of the majority's pressure, the level of 'obedience' also decreases. Another factor fostering autonomization is a group heterogeneity. It is well known that homogeneous groups are more conform than heterogeneous ones. We can presume that the International Space Station crew that are heterogeneous in terms of nationality, gender and profession, will be less exposed to pressure of society than national crews of the past generation of space stations.

Therefore, as we pointed out, in isolation, the pressure both of physical and regulatory social information on isolated small group decreases due to a restricted number of communicators and of a restricted volume and diversity of communication. In this case, the opposition to the external pressure originally related to some operational aspects due to a higher competence of the isolated group in this respect may turn into the opposition to behavioral norms imposed by society. This opposition can be disguised as the so called public conformity, a demonstration of a socially acceptable reaction stereotype of the type "we are all right", while this attitude changes in private contacts with the confidants. In case of a further evolution of a group's inconformity, anti-social behavior can appear (such a degraded hygiene status) all the way to an open protest.

6.4 Unfavorable manifestations of remote communication

The 'psychological closing' and 'autonomy in communication' phenomena identified by us reflect the combined influence of isolation and intra-group and intergroup dynamics on communication. A high degree of 'psychological closing' in communication may lead on to decreased informational flows coming from the isolated group, to the filtering of outgoing information by the group especially with respect to problematic situations and also to a reduction of the number of external communicators with whom the isolated group wants to interact. Extreme manifestations of 'autonomy in communication' mean that the isolated group constantly defends their point of view, tries to impose the in-group beliefs (and even prejudices) onto the external communicators, and confronts them. Under such conditions, the outside group's attempts to regulate the isolated small group's behavior will be regarded by the isolated small group as invasion, aggression which should be immediately fended off.

An extreme evolution of the above phenomena is dangerous because as a result, the support group will not have enough information to take adequate decisions and help the isolated small group. And even the confidants trusted by the isolated crew and thus obliged to be less critical, will have more information but still this information will be distorted by the crew's prejudices. Therefore, some operational proposals and decisions of Earth (Mission Control) based on such insufficient or distorted information, might be inefficient and can aggravate a difficult situation, making the support group's authority seem even lower in the eyes of the crewmembers. More than that, the support group's attempts to interfere with the crew's affairs, being inadequate due to the lack of knowledge of the situation onboard, might aggravate the confrontation and as a consequence, the crew might refuse to fulfill Mission Control's instructions, ignore Mission Control's opinions as this has already happened in long-term space flights (e.g, the 'Skylab' strike).

The USSR practice of space crews communication was organized in the way that principal Mission Control operators communicating with space crews were themselves members of cosmonaut corps. Therefore, space crews mainly communicated with people well known to them who had similar experience in life and profession. This approach ensured a greater confidence and mutual understanding of communicators. However, more complex flight programs expanded the circle of contacts with which space crew had to communicate. Cosmonauts have to speak to scientists and specialists little known to them or completely unfamiliar. So the role of cosmonaut corps members as mediators between space crews and Earth substantially reduced. The problem of ensuring confidence in space crew communication arose again and space crews' refusals to speak to certain interlocutors became more frequent.

Communication through a closed confidential channel has always been an important operational factor in space flight. Private psychological conferences began to be also used in flights on ISS. So cosmonauts and astronauts gained an opportunity to speak about their problems and drain their negative energy outwards without being afraid that this might harm their reputations and carriers. However, like in the above case, the problem of ensuring the full-fledged communication has been resolved only partially. The confidants are bound by written confidentiality obligations to keep secret information received through the closed channel. This does not allow to use such private information to improve a space crew's activity and state and resolve their problems.

At present, the problem of intergroup communication of space crews on ISS is aggravated by the presence of two national Mission Control Centers each of which speak mainly with their national astronauts and cosmonauts onboard. As a result, each MCC has only a part of information and only a partial notion of the whole picture of what happens on ISS, distorted by the national and culture-bound prejudices of their national crewmember. In the long run, such practice cannot but lead on to a confrontation of MCCs since their opinions on one or another issue might be based on somewhat different input data.

6.5 Problem of remote communication in mission to Mars

The problems mentioned above will be especially significant during preparation and implementation of a manned mission to Mars - the most promising of space projects existing now, which attracts public attention worldwide. The key feature of a mission to Mars is the space crew autonomy. It means in the first place that the crew will not receive help from Earth, including an immediate evacuation of a crew member in case of emergency, a resupply of resources (water, oxygen, food, devices etc.). They will have to use only resources available onboard (including informational resources) and fall back on their own strengths and ability to make their own decisions in extreme conditions. The autonomous nature of such mission combined with the well known features of space crews' communication may quite complicate the 'onboard - Earth' contacts.

We think that this together with delays in communication may lead on to a reduction of the Earth's controlling role in the course of the flight. MCC should switch from the function of controlling the crew to the function of consulting the crew. That is to say that in the past 40 years, the dominating strategy of ground services was to daily instruct space crews and set up tasks for them. Now ground services should provide space crews with informational support based on requests coming from onboard and do this in the maximally friendly and unobtrusive manner. The big Mission Control Center and the small crew should find new common goals and try to achieve them on the basis of a full-fledged partnership and not of subordination as this happens now.

Stylistic features of MCCs' communication will be very important for the establishment of equality and cooperation in interaction of MCCs and space crews. First of all, such communication should be based on mutual confidence established before flight and maintained during the whole expedition. Besides that, the Earth's communicative style should be concordant and meet the actual needs of the isolated crew in terms of communication volume and content. All this will require a significant modification of the current concept of the 'onboard - Earth' communication as well as a principally new communication training of Mission Control operators. Operators should be involved in the process of the ground psychological preparation of the crew, participate together with the crew in group trainings of communication, conflict settlement, they should establish solid confidential relationships with the crew.

7. Conclusion

We regard communication as a certain sort of professional activity. During space flights, crewmembers have to be in contact with ground personnel, as well as they have to do their job. Communication is one of the main channels of information from the crew. Still, there are certain regulations of verbal behaviour and professional vocabulary, elaborated for fast information transmission.

Since communication is regarded as a professional activity, we can admit, that its analysis would let us make estimates about its effectiveness - indirectly, without going deeper into operational aspects. Then, it becomes possible to manage informational exchange by means of personnel and crewmembers' communication trainings. Choosing the right staff, from one side, and reducing conflict tension from the other side leads to rise and support of trust and openness in informational exchange. This point is especially important in interplanetary missions, as an effective informational exchange would result in adequate and correct decisions on Earth as well as in the space crews.

Communication process in space flights does not come to pure informational exchange. It is a psychosocial process and a source of information about personality and its mood. Psychological support in the present case is to ensure the psychological comfort through communication process and to obtain data about crewmembers' psychological state.

8. References

[1] Asch S.E. Opinions and social pressures // Scientific American, v. 193, 1955.

[2] Bales, R.F. Interaction Process Analysis: A Method for the Study of Small Groups. Addison-Wesley Press, 1950.

[3] Gazenko O. G., Myasnikov V.I., Uskov F.N. Behavioral Control as a Tool in Evaluating the Functional State of Cosmonauts in Flight. In: Aviat. Space Environ. Med., v. 47, pp. 1226-1227, 1976.

[4] Grigoriev A.I., Kozerenko O.P., Myasnikov V.I. Selected Problems of Psychological Support of Prolonged Space Flights. In: Proceedings of the 38th Congress of the IAF, Papers IAF 86-398, AIAA, Washington, 1986.
[5] Jetten, J., Postmes, T., & McAuliffe, B. J. We're all individuals: Group norms of individualism and collectivism, levels of identification, and identity threat. European Journal of Social Psychology, 32, 189-207, 2002.
[6] Krippendorff, K. Content Analysis: An Introduction to Its Methodology. Newbury Park, CA: Sage, 1980.
[7] Myers D.G., Lamm H. The group polarization phenomenon // Psychological bulletin, v.83, 1976.
[8] Tajfel H. Experiments in intergroup discrimination // ScientificAmerican, 1970, v 223.
[9] Ageev, V.S. Mezhgruppovoe vzaimodeistvie: socialno-psihologicheskie problemy. Moscow, 1981.
[10] Vinokur, T.G. Govoryashii i slushajushii: Varianty rechevogo povedeniya. Moscow, 2007.
[11] Kelly A.D., Kanas N. Communication between space crews and ground personnel: a survey of astronauts and cosmonauts. Aviat Space Environ Med 1993; 64: 795-800.
[12] Gushin, V. Problems of psychological control in prolonged space flight // Earth Space Review. 1995, vol 4 #1.
[13] Gushin V.I., Zaprisa N.S., Kolinichenko T.B. et al. Dinamika communicativnogo vzaimodeistviya ekipazha s vneshnimi abonentami v usloviyah dlitelnoi izolyacii // Aviakosmicheskaya i ekologicheskaya medicina. 1997. #4.
[14] Leonov, A.A., Lebedev, V.I. Psichologicheskie problem mezhplanetnogo poleta. Moscow, 1975.
[15] Distancionnoe nabludenie i expertnaya ocenka: obschenie i communicatsiya v zadachah medicinskogo kontrolya. Ed.: Myasnikov V.I. Moscow, Nauka, 1982.
[16] Myasnikov V.I., Zamaletdinov I.S. Psihicheskoe sostoyanie i gruppovoe vzaimodeistvie kosmonavtov v polete // Kosmicheskaya biologiya i medicina. Vol.3. Chelovek v kosmicheskom polete. Book 2, chapter 19. Moscow, Nauka, 1997.
[17] Problema psichicheskoi astenizatsii v dlitelnom kosmicheskom polete. Eds.: V.I. Myasnikov, S.I. Stepanova. Moscow, 2000.
[18] Orbitalnaya stanciya Mir: kosmicheskaya biologiya i medicina. Vol.1 and 2. Ed.: Grigoriev A.I. Moscow, IMBP, 2002.
[19] Novikov M.A. Psihofiziologicheskie i ekopsihologicheskie aspekty mezhlichnostnogo vzaimodeistviya v avtonomnyh usloviyah // Problema obsheniya v psihologii. Moscow, 1981.
[20] Umansky, L.I. Psihologiya organizatorskoi deyatelnosti. Moscow, 1980.
[21] Shadrikov V.D. Problema systemogeneza v professionalnoi deyatelnosti. Moscow, Nauka, 1983.

[22] Yusupova A.K., Gushin V.I., Popova I.I. Obshenie v konture bort-Zemlya: socialno-psihologicheskie aspect // Aviakosmicheskaya i ekologicheskaya medicina. 2006. Vol.40. #3.

12

Group's Positions and Language Use: The Connection Between *Themata* and *Topic Grounds* (Lexical Worlds)

Laura Camara Lima
Universidade Federal de São Paulo - UNIFESP (Federal University of São Paulo)
Brazil

1. Introduction

This chapter intends to study the way different categories of individuals, implicated in a debate involving a given social object, take position one in relation to the other and each of them in relation to such an object focusing on how they use language to communicate to one another. The link of correspondence consists in associating two concepts: topic grounds (or lexical worlds), which emerge from the method of pragmatic analysis named Alceste (Reinert, 1990, 1993, 1999), as well as themata defined by the Theory of Social Representations (Moscovici & Vignaux, 1994). The goals are: get information about the controversies that intensify the relationships among groups, reveal how these relationships (often asymmetrical) determine the use of the lexicon and the communication and identify the themata which are contained in the lexical worlds. In order to illustrate the validity and the relevance of the transpositions proposed here the results of an empirical study are described.

Keywords: Themata, Topic ground, Social Representations, Alceste, Pragmatic analysis, Intergroup relations;

This paper proposes a conceptual device to social psychologists interested in studying the connections between intergroup relations, inter-individual communication, speech production and the formation of social representations. The referred device is a pragmatic approach to language, conceived to clarify the way in which different categories of individuals, implicated in a symbolic exchange (involving a given social object) take positions, one in relation to the other and each one in relation to such an object. This clarification will be produced through the analysis of the manner in which individuals use language to communicate to one another.

The starting point consists of associating two theoretical concepts: themata and topic grounds. Themata were first defined by Holton (1973), in his philosophical and empirical work on the history of science, and later defined by Moscovici and Vignaux (1994) and Marková (2003), in their social psychological work on communication, language and social representations. Topic grounds were conceived by Reinert (1990, 1993, 1999, 2001a) in his "pragmatist" approach to language and assimilated to the concept of lexical worlds which

Reinert defined (empirically) using the method of pragmatic analysis of text he created and named ALCESTE (Analyse des Lexèmes Cooccurrents dans un Ensemble de Segments de Texte) (Reinert, 1990, 1993, 1999, 2001).

The association, themata - topic grounds, is legitimate and twice relevant: a) it makes possible the realization of a practical application of the concept of themata and b) it allows a better theoretical exploration of the concept of topic grounds. Indeed, until now, these two complementary possibilities have not been sufficiently exploited, considering their potential heuristic power. Furthermore, this connection can be a useful conceptual device, providing means to find out and demonstrate the correspondence between two levels of communication: representational and relational.

Once this connection is established, social psychologists would be able to understand: a) how different individuals or groups take positions in a symbolic exchange involving a given social object; and b) how the different positions taken by the different individuals or groups will reactivate existent themata, adapting them to the present situation (here and now). From this moment onwards, the production of social representations will be triggered.

2. Themata

The philosopher of science Gerald Holton (1973) is the first scientist (in the history of science) to come out (in the seventies) with the conception and definition of themata. Based on his empirical and theoretical work, Holton (1988, p. 13-14) demonstrated that the scientific imagination is often constrained by "fundamental preconceptions of a stable and widely diffused kind that are not resolvable into or derivable from observation and analytic ratiocination". According to Holton (1988, p. 3), themata belong not merely to a pool of specifically scientific ideas, but spring from the more general ground of imagination. They guide the minds of the scientists towards certain theories, rather then others. Holton (1988, p. 16) was able to distinguish three categories of themata influencing the development of scientific knowledge: a) Thematic concepts, which are those having a significant projection on the thematic dimension.

However, purely thematic concepts are difficult to find; they seem to be rare in established science. Holton set up a solution to overcome this difficulty, which consists in taking concepts, such as force and inertia, which have strong components (contingents and thematics) and study them focusing mainly on their thematic components; b) Thematic positions, which are those that guide scientists in the pursuit of their scientific work. These also called Methodological themata (such as preference for analysis or for syntheses), determinate how scientists conceive and do research; c) Thematic propositions, which are those that give the starting point to or form the core of the scientific theories. These, also called thematic hypotheses are, for example: the principles of special relativity or the way in which scientists express the laws of physics (in terms of constancies, or maxima and minima, or impotency). These three categories of themata can be related in the following way: a thematic proposition contains one or more thematic concepts and is a product of a methodological thema.

In the 1990s, Moscovici and Vignaux (1994) redefined the concept of themata, adapting it to the social psychological approach to language they were developing at that time. For

Moscovici and Vignaux (1994, p. 64), the notion of theme designates the configuration of a common field composed of ordinary knowledge and available significations shared by individuals or groups. Themes are epistemic systems, which are related to general and essential properties attributed to categories of objects of the world. In this new epistemological context, the notion of themata will refer to "frames of thinking" which are dependent on "systems of belief", which are anchored in values, traditions and images of the world and of the being. According to Moscovici and Vignaux (1994, p. 35), these "frames of thinking" are composed of "source-ideas" or "force-ideas" which motivate and command the social functioning of the speech, imposing "common ideas" to be adopted or, at least, accepted. Themata function in the same way then as topoï, which are "places of commonsense", which can be anchored: in the perceptible world, in the popular knowledge and in the ritualistic experience (Moscovici & Vignaux, 1994, p. 37). In Moscovici's theory, social representations are defined as being syntheses of knowledge, which are spontaneously produced by the members of a group, grounded on consensus and tradition. Social representations are situated between popular knowledge (comprised of beliefs and know-how, coming from the natural thinking) and scientific knowledge (comprised of systems of explanation, coming from the rational thinking), which are ideologically, logically or methodologically organized by the authorities (political or scientific). Social representations neither trigger off conducts nor guide them directly. They propose "figures and shapes", by means of which concrete social relations can find their expression. Moscovici (1961, p. 304) assumed that the degree of engagement subjects have in relation to different social objects necessarily varies. In his empirical work, Moscovici (1961, p. 314) observed that individuals and groups usually give, in a spontaneous manner, more attention to some particular zones of the lexical environment than others. The language style subjects will employ will change according to: the place from where they are producing their speech, to the particular perspective they are focusing on, to the kind of social relations they have with the other subjects and to whom they are communicating.

The oppositional nature of the mental processes (comprised of perception, thinking, knowledge and language) has always interested the social psychologist Ivana Marková. More recently, she has been investigating social objects such as: AIDS (Marková, 2000), democracy (Marková, Moodie & Plichtovà, 1998) and individual (Marková, Moodie, Farr, Drozda-Senlowska, Erös, Plichtová, Gervais, Hoffmannová & Mulerová, 1998), using the paradigm of social representations. She found out that when some contradictions are explicitly expressed within the social thinking, they are converted into (what she called) fundamental themata. From this moment they become able to generate social representations. We conclude that the production of social representations is dependent on a dynamic exchange of theses, through which themata are (locally or universally) negotiated. These exchanges reactivate the intergroup relations, motivate parts to communicate and increase the production of speech or text, keeping (by these means) the formation of social representations going on. Different theses exist because different individuals or groups take different positions in relation to one another and to social objects. On the contrary, themata are quite often the same establishing families of social representations. As Holton (1988, p. 17) showed, they exist in limited number (a total of fewer than fifty couples or triads) and have a long life, since only occasionally it seems necessary to introduce a qualitatively new one into science. Generally, as Holton observed, the old themata in a new context do surprisingly well.

In short, each family of social representations is related to a "frame of thinking" (themata), which refers to a "place of enunciation", whose topology influence (determinates) the semantic production. These attributes are those that inspired and legitimated the idea of connecting themata to topic grounds.

3. Topic grounds (lexical worlds)

The statistician specialized in semiotics and psychoanalyses, Max Reinert, formulated the concept of topic grounds in the frame of his "pragmatistic" approach to language (which is generally applied to social sciences). Reinert (2001b, p. 34) started from the observation that in every text or speech there are "associative grounds" operating. He decided to call them Topic grounds, because he considered that their "association" was mainly a result of the fact they have the same topic of origin. Topic grounds are kinds of "places" which are original and archaic, functioning as sources of "semiosis" or "sign-activity" (Peirce, 1978). They must be considered, simultaneously, in their "internal coherence" and in their "contrast" in relation to other "places". These places are linked to the activities of the subjects who "inhabit" them. If these subjects are more than one, then these places will be "commonplaces" (marked and highlighted by social inscriptions). The ancient Greek rhetoric used to call these "places" topoï, defining them as "a grouping of strategies or probes for exploring a subject or developing an argument". Commonplaces (in Latin: locus communis; in Greek: koinos topos) signify the orienting experiences or modalities, which serve to anchor or reference different subjects within the experience of making meaning (together). The study of these commonplaces enable social psychologists to reach the cultural core of social representations, which are shared images, scripts, cognitions and singular habits or rituals, which mark the collective practices, generating a singular use of language and a particular choice of vocabulary.

In his pragmatic approach to language, Reinert considers that enunciations (which are contained in a speech act or text production) are kinds of theater scenes, in which three elements are acting: "lexical worlds", "subjects" (of enunciation) and "local logics". Lexical worlds are defined as being, at the same time, vestiges of places of reference and signs of forms of coherence. These forms of coherence, also named "local logics", are linked to the acts of language of the subjects of enunciation. According to Reinert (1993, p. 12) lexical worlds superimpose, in the same "place", different points of view, or different subjects' activities in their different moments. For Reinert (1993) a "point of view" is a position (here and now) of a subject of enunciation (speaker) which is dependent on a "world", but which is more conscious and more immediate than a "world". A "world" being a more stable and more permanent position ("commonplace" or "general view"), which is more unconscious (because automatic) than an individual point of view. So, Lexical worlds are kinds of stable structures (distribution of words into the unities of text), which take form and remain, in spite of the local instabilities, which characterize the single enunciation. Furthermore, topic grounds are dynamic structures, which express conflicts resulting from the opposed positions taken by one or more subjects (of enunciation). Reinert realized that these conflicts leave traces that stay "printed" in the topology of the text, composing the relief of the topic grounds. In order to study this relief, he created the software ALCESTE. This program of automatic lexical analyses was conceived to examine the text, track the traces of tensions, detect the lexical worlds and make their cartography.

The program is capable of identifying what Reinert (1993, p. 13) named lexical worlds and describe as being "spaces of reference, statistically defined, associated to a big number of enunciations". Lexical worlds are dynamic structures, which refer to the movement of alternation between two (or three) antagonistic orientations, each one of which trying to impose a particular "point" to the others. This "point" is not only an opinion or an argument; moreover it is an entire "position", regarding relational issues (which always involve others parts and a prized social object).

In order to investigate the lexical worlds, which are present in the text, ALCESTE's algorithm operates in the following steps. Firstly, it identifies all the "full words" that are present in the text and reduces them to their radical (lexicon). Reinert named "full words" as those that are "full of sense", meaningful by themselves, independently of others' words; namely: names, adjectives, adverbs, numbers, etc. In opposition, he named "tool words" as those words whose sense is dependent on (or relative to) the sense of others' words; namely: articles, propositions, pronouns, auxiliary verbs, etc. These "full words" are counted by ALCESTE and used for calculations with which it comes across the clusters and the factorial plans. The "tool words" are not considered in the calculations, but they are projected in the clusters and factorial analyses, in order to give complementary information. Secondly, the algorithm splits the text in many equal size parts, which Reinert called as "unities of context". In order to establish, empirically, the best size of these unities we must have, as ALCESTE does previously, some estimations. The definition of this ideal size (tailored to fit the text) is done automatically, based on two criteria. The first criteria, consists of using the punctuations marks, which the text come with, and the breaks which separate phrases, paragraphs, chapters of the texts and different texts. The parts resulting from this first fragmentation, Reinert calls, the "initial unities of context" (i.u.c.). The second criteria, consists in counting a certain number of full words (determined by means of tests), in order to split the text into parts. Crossing these two criteria, Reinert obtains what he named "elementary unities of context" (e.u.c.) and defined as being the smallest statistical unities the program uses to operate the statistical calculations. Thirdly, the algorithm verifies the presence of "full words" in these "elementary unities of context" and considers their relative distribution by mapping groups of words. Finally, making specific statistical calculations, ALCESTE detects the clusters and the factors (related to theses clusters), which better represent the lexical topology.

In sum, the algorithm's capabilities are the following: a) it studies the distribution of full words and comes out with a cartography of them b) it detects the zones of greatest contrast; and c) it identifies the full words that better characterize the vocabulary employed by different subjects in different localities of the text (these localities being very similar to the "commonplaces" referred by the classic notion of topoï). ALCESTE's output is a report that can be very useful. It contains resources that facilitate the visualization and the knowledge of the topology of the text: a) graphics that represent the structure of the clusters (lexical worlds) based on how and where they get apart one from the other; b) a summary of the lexical contents of each cluster (lexical world); and c) a factorial plan that summarizes the opposition of each factor (axes) is composed and the dynamic relations that keeps the multiple factors apart and perpendicular to one another. The most important advantage the program presents (in relation to others), is the possibility to establish a correspondence between the relational and the lexical levels. This possibility comes from the acknowledgment of two kinds of isomorphism: a) between lexical worlds and subjective positions: both isotopic; b) between factors and themata: both bipolar. For all these capabilities, ALCESTE can be considered a helpful tool to social psychologists interested in mapping and understanding the lexical topology of a text.

4. Themata and topic grounds: The same properties

Themata have topological properties: a) they can be assimilated to fields (of knowledge) and to topoï (places of commonsense); b) they behave according to a geometry of position (mostly, than a spatial one); so, in order to approach them adequately, the researcher must consider: the relations between all the elements, the morphological proprieties of the sets and the analysis of the situation; c) they have a topological orientation mainly; so, in order to identify and understand them, the researcher must analyze the contrasts and the tensions between groups of words (more than the distances between single words). Topic grounds, as they were named and defined by Reinert, have topological properties as well. They are kinds of "places" or more exactly "commonplaces" which compose the topology of the text.

Themata are primitive conceptions, images and categories, which are culturally shared in social and historical contexts and can be transmitted, from a generation to the next, during a long period of time; this transmission has been done through the collective memory (Markovà, 2000). Topic grounds are "places" that are "archaic", "original", "linked to the topic origin" (Reinert, 1993, 1999). These two concepts emanate from the deepest level of language's production, where sense and knowledge are one (and the same). Both have epistemic properties.

Themata are dynamic structures, which are composed of two opposed sides, defined one in relation to the other. Topic grounds also have a dynamic nature. The presence or absence of a lexicon (full word) in a statement (unity of context) or the way in which subjects use words in different statement sets (simultaneously, successively or alternatively), can modify the formation of topic grounds. Both concepts are sensitive to the slightest change in the lexical context.

Themata are axes composed of two opposed poles; their dynamic force comes from the alternative domination of one pole in relation to the other. In their turn, topic grounds are also founded on the dynamic movement of alternation between antagonistic orientations, which are repeatedly reiterated in the speech or text. Both concepts are dyadic.

There is a movement, in the basis of themata, whose dynamism is created by the materialization of some forms (constantly reiterated) and by the emergence of some postulates. Moscovici and Vignaux (1994, p. 68) explained that these postulates are anchored in beliefs, which operate and express themselves by means of couples of notions which integrate two opposed visions into one. Reinert got to the same conclusion in relation to topic grounds. He observed that their dynamics is created on the basis of confrontations of two or three antagonistic orientations of the subjects of enunciation.

5. An example of empirical research: EDF and its "deprived clients"

The demonstration of the common characteristics of the concepts, done above, constitutes sufficient evidence of the pertinence of the connection between themata (collective imaginary level) and topic grounds (language level). Now, it is time to explain how this connection can be applied to the study of a specific speech or text, produced in a definite social reality. The outcome of an empirical research will be presented here in order to illustrate the mentioned connection. This particular research was chosen because its results are exemplary, for the purpose of the demonstration that must be done. The example is deliberately a very simple one, because the goal is not to report the results of this particular study, but to explain the method and the form of the pragmatic analysis that was done. The text is relatively small, the object is not complex and the method is not sophisticated. The reason for taking this option is that simplicity allows to see, more clearly, the main lines of the demonstration and to increase the possibility to reach a systemic comprehension.

The referred research was realized in a specific institutional context, which is: the Research & Development (R&D) division of a French national company called Electricité de France (EDF). This important multi-national is responsible for the totality of the production, transportation, distribution and commercialization of electric power in France. EDF was, in its beginnings (in the fifties), a national company of public service. More recently, in 2004, EDF (the company) became an anonymous society and EDF (the group) opened its capital to international investments and to the Stock Exchange Market.

The data (that are presented here) are the results of an investigation, realized in 1998, in the sociology department of the Research & Development division. This department, called (at that time) GRETS, was specialized in internal research concerning social psychological issues that are related to agents and clients of the company. At that occasion, the sociologists of the GRETS were studying how a new service was valued by a particular population of clients, for whom it was created. These clients were identified as being the "impoverished" clients (clients démunis), because they did not afford to pay the electricity bill (for different reasons, comprised of: unemployment, illness, debts, or other financial or personal problems) and contracted debts in relation to the company. The sociological profile of these clients was as follows: Most of them belonged to a non-favored population of individuals having: low levels of study, low qualifications, no money, no stable job or no job at all. They could not count on their parents or families and they did not have other means of getting financial resources to help them pay their debts. Some of them had some kind of allowance or social benefit, but most of them would have liked to have more financial support and more assistance to come out of this deficient situation. The service of "electric power maintenance" (SEPM) was instituted in 1994, to give these "impoverished" clients a minimum provision of electric power in order to avoid power cuts. Actually, the families who had passed through power cuts before remember them as very unpleasant. So the service was conceived to maintain only a minimum of electric power provision, to keep rooms lit and electrical devices working. The limitation was that the high consumption devices (for example: the electrical shower or the washcloths machine) could not be used at the same time otherwise the electric power provision was interrupted. This was a way to restrain the amount of electric power that they used. So, with the purpose of knowing the "impoverished" clients better, the sociologists created a questionnaire in order to discover their clients' "needs", to obtain their "image" of EDF and its services in general and to obtain their "evaluations" of the "electric power maintenance" service. They also intended to find out how they had experienced, if it was the case, the situation of having an electric power cut in their place. The questionnaire was composed of 50 questions (of which 6 were open responses and 44 were multiple-choice ones), which were thought to accomplish two goals basically: a) to measure how informed these clients were about technical subjects, such as the electric power consumption of the electrical devices, the price of electric power, the different rates during day and night, or the good habits to acquire in order to save electricity; and b) to measure how satisfied these clients were with EDF, in terms of the efficiency of its services, the availability of information, the accessibility of its agencies and the methods and policies of the company. Every year, the sociologists employed a survey institute (called Laval) to send interviewers to interrogate these clients, using the questionnaire they conceived for this purpose. In 1998, a sample of 567 subjects was interviewed, which was representative of the population of "impoverished" clients. The data treated in this paper comes from this survey.

The results described below are only a part of the output of the inquiry. They concern, exclusively, to the answers given to the very last question of the mentioned questionnaire; the other questions of the questionnaire were not considered because they are not needed for the demonstration that we are interested in doing here. This final question was an open response one, which was formulated like this: "Finally, I invite you to make all remarks or suggestions that you would like to make, in particular to those regarding the services offered by EDF". The researchers of the sociology department were disappointed because they didn't have the feedback they were expecting to, neither in terms of form, neither in terms of content. They thought they were giving to their clients the "opportunity" to express their opinions, needs and evaluations. Instead, the answers given to the questionnaire in general and also to this question were very short, most of them laconic. This is the reason that explains why the corpus (containing the totality of the responses) is a relatively small one, counting 57000 characters and 13634 words. Besides, the responses were poor, in terms of the contents. The two most frequent replies given were: "I don't know", "I don't have anything else to say about it", which probably indicate that (when questioned) the subjects did not feel like communicating their opinion (either showing their lack of interest or knowledge) on the matter. This resistance could come from the end-of-questionnaire effect, which made the subjects to concentrate less and thus less collaborative. However, we had the occasion to find out empirical evidence to prove that these are not the only reasons for the presence of this negative attitude towards the interviewer and its questions.

The mentioned occasion was that, being specialists in text analyses using the program ALCESTE, we were invited by the sociologists of the GRETS to sign a temporary research contract with EDF. Our mission was to realize a pragmatic analysis of the answers given by the deprived clients to the six open questions of the mentioned questionnaire. However here we are discussing only the responses to the last question (as described above). Having studied ALCESTE's output (clusters and factorial graphics), we were able to understand that what "prevents" these "deprived" clients to provide longer and more detailed information about their difficulties, their situation, or their opinion is the asymmetry that characterizes the relations they have with EDF. The analyses described below will substantiate and explain this statement.

6. Results

The corpus (in the basis of which the analysis commented here were done) was composed of a set of short answers, which were given by the 567 "deprived" clients interviewed to the last question of the questionnaire (mentioned above). The program found out three stable clusters. Together these clusters explain what occurs within 72% of the elementary unities of context of the corpus text. This percentage indicates that it is a good analysis, since only less then a third part of the elementary unities of context is not explained by the output (clusters and factors).

The graphic below shows the results of the analysis. The lines of the diagram represent the moments in which they get apart (in relation to a ruler on top). The cluster number two is separated from the cluster numbers one and three. The number of elementary unities of context (euc) indicates the size of each one: the larger one (322 euc) is twice bigger than the two others put together; the two smaller ones have more or less equivalent sizes (85 and 72 euc).

```
                     |----|----|----|----|----|----|----|----|----|----|
Cluster 1  (85 euc)  |---------------+
                                     |-------------------------------+
Cluster 3  (72 euc)  |---------------+                               |
                                                                     +
Cluster 2  (322 euc) |-----------------------------------------------+
```

Graph 1. The three clusters detected by ALCESTE; the corpus was composed of the responses given by 567 «impoverished clients», to the last question of the questionnaire formulated by EDF in 1998.

With the intention of having a right comprehension of these clusters and to produce a correct interpretation of their sense, we followed the enlightenments of the program's creator. According to Reinert's (2001a, p. 10), the clusters (lexical worlds) can be analyzed from three different points of view: a) They can be considered as contents, when one observes the list of specific words that they enclose; b) They can be considered as activities, when one becomes conscious of the undercover tensions that made them separate, one from the other; c) They can be considered as representations, when one realizes that each one of them reflects a certain stabilization of the subject's activities and that the three of them form a system. This possibility of triple interpretation is an evidence of the complexity and richness of the lexical worlds (or topic grounds). This is the link that makes it possible to operate the connection between topic grounds (that Alceste will find) and themata (social psychologists are looking for): themata have the same three dimensions - semantic, dialectic, systemic - that of the lexical worlds (or topic grounds). Themata are contents, because they are equivalent to the properties (general and essential), which are attributed to the categories of objects of the world. Themata are activities because they determinate classes of argumentation. Themata are (linked to) representations because they are places of commonsense, frames of thinking and systems of belief.

7. The contents of the clusters: The lexical worlds

In order to examine the three clusters from the point of view of their contents, we checked out the list of words, which each one of them contain, giving special attention to the most significant ones (those with highest chi²). Having studied these lists of words we were able to acquire a comprehension of the different lexical worlds and to give them a name.

The first lexical world contains these words related to the consumption of electric power; the words are translated in English from the French form (without accent) cited in italic in parentheses; they are cited in decreasing order of importance in relation to their chi^2: "to count" (compter) (71), "electrical devices" (appareil) (37), "verifying" (verifier) (28), "hour" (heure) (27), "installation" (installation) (27), "reading the meter" (relever le compteur) (24), "gas" (gaz) (18), "to reduce" (reduire) (18), "to do" (faire) (15). So, this lexical world received the name Consumption accounting. In this cluster we found out the following dichotomies: "full" (plein) (19) - "empty" (creux) (19), which are the qualities of the hour of the day which determine the rate of the electrical power; "pay attention to" (attentif) (46) - "not pay attention to" (pas attentif), the consumption; "expensive" (cher) (31) - "not expensive" (pas cher), the price of the electric power.

The second lexical world contains the following words, cited in the decreasing order of chi^2: "service" (service) (15), "EDF" (11), "people" (gens) (11), "to be kind" (aimable) (9), "to find out" (trouver) (9), "solution" (solution) (9), "contact" (contact) (9), "problem" (probleme) (8), "understanding" (comprehensif) (8), "help" (aide) (8), "telephone" (telephone) (8), "social" (social) (7), "to try" (essayer) (7), "to pay" (payment) (7), "human" (humain) (6), "to cut" (couper) (5), "to accept" (accepter) (5), "to go" (aller) (5). These words are related to the way (frequently negative) in which the impoverished clients experience their relations with the agents who receive them at the agencies of the company. It is to them that they have (between other things): to explain their personal problems, to complain about a technical problem and, eventually, to negotiate their debts and to claim back a suppressed service. In a big number of cases, the clients blame the agents, complaining about their lack of respect, attention, comprehension, mind opening. What these clients really expected EDF (and its agents) to do was to show more "goodwill" in relation to the search of alternative solutions, since they feel themselves incapable of finding other resources. The solutions that the impoverished clients would expect that EDF propose to them were (basically): more delay to pay the debts, more financial help from social and assistance funds, or still a big discount on their electric bills. So, this lexical world received the name of Contact agent - client. In this cluster we found out the following dichotomies: "social" (social) (7) - "financial" (financier) (2), "human" (humain) (6) - "inhuman", "personal" (personnel) (3) - "impersonal" (impersonnel).

The third lexical world contains words linked to the disproportion between the high price of the electric bill and the low income of the impoverished clients, such as (cited in the decreasing order of chi^2): "month" (mois) (100), "bill" (facture) (71), "to pay" (payer) (56), "to spend (depenser)" (45), "end" (fin) (34), (revenu) (31), "to go out" (sortir) (29), "really" (vraiment) (29), "to know" (savoir) (27), "to want" (vouloir) (14), "to love" (aimer) (13), "debts" (dettes) (11), "price" (prix) (11), "to exceed" (depasser) (11), "to display" (etaler) (11), "to allow" (permettre) (11), "to receive" (recevoir) (10), "to look for" (chercher) (10), "level" (niveau) (10). So, this lexical world received the name of Big bill, little income. In this cluster we found out the follow dichotomies: "big (gros) (18) - small (petit) (21)", "to pay (payer) (56) - to consume (consommer) (45)".

8. The dynamics between lexical worlds: The factors

In order to examine the three lexical worlds from the point of view of the activities, we studied the position of the clusters in relation to the two factors, which compose the factorial plan. In relation to the first one (horizontal), the cluster Contact agent - client is in the left side and the two other clusters are in the right side. So this factor was named Relational - Material factor. In relation to the second one (vertical), the cluster Consumption control is in the top side and the cluster Big bill, little income is in the bottom side. So this factor was named Material factor. This factor results from the tension between the two positions that the impoverished clients can take: paying attention to reduce the consumption or having a big bill to pay which the income cannot afford.

Now, it is time to examine in detail these three lexical worlds, in order to detect the themata that are acting through them. The words that we decide to comment on here are those that have a significant role in the constitution of the topology of the topic grounds. These words are those in the graphs that are placed on the extremities of the factors. These words (located in the furthest point in relation to the opposed side) are those which represent better their own cluster and which represent the biggest possible contrast in relation to the other clusters. If the preference was given to two kinds of words it is because, in this corpus, they express dichotomies that are important to the comprehension of the themata which are acting within it.

The graph below shows the distribution of some of these dichotomies. Their allocations, in relation to the factors, provide precious information. The results presented and discussed here are those related to the use of modal verbs and pronouns. These two classes of words were chosen because they illustrate the demonstration of the kind of systemic view social psychologists can get when they operate the connection between lexical topologies and intergroup relations.

Observing the location of the modal verbs in the graphs, we observed that in relation to the horizontal factor, they are distributed like this: in the left side, there are the modal verbs "to know" (savoir) (-30, 10), "to say" (dire) (-25, 10), "to ought to" (falloir) (-20, 2) while, in the right side, there is the verb "to have" (avoir) (30, -10). In relation to the vertical factor, they are distributed like this: in the topside, there is the verb "must" (devoir) (-20, 15) while in the bottom side, there are the verbs "want to" (vouloir) (30, -16) and "be capable of" (pouvoir) (10, -20). Observing the location of the pronouns in the graphs, we observed what follows. In relation to the horizontal factor: in the left side, there are the pronouns "them" (eux), "they" (ils), "their" (leur) while, in the right side, there are the pronouns "we" (on), "my" (mon). In relation to the vertical factor: in the topside, there is the pronoun "you" (vous) and "us" (nous) while and in the bottom side, there is the pronoun "I" (je) and "me" (moi), "my" (ma, mes). This first axis is clearly the one which epitomize the social categorization which characterizes the relation between EDF's agents (them) and the "impoverished" clients (we) in general; and between the needs and the problems of the individual (my) (such as: installation, consumption, heating, etc.) and the lack of comprehension of the agents (their), more specifically.

9. The relational – Material factor

In the left side of this factor there are the verbs "to know" (savoir), "to say" (dire), "must" (devoir). Afterwards, when we were able to go back to the text to verify manually how these verbs were used, we saw the following. The verbs "to know" (savoir) and "to say" (dire) were used, most of the times, in the negative form: "anything to say" (rien a signaler, rien a dire). The expression "I don't know" (je ne sais pas) was used 57 times, which means that 10% of the subjects gave that answer. This verb (in its infinitive and negative form) is associated with the following objects: "prices" (prix), "timetables" (horaires), "rates" (tarif), "how to save electric power" (comment faire des economies), "what to do in case of

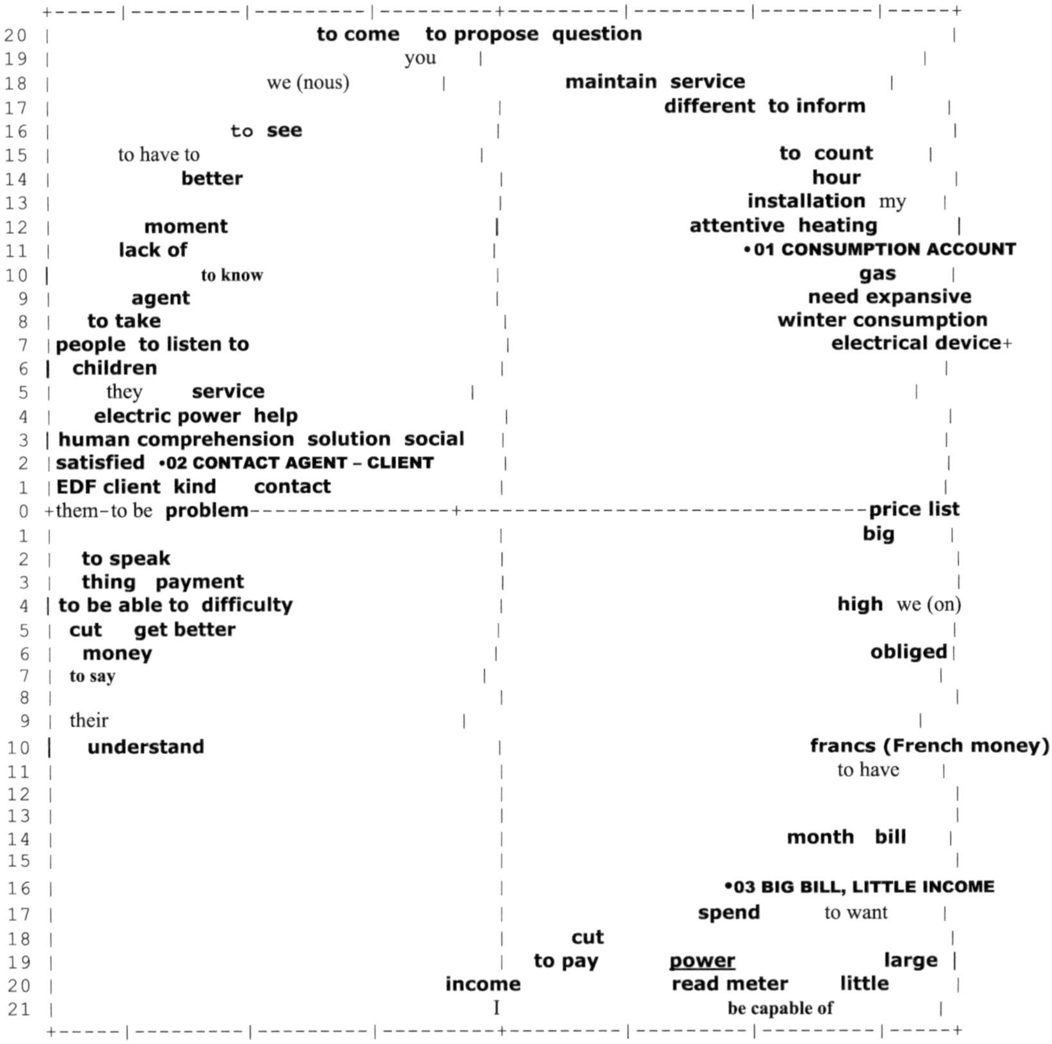

Projection of the analyzed words on the plan 1 2 (correlations)
Horizontal axes: First factor: V.P. =.3798 (58.78 % of the inertia)
Vertical axes: Second factor: V.P. =.2664 (41.22 % of the inertia)

Graph 2. Projection of the analyzed words on the plan 1 2 (correlations)

problems" (quoi faire en cas de probleme). Checking (manually) the use of the verb, "must", we observed two possibilities. When the "impoverished" clients applied it to themselves, the verb takes the following sense: "EDF (and its agents) thinks I must have money to pay the electricity bill, but actually I don't have". When the "impoverished" clients applied it to the company, the verb expresses what they think that EDF (and it agents) were in the obligation to do in respect to them; and this, in relation to four points mainly: a) the high cost of the bill (in relation to their income); b) the maintenance of the electric power provision (whatever); c) the preservation of the respect and of the humanity in the contacts (between clients and agents); d) the quality of the services. The use of the form "should" (devraient) is applied, specially, to what they would like EDF to do for them: a) more contact with the agents who receive them and the technicians who do the services for them; b) more access to simple information about the services and its possibilities; c) payment facilities or less expensive bills.

In the right side of the horizontal factor we found the verb "to have" (avoir). The use of this verb was also studied in detail. In the infinitive form, it refers to three categories of social objects: a) The first of which is composition of concrete objects, such as: "consumption" (consumation), "heating" (chauffage), "financial resources" (ressources financieres), "bill" (facture), "costs" (couts), etc.; b) The second of which is composed of services offered by EDF, such as: "information" (information), "agents welcome" (accueil des agents), "appointments" (rendez-vous), "rights" (droits); c) The third of which is composed of the advantages which come out of the "good" contact: "facilities" (facilites), "participation" (participation), "procedures" (systeme), "patience" (patience). The verb is also used as the first person, in the positive or negative form related to four categories of objects: a) (I have) remarks or comments coming from the agents (j'ai des remarques de la part des agents); b) (I don't have) money to pay (je n'ai pas d'argent pour payer); c) (I have) problems and difficulties (nous sommes personnes en difficulté); d) (I don't have) the right to have (or not) information, electrical power provision (or cut), service of "electric power maintenance".

10. The material factor

In the topside, there is the verb, "must" (devoir), which is used 42 times, in the conditional form; 16 of which in the third person of the plural "they would have better" (ils devraient). Here the impoverished clients express what they think should be EDF's duties in relation to their specific needs and situation. The objects of disagreement are: cuts in the electrical power provision (specially when in certain difficult conditions like "winter" (hiver), "children" (enfant), the high price of the electricity bill in relation to the low level of the income, the high cost of the phone calls made to EDF (which these clients would expect to be free for them). Furthermore, the clients complain about the complexity of their bill and about the indications of their consumption. They would like to have more clear information and better treatment when received by the agents, at the company's agencies.

At the bottom, two modal verbs are present. The verb "want to" (vouloir) is used many times, a great part of which related to the verb "to pay" (payer) (sometimes in the conditional form: "I would like to pay, but..." ("j'aimerais payer, mais..."). The verb "be capable of" (pouvoir) is used most of the time in the negative form, signifying the impossibilities these clients have, which are: a) they cannot pay the electricity bill; b) they cannot live without electric power; c) they are not informed about the rates, prices, services, etc.; d) they are not successful in communicating to EDF's agents.

Considering the employment of these two verbs "must" (devoir) and "to want to" (vouloir) together, we conclude that the "impoverished" clients felt twice frustrated. What they would like to do (pay their bill, have heating in winter time, have electrical power and electricity) they cannot afford; while what they can hardly stand (staying without electric power, being uninformed about prices and costs, having difficulties to communicate to any agent) they are subjected to, in their experience.

So, after analyzing all these results, the conclusion is that the way the verbs are used in this specific lexical context translate an implicit tension between the "impoverished" clients in one side and EDF and its agents in the other: the first ones being powerless, the second ones being powerful.

Other "sign" of this asymmetric relation (clients-agents) is the dissimilarity of technical knowledge between the lack of knowledge and information of the "impoverished" clients and the excess of knowledge and information of EDF and its investigators, which comes out with a fifty questions questionnaire, full of technical details. While what they "know" (experience) is that they need some help.

11. Syntheses of the empirical research

The method ALCESTE, gives the means to capture the deepest sense attributed to the words, which is unique since linked to the specific lexical context, in the moment of the expression of a particular relation between subjects of enunciation. The specific use of certain words, in certain moments or locations of the speech, is an evidence of a topic ground and the presence of a themata. The use of certain chosen terms in the speech that we just analyzed, offer a good demonstration of how a unique lexicon may unify charges that are opposed, representing a pair of antagonistic forces. In a particular relational context, the words take a very particular sense, which combine many senses in the same word. Actually, this condensation (more than one meanings transmitted by only one word) gives to these "chosen" words a thematic quality.

In this particular case we are discussing here, we noticed the phenomena of meaning condensation in relation to the dialectical peer: "to have the power of" or "not to have the power of" doing something. The term "power" combines in one single word all these meanings: "electrical power", "financial power" and "personal power" (capability of doing something). The asymmetry of the relation is explicit in the way the different groups place themselves, in relation to the utilization they do of the opposed means of the vocabulary. The "impoverished" clients see themselves still more "powerless" ("I can not pay the bill"), because they are comparing themselves to (or putting themselves "against") a "powerful" company, which they see as having many possibilities at its disposal ("They could do something to help us"). On one side, EDF has 'plenty' of powers and on the other, the clients are 'empty' of these powers (electrical, financial and personal). In relation to EDF's superpower, the impoverished clients feel completely powerless. The EDF sees them from a materialistic perspective as "clients" and in relation to what they do not have and they see themselves as "people" with big difficulties.

The same concentration of meaning occurs in relation to the term "anything" (rien), which condensate the sense of the EDF's agent's speech when they express a kind of refutation like that: "I can't do anything for you" (je ne peux rien faire, il n'y a rien que je puisse faire pour vous) and the sense of the clients speech, when they reply to the interviewer who was representing EDF: "I don't have anything to say to you" (rien a declarer, rien a dire). It is like if they were reasoning in function of a kind of private "vengeance" that could be formulated like: EDF and its agents refuse to do something to help them, so they refuse to answer the questions the investigators sent by EDF come to ask them.

This asymmetric relation between the giant EDF and the "impoverished" clients recalls the disparity that once existed between David and the giant Goliath. However, in the Biblical example, the difference of size was compensated by the difference of intelligence; the lack of strength compensated by the force of invention. Unfortunately, in the case treated here, the destiny of the weak personage is less fortunate than in the Bible's adventure. The relation the "impoverished" clients have with EDF (and its agents and interrogators) is twice asymmetrical. And we can suppose that as long as the same conditions are maintained (the existence of tensions between the verbs "to be" (etre), "to say" (dire) in one side and "to have" (avoir) in the other; "duty" (devoir) and "knowledge" (savoir) kept separated from "desire" (vouloir) and "capabilities" (pouvoir) the asymmetry will remain and the agreement field between clients and agents will stay unoccupied.

To change that it would be necessary to find a way of overcoming the tensions and integrating the oppositions in a higher-level synthesis.

12. Conclusion

In sum, the possibilities of connecting two key concepts and using an adapted program to make a pragmatic text analyses, provide enough information to unable social psychologists to conceive a system of explanation which is capable to consider, simultaneously, symbolic exchanges and relational issues. Among all the possibilities of meaning that the terms of the language offer to the speakers, there will be always some that will be highlighted with a specific context, because they will be vectors of a meaning condensation, sign of a lexical world where themata were recently activated. That is exactly the phenomenon that the pragmatic approach presented here allows to discover in the unities of context of the text.

After all theses considerations we are allowed to affirm that the particular structure of the sense within the language, the particular distribution of the lexicon within the speech and the original production of social representations within the communication are "isomorphs" with the asymmetry which defines intergroup relations. The forms the symbolic level can take (comprised of speech acts, practice of language and production of social knowledge and construction of social representations) are directly linked to the forms that the relations can take (comprised of: symmetric or asymmetric, dependence or independence, domination or submission, inclusion or exclusion, etc.). In spite of contextual variations, the principle is always the same: the experience of a kind of relation determines the use of a certain kind of vocabulary.

13. References

Holton, G. (1978). The Scientific Imagination: Case Studies. Cambridge: Cambridge University Press.

Holton, G. (1988). Thematic Origins of Scientific Thought: Kepler to Einstein. Cambridge MA, London UK: Havard University Press (copyright 1973).

Marková, I. (2000). Des thêmata de base des représentations sociales du SIDA. In C. Garnier (Ed.), Les formes de la pensée sociale (pp. 55—77). Paris: Presses Universitaires de France.

Marková, I., Moodie, E., Farr, R., Drozda-Senkowska, E., Erös, F., Plichtová, J., Gervais, M.-C., Hoffmannová, J., Mullerová, O. (1998). Social Representations of the Individual: A Post-Communist Perspective. European Journal of Social Psychology, 28, 797-830.

Marková, I., Moodie, E., & Plichtovà, J. (1998). The social representations of democracy: stability and change in word meanings. In A.-V. Rigas (Ed.), Social representations and contemporary social problems (pp. 155–177). Athens: Ellinka Grammata Publ.

Marková, I. (2003). Dialogical triads and three-component processes. In Dialogicality and Social representations, the dynamics of Mind (pp. 147–176). Cambridge: Cambridge University Press.

Moscovici, S. (1961). La psychanalyse son image son public. Paris: PressesUniversitaires de France. (second edition 1976).

Moscovici, S., & Vignaux, G. (1994). Le concept de Thêmata. In Ch. Guimelli (Dir.), Structures et transformations des représentations sociales (p. 25–72). Neuchâtel: Delachaux et Niestlé.

Peirce, C.S. (1978). Écrits sur le signe. Paris: Seuil.

Reinert, M. (1990): Alceste, une méthodologie d'analyse des données textuelles et une application: Aurélia de Gérard de Nerval. Bulletin de Méthodologie Sociologique, 26, 24–54.

Reinert, M. (1993): Les «mondes lexicaux» et leur «logique» à travers l'analyse statistique d'un corpus de récits de cauchemars. Langage & Société, 66, 5–39.

Reinert, M. (1999): Quelques interrogations à propos de l'«objet» d'une analyse de discours de type statistique et de la réponse «Alceste». Langage & Société, décembre, 90, 57–70.

Reinert, M. (2001a). Processus catégorique et co-construction des sujets et des mondes à travers l'analyse statistique de différents corpus. In M. Arrivé. & C. Normand, Linguistique et Psychanalyse (pp. 385–398). Paris: In Presse.

Reinert, M. (2001b): Alceste, une méthode statistique et sémiotique d'analyse de discours. Application aux «Rêveries du promeneur solitaire». La Revue Française de Psychiatrie et de Psychologie Médicale. Tome V, 49 (10/2001), 32–36.

Section 6

Social Psychology

13

Minority and Majority Influence on Attitudes

Nina Dickel and Gerd Bohner
University of Bielefeld, Germany

1. Introduction

1.1 What is an attitude?

In a complex world a quick evaluation of objects and situations is very helpful. It can guide our attention and behavior toward the things that matter to us. Attitudes are such evaluations. They can refer to anything one can conceive of: individuals and groups, products, music, or even smells, as well as suggestions and ideas. For example, when we meet someone new, we form an attitude toward our new acquaintance within seconds. Often, we do not know where this affective reaction comes from.

Attitudes can be formed in various ways: Imagine you are browsing the Internet for a holiday destination. You will find hundreds of different offers for package tours: how do you decide which one to book? You may like the pictures of the sea or of people relaxing in a bar. Maybe the web advertisement claims that 89% of costumers were highly satisfied with the holiday. Or, if it is very important to you not to spend too much money, you will elaborate carefully on which services are included. Eventually, you will come up with a summary evaluation regarding which offer is the best, and, if you consider the price to be appropriate, perhaps buy it. As this example illustrates, many different aspects can impact the evaluation of an object. A spontaneous affective reaction is immediately activated (in this case that could be a positive reaction to sunny pictures), heuristic inferences are made, for instance, "if 89% were happy it must be quite good", or very systematic thinking about the concrete features of the offer results in a judgment of whether this holiday suits you or not (see Erb, et al., 1998, expt. 2).

1.2 How to measure attitudes?

Social psychologists invented a large range of measurement paradigms that tap into different aspects of attitudes and attitude change. The simplest way to assess an attitude is to just ask people how they like something, on a scale, for instance, from "not at all" (1) to (7) "definitely like it," or to ask whether or not they agree with statements in favor or disfavor of the attitude object (Likert scale; Likert, 1932). Those are examples of self-report measures of attitudes that will be referred to as explicit attitudes in this chapter. When attitudes are measured by asking people explicitly how the object of interest is liked, respondents are usually able to answer this question. However, the outcome is also subject to impression management and may not cover all aspects like spontaneous affective reactions. To eliminate effects of social desirability on attitude measures social psychologist developed several "tricks".

They used feigned lie detectors (bogus pipeline, Jones & Sigall, 1971), word fragment completion tests (Gilbert & Hixon, 1991), and numerous other paradigms.

A relatively new class of attitude measures concentrates on reaction time effects of attitude stimuli. In a nutshell, attitudes are inferred from effects of interference or facilitation on very fast evaluative responses. These paradigms allow to measure spontaneous, difficult-to-control reactions that will be referred to as implicit attitudes in this chapter. Two paradigms have been predominantly applied: the implicit association test (IAT, Greenwald, et al., 1998) and the evaluative priming task (Fazio, et al., 1995; for a review see De Houwer, et al., 2009). When answering an IAT, participants classify stimuli via key-presses with respect to a target category or to their valence. Two sorts of experimental blocks are conducted with several trials each: in a "compatible" block, the target categories and positive or negative answers share response keys according to their presumed association. For example, participants press the left key for insects or negative stimuli, and the right key for flowers or positive stimuli. In an "incompatible" block, one of the key-assignments is reversed (insects or positive - left; flowers or negative - right). Differences in response times between the two blocks (incompatible minus compatible) indicate the difference in implicit attitudes toward the two concepts. More positive implicit attitudes toward flowers (versus insects) result in shorter reaction times in the compatible block and longer ones in the incompatible block, thus resulting in a positive difference. For more information about implicit measures of attitudes we refer the reader to other volumes (see e.g. De Houwer et al. 2009; Gawronski & Payne, 2010), as a full discussion would exceed the range of this chapter.

In sum, we have seen that attitudes can be measured in different ways. Attitudes have consequences on how we think and act (Allport, 1935). Thus, measuring different aspects of attitudes can help to predict how people eventually act. The prediction of both spontaneous and deliberate aspects of behavior may improve when applying both implicit and explicit measures of attitude (Friese, Hofman, & Wänke, 2008).

2. Attitudes and attitude change

As in other fields of social cognition, the notion of automaticity was central to attitude research within the last two decades (Bargh, 2007). Although implicit measures are probably not the "bona fide pipeline" (Fazio, et al., 1995) to attitudes, they do provide the means to investigate automatic evaluative responses that are often not easily accessible to introspection - and therefore cannot be easily reported in questionnaires. A great number of studies employing several variants of implicit measures of attitudes aimed to disentangle the processes underlying spontaneous attitude formation and change (e.g. Conrey, et al., 2005). Concerns, with respect to internal and construct validity of implicit measures have been extensively discussed (e.g. Rothermund & Wentura, 2004; Moors & De Houwer, 2006). Meta-analysis suggests that implicit and explicit attitudes are generally related, but higher levels of elaboration can reduce correlations (see Hofmann, et al., 2005). For the purposes of this chapter we will assume that implicit measures tap more or less into spontaneous affective reactions, while explicit measures reflect more effortful thinking including self-presentational issues.

Several models have been proposed to integrate results from implicit and explicit measures, including the meta-cognitive model (Petty, et al., 2007) and the reflective-impulsive model

(Strack & Deutsch, 2004). We will concentrate here on one of the most influential models, the associative-propositional evaluations model (APE model, Gawronski & Bodenhausen, 2006a).

2.1 Explicit attitude change: How many routes to persuasion?

An early explanation for attitude change was cognitive dissonance theory (Festinger, 1957). Cognitive dissonance emerges when interrelated cognitions contradict each other. For example, if I drink a coffee with my colleagues after every lunch although I do not like coffee in general, this would give rise to dissonant feelings about coffee. On the one hand, I don't like the taste, but on the other hand, I drank it, so I must like it (Bem, 1972). When individuals have a reason to which they can attribute their behavior, this reason can be added as dissonance-reducing cognition and no attitude change is necessary. In the coffee example, such additional cognitions could be "it's nice and sociable to have a coffee together" or "drinking a coffee makes me alert enough to concentrate on my work". When no external justification and no other way to resolve dissonance can be found, attitudes are often changed to regain cognitive consistency. In this example, the attitude toward coffee would become more positive. This effect was shown with participants who were asked to tell another participant that a boring experiment they had just attended was in fact exciting (Festinger & Carlsmith, 1959). They were either paid 1 $ or 20 $ for lying. The group who received the large amount of money did not change their attitude toward the experiment, whereas the group who received only 1 $ liked the experiment more. Here, the relatively large amount of money served as external justification for the positive statement about the experiment. If only little money was received this was not sufficient to resolve dissonance, so attitudes were changed.

Dual-process models of persuasion - the elaboration likelihood model (ELM, Petty & Cacioppo, 1986) and the heuristic-systematic model (HSM, Chaiken, 1987) - emphasize that attitude change can be due to low-effort or high-effort processing, termed peripheral and central route in the ELM and heuristic and systematic processing in the HSM. Which processing style occurs depends on a person's current motivation to hold a correct attitude and limits to processing capacity. Low motivation or scarce capacity will result in peripheral/heuristic processing, whereas high motivation and ample capacity lead to central/systematic processing of the arguments. The ELM emphasizes that any variable in the persuasive setting can function in "multiple roles" (Petty & Wegener, 1998). Take, for example, the presentation of a car by an attractive model: People may either process effortlessly, misattributing the positive affect elicited by the model to the car, or they may apply more processing effort, thus realizing that the attractiveness of the model does not say anything about the quality of the car. Moreover, the attractiveness of the model could also trigger motivation to associate oneself with her by liking the car she drives and thus motivation to find reasons to like the car by increased central processing. The ELM also predicts that the amount of central processing an individual engages in is positively related to the strength of resulting attitudes (Petty, et al., 1995).

The HSM assumes that both heuristic and systematic processing may serve multiple motives: accuracy, impression, and defense motivation. Accuracy-motivated individuals strive to hold correct attitudes, thus systematic processing is increased. When the impression motive is high, social needs will be served through expressing socially acceptable views; thus, impression-motivated processors will need to determine which attitude is most socially desired. Defense-motivated processing tends to confirm a person's self-relevant views and to avoid or reject opposing views. The HSM also features hypotheses about the co-occurrence and interplay of heuristic and systematic processing (Bohner, et al., 1995; Chaiken, et al., 1989): The *bias hypothesis* predicts that heuristics may lead to systematic processing in line with the valence of a heuristic cue. For instance, Chaiken and Maheswaran (1994) found that, under conditions of high task-importance, systematic elaboration of ambiguous arguments was biased by source credibility cues. Thus, readers' evaluation of a fictitious answering machine was more positive when ambiguous reasons to buy came from an independent test magazine rather than when the same arguments were stated in a retail chain's advert. Evaluative judgments were mediated by the valence of listed thoughts, indicating that systematic processes were indeed biased by cue information. A mirror-image of the bias hypothesis is the *contrast hypothesis*, which assumes that source cues can bias message processing in a direction opposite to the evaluative implications of cue valence. This effect was shown with expert and lay communicators giving strong versus weak arguments on a tunnel project (Bohner, et al., 2002). When experts promoted the tunnel with only weak arguments, participants' attitudes were less favorable than when the same weak arguments came from a lay person. Conversely, strong arguments presented by a lay person (vs. an expert) tended to be more persuasive. Presumably, when argument quality violates expectancies derived from source information, the result is a contrasting evaluation of the topic.

Despite their ability to predict attitude change in persuasion research, dual-process models of persuasion were challenged by the unimodel (Kruglanski & Thompson, 1999). The unimodel claimed that differential effects for cue versus message processing were due not to qualitatively distinct *processes* but rather to the different *nature of the information*. In typical persuasion experiments, cues were relatively short and easy to process, whereas arguments typically consisted of longer texts that consume more effort and time to read. Therefore, unsurprisingly, it takes more effort to process lengthy message arguments than, for instance, a short sentence about source expertise. Moreover, in research on dual-process models, persuasion cues were typically presented at the beginning, and arguments followed later. Kruglanski and Thompson (1999) argue that all processing of attitude-relevant information could be conceptualized better via a single underlying mechanism of syllogistic reasoning: When a recipient reads a persuasive message, she will compare the information with available relevant knowledge. For instance, if an expert from a renowned 'Institute for Natural Energy Resources' claims that oil is becoming scarce, every part of the sentence will run through a check-up with relevant knowledge. A major premise (i.e. prior knowledge) in this case may be "experts know a lot about their field and are usually right", and the minor premise taken from the persuasive information could be "this is an expert on the topic", and the conclusion will then be "... so she is probably right, and oil is indeed becoming scarce". Similar inferences can be made about specific arguments of the message. In this case, one of the arguments could be that oil prices are constantly rising, which can be related to knowledge about price increases following the scarcity of a product. The unimodel postulates that some parts of information may be processed relatively easily, whereas some inferences may require relatively large amounts of effortful thinking. How much effort is put into processing of a persuasive message is determined by motivation and capacity to process. If motivation or capacity to process is low, elaboration will end relatively early. Consequently, information that is presented first - like cue-information in studies on dual-processes in persuasion - will affect the evaluative judgment more strongly than identical information that is presented later. In sum, the unimodel does account for evidence that had been interpreted in terms of dual-process models; moreover, it explains additional effects of order of presentation (see e.g. Erb, et al., 2007), which dual-process models could not easily explain.

As models of persuasion were primarily concerned with the explanation of effects on explicit evaluative judgments, they cannot be directly applied to findings from studies employing implicit measures of attitudes (but see Petty & Wegener, 1998). The next section will introduce a model that integrates findings from explicit and implicit attitudes.

2.2 Integration of implicit attitudes and explicit attitude change

Based on a constructionist concept of attitudes (Schwarz & Bohner, 2001; see also Bohner & Dickel, 2011), the APE model (Gawronski & Bodenhausen, 2006a) discusses the interplay between changes on implicit and explicit measures. It proposes two general, distinct processes of attitude change: associative change, i.e. change in the automatic activation of cognitions associated with an attitude object, which is largely reflected in changes on implicit measures, and propositional change, which is characterized by the process of consciously ascribing a truth value to a thought about an object; the latter is captured mostly by explicit attitude measures.

Associative structure is modeled based on connectionist theory (for connectionist conceptualizations of attitudes see Conrey & Smith, 2007; Monroe & Read, 2008; Smith, 1996). "Connectionism is an approach to cognitive modeling that uses linked networks of concepts to represent cognitive structures. In these networks, activation flows between nodes and changes the activation of individual cognitions" (Monroe & Read, 2008, p. 735). The APE model assumes that *associative change* - as captured by implicit attitudes - relies either on changes in the associative structure or on changes in the activation pattern of associations. When a stimulus is perceived, associated cognitions are activated automatically, irrespective of the personal approval of an association. According to the APE model, the prototypical case of change in associative structure is evaluative conditioning, a procedure by which an originally neutral stimulus acquires valence when perceived together with a positive or negative stimulus. For example, in a study on evaluative conditioning with children, unknown cartoon characters were repeatedly presented paired either with ice cream or with Brussels sprouts (Field, 2006). Afterwards, the children liked the characters more when they had been presented together with ice-cream than when they had been presented with Brussels sprouts. The APE model assumes that procedures like this change the associative structures and therefore produce change on implicit attitudes. Associative change can also occur due to changes in pattern activation, this means, accessible parts of the associative structure are activated situationally. For illustration, consider a consumer who usually buys the same brand of a chocolate bar, because he likes the sweetness, color of packaging, texture, etc. When he is on holiday he might associate completely different aspects related to chocolate than usual, which have become more accessible through the unfamiliar situation. For instance, when it is hot, chocolate might be considered to melt easily, or different product alternatives might be available. Depending on the context - home versus holiday - different aspects are highly accessible: at home the usual association of the bar as being smooth and sweet is likely to be activated, whereas on holiday, when it is hot, the sticky aspect of melting chocolate might take priority. After all, our consumer will perhaps buy some olives instead. Hence, different contexts can render certain aspects accessible, i.e. the pattern of activation can differ depending on the context. A research example for context-effects on implicit attitudes is an IAT-study by Foroni and Mayr (2005), who showed a reversed pattern of liking for insects and flowers after participants imagined a fictional post-nuclear war scenario, where insects were the only healthy nutrition and flowers were contaminated (for more evidence of context-sensitivity of implicit attitudes see e.g. Barden, Maddux, Petty & Brewer, 2004). The APE model emphasizes that associations are activated automatically independent of personal approval.

In contrast, *propositional change* of attitudes, according to the APE model, is based on careful thinking about a topic. Every thought is given a positive or negative truth value. Consequently, the set of considered propositions can be consistent or inconsistent. Evaluative implications of automatic associations are set into proportion to propositions and will be either approved or rejected. The amount of propositions that is generated or considered is determined by motivation and opportunity to process. Longer engagement in propositional evaluation will result in more propositions, which, in turn, increases the likelihood of imbalance within the set of propositions. In our example on oil prices, additional thoughts like "distributors may have deliberately flowed less oil to increase prices" could weaken our earlier reasoning that rising oil prices allude to significant scarcity of natural oil resources, and would call into question the expertise of the communicator and her statement. These new propositions are added to the set of considered propositions and might result a higher degree of inconsistency. Individuals can adopt several strategies to reconcile inconsistent propositions (see Festinger, 1957). Inconsistency can be resolved either by rejecting an inconsistent proposition as false or by finding new propositions that resolve the inconsistency. Only the first strategy will result in explicit attitude change.

According to the APE model, attitude change can occur independently via both processes, and one process can also be mediated through the other, respectively. However, the default case is approval of the associative evaluation, as individuals usually invest as little cognitive effort as possible (see also the "cognitive miser", Fiske & Taylor, 1991). If motivational factors lead to further elaboration, automatic evaluations can be rejected, or systematic thinking can bring propositions to mind that reflect on associative structure, for instance with the activation of incidents like the crash of the oil rig "deepwater horizon", which was associated with destruction of nature, thus presumably activating negative associations.

The assumption that processes of implicit and explicit change differ qualitatively from each other has been questioned (Kruglanski & Dechesne, 2006) - a discussion resembling that between dual-process models and the unimodel in persuasion research. In particular, the view that activation of an association is independent of assigning a truth value to it, and that evaluative conditioning is a paradigmatic case of associative change has been much debated (Kruglanski & Dechesne, 2006; Mitchell, et al., 2009). Against the view that the activation of associations can be thought of as rule-based ("if ... then rules" like in the unimodel, Kruglanski & Thompson, 1999), Gawronski and Bodenhausen (2006b) hold that associative pattern activation may well follow rules, but these do not have to be consciously represented by individuals; instead, they can be inferred by researchers observing behavioral data. With respect to evaluative conditioning, a recent approach postulates a merely propositional process to underlie evaluative conditioning (De Houwer, 2009).

Despite these controversies, for our analysis it seems crucial that implicit measures of attitude capture very quick reactions that reflect more difficult-to-control affective reactions to an object (Hofmann, Friese, & Strack, 2009), whereas explicit measures of attitude capture more reflective, controlled evaluations (see also Strack & Deutsch, 2004).

Having introduced major theories of attitude concepts and attitude change in general, we will now turn to a highly interesting special case of attitude change - social influence on attitudes exerted by minorities and majorities. On the one hand, it will be very helpful to have theories of attitude change as a background for analyzing effects of minority and majority communication. On the other hand, sometimes paradoxical findings in minority and majority influence research provide the chance to test the applicability and limits of recent attitude change theories. In the last part of the chapter this discussion will converge into a new model of consensus effects.

3. Minority and majority influence

Although the origins of majority and minority influence research started with the investigation of the malleability of perceptual judgments, most studies conducted since the late 1980s have concentrated on how attitudes are influenced by minority and majority sources. We will nevertheless start with a short discussion in honor of the seminal works by Solomon Asch (1952, 1956) and Serge Moscovici and his colleagues (1969, 1980), because most studies still refer to the methods and assumptions introduced by them.

3.1 The roots of social influence research: Conformity and nonconformity in perceptual judgments

3.1.1 Nothing but conformity?

Under the impression of the Holocaust, social psychology used to focus very much on effects of group pressure. Solomon Asch asked whether we may "simply conclude that [groups] can induce persons to shift their decisions and convictions in almost any desired direction [...]" (Asch, 1956, p. 2). In his seminal studies on conformity (1956, Exp. 1) he investigated whether even simple perceptual judgments could be affected by a contradictory majority claim. A confederate majority of eight students and a minority of one participant engaged in a line judgment task that compared the length of a standard line to a set of three comparison lines. The line of equal length should be identified and stated out loud. In critical trials, the majority unanimously gave an evidently wrong answer. Compared to a control condition, where participants and confederates wrote down their answers silently, the likelihood of wrong answers in critical trials increased dramatically when participants answered in public.

Asch's work started up a whole field of research in social psychology. Many studies investigated the circumstances that cause conformity and the processes that underlie conforming behavior. A meta-analysis conducted on 133 studies that employed the line judgment task (Bond & Smith, 1996) showed conformity to be stronger in collectivist countries than in individualist countries. Other moderators of conformist behavior were (a) type of stimulus material: the more ambiguous the material the greater the influence by the majority (e.g. Crutchfield, 1955), (b) out-group versus in-group status: out-group majorities had significantly less influence than in-group majorities (e.g. Abrams, et al., 1990), and (c) the proportion of female respondents: a larger proportion of females in the sample increased the size of the majority effect (see Bond & Smith, 1996, p. 120).

In summary, although at least half of Asch's sample can also be said to have acted sensibly by just occasionally giving in to signal their willingness to cooperate with the majority (see Hodges & Geyer, 2006), most researchers in the 1950s to 1970s including Asch himself saw overwhelming evidence for non-rational conformist behavior (Milgram, Bickman, & Berkowitz, 1969; for a review see Cialdini & Trost, 1998). This prevailing perspective provoked Moscovici and his colleagues to challenge the one-way reasoning on social influence processes by investigating how minorities can exert influence on majority members.

3.1.2 The rehabilitation of the minority

If conformity were the dominant principle in groups and societies, a complete synchronization of thoughts, actions and attitudes would result, and no societal change would ever happen. Thus, new ideas that are usually supported by minorities at the beginning would never succeed. However, there are numerous examples from history that social change is possible, and hence minorities do exert some influence. A very successful social movement that was supported by a minority of people at the beginning was, for example, the environmental movement. Thirty years ago the use of recycling paper and saving energy was rather exotic, but today has become rather common.

Moscovici and his colleagues wanted to find experimental evidence that minorities also could exert substantial influence on majority members' judgments. For this purpose, a perception task was used (Moscovici & Personnaz, 1980): Predominantly blue slides with little proportions of green were projected on a white wall. A confederate and a participant were asked to publicly name the color of the slides and then, in private, to name the color of the afterimage that appeared on the white background after the stimulus had disappeared. Due to features of human vision, the color of this afterimage is complementary to the originally perceived color. The confederate answers (always "green") were allegedly either associated with a minority of 18% or with a majority of 82% from earlier experimental trials. As a result, public responses on the color of the slide did not differ between the minority and majority condition. However, color judgments of the afterimage given in private tended to be closer to the afterimage of green in the minority condition than in the majority condition (Moscovici & Personnaz, 1980). Studies on the afterimage effect constituted the core endorsement of Moscovici's conversion theory (1980), which assumes that minority and majority influence engender two different processes: individuals confronted with a majority engage in a comparison process, which compares their own tendency to answer with the majority's response, but do not consider in detail the reasons behind the majority statement. The detection of differences between one's own answer and the predominant answer results in public compliance, but not in private change. Minority positions, in contrast, due to their distinctiveness, set off a validation process that strives to understand why the minority's response is different. Minorities, thus, can cause private change that is usually not stated publicly, as people do not want to be associated with a minority (see Mugny, 1982).

The afterimage studies and conversion theory have been most influential in social influence research and induced several research projects on the impact of minorities (e.g. Mugny,

1982; Nemeth, 1986). However, despite its large influence, the original studies turned out to be difficult to replicate (see Wood et al., 1994, who found authorship effects with higher levels of indirect minority influence for studies conducted by Moscovici or his students as compared to other research groups, p. 335). Several criticisms concerning the methodology of the after-image studies lead to rejection of the evidence from the afterimage paradigm (see Martin & Hewstone, 2001). Still, - much like conversion theory itself assumes - the afterimage studies and their precursors, initially being a minority position in the scientific field, directed attention toward the impact of minorities and have stimulated a lot of research, of which a selection will be reviewed in the next section.

3.2 How many routes to minority and majority effects on explicit attitudes?

Much like in persuasion research generally, there are two lines of modeling processes of minority and majority influence. On the one hand, approaches based on Moscovici's conversion theory assume two distinct cognitive processes underlying minority and majority influence (e.g. Crano & Alvaro, 1998; Nemeth, 1986). While minorities urge people to think carefully about the positions and agree rather privately than in public, majorities cause public conformity without much systematic thinking. On the other hand, some models posit the same underlying process for minority and majority influence, with power of influence proportionate to the level of support (e.g. Doms & van Avermaat, 1983; Kruglanski & Mackie, 1990). Although the implementation of paradigms from persuasion studies in minority and majority influence research (e.g. Baker & Petty, 1994; Erb et al., 1998; Maass & Clark, 1983; see also Bohner, et al., 1995) allowed for a more direct assessment of the amount of processing that was triggered by each source, as we will see, the findings are mixed (see Wood et al., 1994). This is mainly due to different experimental designs and operationalizations, which will be discussed.

3.2.1 Dual-process accounts

Most of the dual-process models of minority and majority influence assume that minorities - due to their distinctiveness - attract larger amounts of attention toward their positions (Moscovici, 1980; Nemeth, 1986). If not derogated per se, e.g. because the minority belongs to an out-group (Mugny, 1982), minority statements will be elaborated more intensely than majority issues (Crano & Alvaro, 1998). More intense elaboration of strong arguments should result in greater change, especially when no prior judgment has to be defended (Crano & Hannula-Bral, 1994; Petty & Cacioppo, 1986). This change, however, is often not expressed as people often do not want to be associated with a minority. Change on the focal judgment can also be blocked and transferred to indirectly related judgments. In a series of studies, Crano and his colleagues (Alvaro & Crano, 1997; Crano & Alvaro, 1998) employed an indirect measure of minority and majority influence. Attitude change following in-group minority communication emerged on topics that were only indirectly related to the focus of persuasion, with the participants being unaware of this relation (cf. Mackie, 1987, who found change on related topics following both minority and majority communication).

Since the formulation of dual-process models of persuasion, pronounced parallels to social influence research have become evident (Bohner, et al., 1995; Maass & Clark, 1983; Nemeth, 1986). Both systematic processing (HSM) and the central route to persuasion (ELM) comprise careful scrutiny of available information, which can be seen as similar to the presumed validation process triggered by minority communication. Also, low effort processing modeled by HSM and ELM are comparable to low-effort compliance to majority statements. Thus, minority and majority influence research could benefit from methodological advancements, such as systematic variations of argument quality, to investigate more directly the processes at play.

In an experiment using a thought listing technique, Maass and Clark (1983) assessed which kind of processing route (in terms of the ELM) participants would engage in after minority and majority communication. Following simultaneous exposure to minority and majority argumentation on gay rights (with positions counterbalanced across experimental groups), participants completed a questionnaire either in private or in the expectation that it would be presented publicly to a discussion group. Much in line with conversion theory, attitudes moved toward the majority if expressed publicly and toward the minority if recorded privately (exp. 1 and 2). Thought listings on the topics showed - interestingly - the same level of cognitive activation (i.e. number of thoughts) for both minority and majority sources. As predicted by conversion theory along with the ELM, persistent attitude change was mediated by level of cognitive activity (central route processing), but compliance was not (expt. 2).

Inspired by the HSM (Chaiken, 1987; Chaiken, et al., 1989) and attribution theory (Kelley, 1967, 1973), Bohner, et al. (1996) conducted a study which addressed the role of distinctiveness information in minority and majority influence. Conversion theory (Moscovici, 1980) promotes distinctiveness - besides consistency - as one of the central factors that exclusively increase minority persuasion because it attracts attention to the issue and the minority's position, which should be scrutinized more systematically as a consequence. However, distinctiveness in terms of conversion theory (Moscovici, 1980) differs substantially from distinctiveness as employed by attribution theory (Kelley, 1967): Moscovici concentrates on the salience of the minority members, whereas Kelley focuses on which opinion is salient. The framework of the covariation model, hence, predicts high levels of persuasion when distinctiveness, consistency, *and* consensus are high. Under these conditions high levels of persuasion are mediated by entity attributions (to the facts concerning the persuasive topic). Predictions by attribution theory were supported, showing a disadvantage for minority (as compared to majority) persuasion if distinctiveness and consistency are constant for both conditions. Ironically, Moscovici was right to identify distinctiveness and consistency as powerful mediators of persuasion, although, this applies to both minority and majority sources. However, these results do not speak to the question of whether high levels of distinctiveness lead to more systematic processing. This was further clarified by another experiment (Bohner, Frank & Erb, 1998) which found independent main effects of argument strength and distinctiveness, indicating that distinctiveness in itself did not affect the level of systematic processing.

Evidence by Nemeth and colleagues suggests that it is rather the *type* of thinking than the amount of attention which is guided by consensus information (Nemeth, 1986). In a figure-comparison task where all patterns that contained a standard figure should be identified, participants found more alternative solutions after they had seen a minority (rather than a majority) member find a solution that differed from the most obvious solution (Nemeth & Wachtler, 1983). Thus, following minority influence participants found more alternative solutions, which Nemeth (1986) interpreted as due to a *divergent thinking* style, whereas majority influence prompted mere reproduction of the demonstrated solution, which Nemeth interpreted as due to *convergent thinking*. Further results indicating divergent thinking following dissent were found with other dependent variables like word-associations (Nemeth & Kwan, 1985) and free recall (Nemeth, et al., 1990). Evidence for divergent thinking was also found by Erb and colleagues (1998), who analyzed the content of thought listings following minority communication in a persuasion paradigm: Independent of valence, consensus information predicted the novelty of thoughts. Nemeth (1986) attributed the larger creativity to the fact that being confronted with a minority is generally less stressful than being confronted with a majority. Moreover, when levels of stress are high, more attention is driven to the central task, peripheral aspects are neglected. Thus, the lower levels of stress experienced when confronted with a minority widens the focus and allows for more creative solutions (see also Gawronski & Bodenhausen, 2006a, p. 700). According to the mere consensus approach, a more general explanation for increased levels of divergence following minority communication may be priming unusualness. Minorities - due to their inherent property of being unusual - will make more creative solutions more accessible.

In summary, the adoption of persuasion paradigms by social influence studies has ruled out largely the assumption of high- versus low-effort processing as attached to minority and majority communication. Rather, minority sources (as compared to majority sources) elicit a different focus of thinking: Minority communication seems to widen the focus of the addressee whereas majority communication narrows the focus. Alternatives to social influence models that assume two different modes of processing have proposed a single modus at operation irrespective of the minority versus majority status of the communicator.

3.2.2 Single-process accounts

Single process accounts assume a general influence process for both minority and majority sources (Doms & van Avermaet, 1980; Latané & Wolf, 1981; Tanford & Penrod, 1984). With their social impact model, Latané and Wolf (1981) criticized that minority and majority influence could not be compared validly in many studies to that date, because the direction of influence was either from an active majority to a passive minority or vice versa and was often confounded with power of the source. They proposed that the influence of both sources should instead be studied simultaneously and be defined merely by their numerical differences. As a result, consensus is disentangled from power and other factors that may affect level of influence. The remaining difference in support for a topic can be estimated as a function of numerical group size. Hence, a unitary influence by majorities as well as minorities is predicted by three factors: strength, closeness, and size of a group (Latané & Wolf, 1981). A study on social impact in electronic groups (Latané & L'Herrou, 1996), investigated how spatial relations between people affect the spread of influence and maintenance of diversity. It showed that complex geometries (with clustering in families, etc.) and boundaries to communications (like rivers, walls etc.) promote influence by minorities, whereas open social networks without spatial boundaries foster larger majority influence.

In her studies, Mackie (1987) specifically questions the core assumption of most dual-process accounts, that majority sources elicit less elaboration of the topic than minority sources do. She argues that high consensus usually indicates correctness, and hence, if it differs from one's own position it is worth spending some thought on the majority's statement (see also Bohner, et al., 1998). She had participants listen to tape-recorded discussions with arguments for both sides. Arguments were counterbalancedly attributed to either a minority or a majority; consequently participants were exposed to minority and majority position simultaneously (exp. 1 and 2). Attitudes toward the topic were assessed privately both before and after the message and again with a week's delay. In addition to the focal attitude, related topics were tested. Those participants who had been opposed to the majority's opinion significantly changed their mind in the direction of the majority position, whereas all others did not. Majority-induced attitude change generalized to related topics. Also, the recall and amount of elaboration of arguments predicted immediate attitude change. Thus, participants did process systematically what the majority said. In a similar vein, Baker and Petty (1994, Expt. 2) found that both processing of minority positions and of majority positions can be enhanced when their arguments contradict source-related expectations. That is, majorities that claimed positions opposed to prior attitudes held by participants as well as minorities stating the participant's position were surprising and thus gave rise to scrutinity.

In response to this challenge to dual-process explanations, it could be argued that single-process approaches did not include measures of latent influence that should emerge primarily following minority positions, and therefore the differential impact of minorities (compared with majorities) could not be detected (Maass & Clark, 1984; Nemeth, 1986). Some studies (e.g. Mackie, 1987) considered this aspect by including measures of indirect attitude change, but still did not confirm a duality of processes.

3.2.3 Discussion of both approaches

Kruglanski and Mackie (1990) offered a framework for examination of whether minority and majority influence are driven by distinct processes or rely on the same principles. According to their analysis, strongest evidence for process distinctiveness would be given if a factor affected minority influence in a different way than majority influence. For example, if high behavioral distinctiveness increased only minority influence but decreased majority influence, two different mediating processes could be assumed. As we have seen, however, distinctiveness does not moderate minority versus majority influence (Bohner et al., 1996; Bohner et al. 1998). Factors that necessarily covary with relative source size and mediate the persuasive outcome would also support the duality assumption. In their review, Kruglanski and Mackie (1990) identified only one variable that is necessarily tied to consensus information, namely the applicability of the consensus heuristic ("majorities are usually right"). No other strong cases for process distinctiveness were observed. However, even in cases when source impact moderates the outcome, it is not compulsory to assume two processes at operation (see also Kruglansi & Thompson, 1999, and Miller & Pederson, 1999).

In their meta-analysis, Wood and her colleagues (1994) found mainly quantitative differences between minority and majority influence. Solely for studies with perceptual measures of social influence, a superior minority influence could be shown. However, as mentioned above, due to their methodological flaws these studies should not be counted as evidence for duality of processes in minority and majority influence. A large variety of experimental designs makes direct comparison between studies on minority and majority influence difficult. Minority and majority status was sometimes implemented in combination with power (Mugny, 1982), prior attitudes were either moderate or opposed to the persuasive message (e.g. Mackie, 1987), sources had in- or out-group status (David & Turner, 1999), and other factors were varied (see Wood et al, 1994). At the same time various operationalizations were used, including fictitious (Erb et al., 1998) versus real topics (Maass & Clark, 1983; Alvaro & Crano, 1997), or real groups (Moscovici, et al., 1969) versus reported poll results (Thoben & Erb, 2010). These diverse paradigms complicate a generalization of findings across studies.

However, with their mere consensus approach, Erb and Bohner (2001, 2010) propose to study minority and majority influence detached from all other factors. They argue that "… even if messages are not discrepant and influence groups are not socially relevant to individuals, consensus can have profound effects on message-related processing and subsequent attitude judgments" (2001, p. 43). Responses to high consensus are predicted to be usually more positive than responses to low consensus. This initial evaluative response is said to bias processing of the message. Message processing might also be biased with regard to novelty of thoughts. With messages that comprise several intermediate arguments and few weak and strong arguments, and thus vary argument quality within participants, the biasing effect of consensus information on message processing can be detected more sensitively (mixed-message method, Erb, et al., 2005). Erb and colleagues (1998) report biasing consensus effects even with a pure numerical definition of minorities and majorities, and with fictitious topics where no prior attitudes exist. Majorities do evoke more positive evaluations of attitude objects and cognitive responses. Consequently, consensus in and of itself has a profound influence on social judgments, independent of conflict, power, or prior attitudes.

Of all things, distinctiveness and consistency do not seem to enhance minority influence exclusively (Moscovici, 1980); instead, these factors generalize to majority influence as well (Bohner, et al., 1996; see also Doms & VanAvermaet, 1980). Still, there are factors that seem to moderate whether minority or majority influence prevails: opinion discrepancy (Baker & Petty, 1994; Erb, et al., 2002), in-group versus out-group status (Crano & Alvaro, 1998), need for uniqueness (Imhoff & Erb, 2009), risk priming (Erb, et al., 2009), and motivational states (Bohner, et al., 2008). According to our analysis, these moderating effects of motivation and context are rather due to activation of different aspects that are associated with minorities and majorities than to distinct underlying processes. This idea will be discussed in the remaining sections.

4. Automatic to systematic consensus influence (ASCI) model

With our model of minority and majority influence on implicit and explicit attitudes we argue that introducing automatic processes to minority and majority influence can open a new perspective to the field and generate new predictions. Drawing on the associative and propositional evaluations (APE) model (Gawronski & Bodenhausen, 2006a) and on assumptions about the impact of motivational states on systematic processing, as proposed in the heuristic-systematic model (e.g. Bohner, et al., 1995), we assume that evaluation of minority and majority positions is shaped by the context of presentation and inner motivational and emotional states (see also Kruglanski & Mackie, 1990), at both an implicit and explicit level of information processing.

Figure 1 depicts a schematic illustration of the ASCI model. We will elucidate from the perspective of the ASCI model how information from persuasive settings with minority or majority sources is processed. The level of explicitness is conceptualized as continuous rather than dichotomous, ranging from very fast, spontaneous (or automatic) reactions over the effortless application of heuristics to any desired level of effortful thinking ('continuum of explicitness' in Figure 1). When a perceiver first sees the text with a minority or majority cue and the persuasive message, external input and internal states determine automatic activation of concepts related to the text. External input could be consensus information, message content, the way and the situation in which the text is presented, etc. Internal states can facilitate processing of matching external input as well as activate concepts from memory. For instance, the need to affiliate with others is likely to render majority sources more positive as they provide a larger basis of social support. Other motivational states include the need to be accurate or for a positive self-concept. Automatically activated concepts related to majorities could be: 'safe', 'correct', 'boring', or even 'repressive', etc. For minorities, concepts like 'rare', 'deviant', 'alternative', or 'risky' might be activated. The affective component of automatic associations is assessed via implicit measures of attitude.

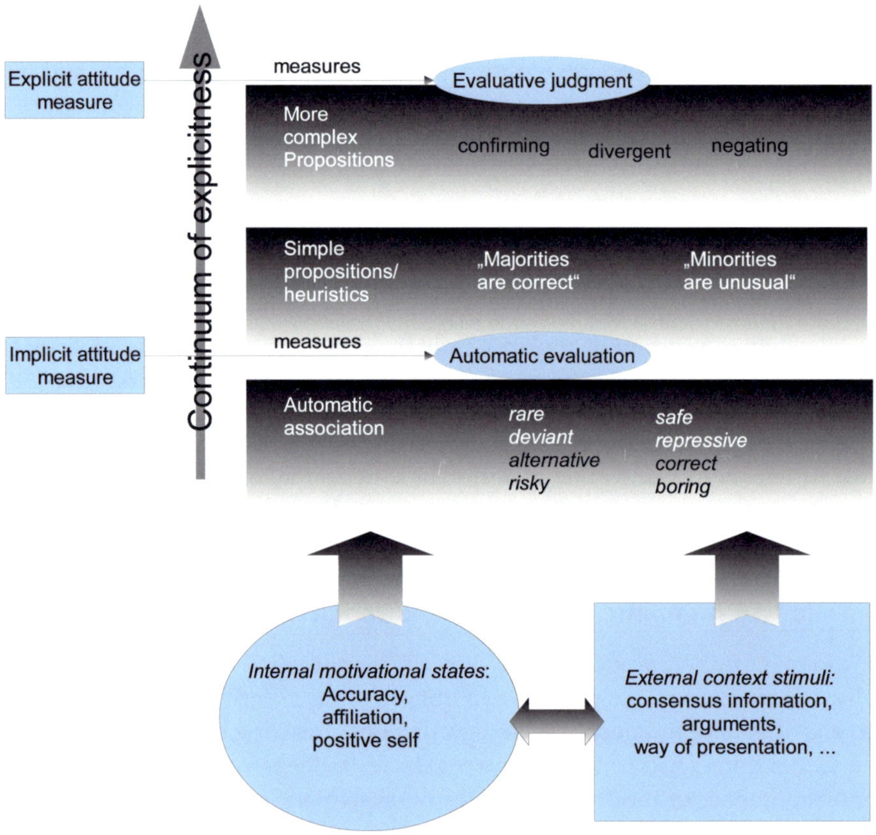

Fig. 1. Motivational states and external context determine automatic associations, simple heuristics and systematic thought about consensus information and persuasive content.

When the level of elaboration increases, simple propositions or heuristics are built upon the activated associations. When motivation to process is high enough, more complex inferences about the relation of consensus information, message content, and other relevant evidence will be built. At all levels of explicitness, evaluative processing is shaped by external input and inner motivational states. Evaluative judgments measured with self-report questionnaires are assumed to reflect high levels of elaboration about the persuasive setting. Moreover, processing of information can be either broad or narrow; we assume that minority cues trigger divergent processing of information at all levels of explicitness. These assumptions by the ASCI model will be outlined and illustrated in the following sections.

4.1 Implicit minority and majority influence

Implicit measures of attitudes provide the possibility to tap (more or less) into effortless, difficult-to-control or automatic manifestations of attitude change (e.g. Moors & DeHouwer, 2006). So far, implicit reaction-time based measures of attitudes have been applied only in very few studies on minority and majority influence. Extending on mere consensus studies (Erb et al., 1998), we added an implicit measure of the target attitude to investigate whether minority or majority persuasion would emerge at an automatic level (Dickel, 2011). Either a minority of 14% or a majority of 86% recommended a fictitious holiday area (the 'Curutao Lake') quoting several arguments of mixed strength (see Erb et al., 2005). Later, participants engaged in an evaluative priming task, where they categorized target words via left-hand and right-hand key-presses according to their valence. Target words were preceded either by the standard primes 'rain' or 'sun', or by the name of the recommended holiday region 'Curutao'. Interestingly, although explicit attitudes were more positive in the majority condition (compared to the minority condition), the implicit measure of the target attitude was not affected by source status. That is, the 'Curutao' prime did not facilitate responses to positive target words or negative target words in either condition. Yet, automatic evaluation of standard evaluative primes ('rain' versus 'sun') was reversed in the minority condition, i.e. participants that had read the minority position on the lake, responded faster to positive targets that were preceded by the 'rain' prime, indicating, that they evaluated 'rain' positively, whereas 'sun' was automatically evaluated negatively. Following majority communication, the usual evaluation of sun and rain was found at an automatic level. This pattern was interpreted as divergent processing at an automatic level (see also Nemeth, 1986) which could be grounded in a creative mindset (see Galinsky & Moskowitz, 2000) activated by minority cues. To corroborate our view, further studies have to be conducted.

To assess automatic evaluation of minorities and majorities per se, Mucchi-Faina, Pacilli, and Pagliaro (2011) had participants complete an implicit measure of attitudes. In a lexical decision task participants decided via key-presses if a letter string was a word or not. Letter strings were preceded by very short (15ms) masked presentation of the labels "minority" and "majority". Response to positive words was facilitated by majority primes, whereas minority primes did not affect target classification. The results indicate a positive connotation of the word "majority", whereas the word "minority" is not unitarily evaluated.

On the basis of these preliminary results from implicit measures and recent theorizing on attitude change, we propose a theoretical reframing of studies that showed an increased impact of consensus information under conditions of low processing effort. Traditionally, such results have been interpreted in terms of heuristic processing. For instance, when argument quality is not considered by participants, indicating that elaboration effort was low, consensus information becomes more predictive of thought valence and evaluative judgments (e.g. Erb et al., 1998). The application of heuristics like "majorities usually hold correct opinions" would require active thought or – in terms of the APE model – propositional thinking. However, increased impact of minority versus majority status when processing effort is low could also be explained by assuming (partial) implicit or automatic processing and evaluation of consensus information. The positive automatic reaction to the majority would then mediate the positive attitude toward the persuasive topic.

Moreover, recent studies (Bohner, et al., 2008; Erb, et al., 2009; Imhoff & Erb, 2009) found low effort influence by minorities and majorities on attitudes that was affected by context information or current motives of the perceiver. For example, when participants' need for uniqueness (Snyder & Fromkin, 1977) was high, participants judged minority positions to be more and majority positions to be less attractive even when there were no explicit arguments (Imhoff & Erb, 2009, exp. 1). Here, in our view, the current motivational state shaped processing of consensus information to serve the need for uniqueness – even at an automatic level. As being affiliated with minority sources provides the possibility to enhance one's own unusualness, minority stimuli were automatically evaluated more positively. Finally, the evaluative judgment was based on this positive automatic evaluation of consensus (see APE, case 1). In another study, minority positions were more attractive when participants had been subtly primed with risk-related concepts (Erb et al., 2009). As statements endorsed by minorities are more risky in the sense that they are not as socially approved as majority positions, participants can gain the valuable position of being one of the few 'clever ones' who were correct – but this outcome is fraught with uncertainty. Consequently, minority positions should be more attractive when people are in a "risky" mindset (Erb et al., 2009). Because participants were not aware of the risk-priming, it is plausible to assume that the priming shifted the automatic evaluation of consensus information. The explicit measures employed in the research just described do not speak to the potential impact of automatic evaluations, but, they may well reflect a blend of automatic and heuristic processing.

In the following sections we will take a closer look at how implicit evaluations of consensus information are formed and changed and how they can impact on more explicit evaluative judgments. Building on the APE model, we assume that the pattern of spontaneous activation of concepts (see e.g. Smith, 1996) related to consensus and the persuasive topic is shaped by contextual input and internal motivational states. Which aspects are activated depends on the current accessibility of concepts, which in turn depends on the context of presentation and on motivational or emotional states within the perceiver. Applied to minority and majority influence, context will render specific aspects of consensus information (or parts of information from the arguments) more accessible. For example, in the context of elections large majorities of more than 90% would likely be associated with cheating, whereas in online customer evaluations a consensus of 99% is quite usual and associated positively. In a study that investigated the effects of large minorities and small majorities – at least outside the context of elections – Erb, et al. (2006) found increased minority influence and decreased majority influence when explicit consensus information was larger for minorities (e.g., 48%) and smaller for majorities (e.g., 52%) than the consensus inferred in conditions where no explicit percentages were provided.

Presumably even more powerful than contextual input, internal motivational states can also shift automatic activation of associations (Ferguson & Bargh, 2004). Aspects that are functional to reach current goals will be highly accessible. For example, when a person's need to be unique is high (Fromkin & Snyder, 1977), associations toward minority cues such as "special" or "rare" might be rendered more accessible because they are goal relevant in the sense that being associated with a minority makes a person more unique (Imhoff & Erb, 2009). Hence, high accessibility of positive aspects related to minorities will result in a more positive implicit attitude toward them. In the same vein, when people are highly accuracy motivated, associations between high consensus and correctness (Bohner et al., 2008; Mackie, 1987) will become more accessible and lead to a positive implicit attitude toward majorities.

To organize the motivational impact on automatic activation of associations toward minorities and majorities we will adopt a catalogue of goals by Cialdini and Goldstein (2004): accuracy in ones judgments, affiliation to others, and maintaining a positive self-concept. When motivation to hold accurate attitudes is high, presumably valid and important information in the persuasive setting is functional to reach the goal, thus, corresponding concepts are activated (e.g. majorities = correct; scientific study = approved). High motivation to affiliate with others will highlight socially relevant aspects that help to reach the goal of affiliation. For example, the aspect that majorities comprise a large source of support might be activated automatically. Ingroups should be evaluated even more positively under high affiliation motivation. When the motivation to maintain a positive self-concept is dominant, aspects that support own held beliefs will be more accessible.

Research from the domain of stereotype reduction (Sassenberg & Moskowitz, 2005) suggests that automatic perception of minority and majority cues might not only impact accessibility of concepts related to consensus information, but could also be capable to affect the *way* in which information is processed (Nemeth, 1986) - even at an automatic level. A creative (versus thoughtful) mindset was activated when participants described three instances where they had been creative (versus thoughtful). Subsequently, a lexical decision task with facial primes of African and European Americans was completed to reveal racial stereotypes of African Americans. Stereotype activation was significantly reduced for participants in a creative mindset (Sassenberg & Moskowitz, 2005). Relating this to our finding, discussed above, that the automatic evaluation of standard words was reversed following minority communication (Dickel, 2011), we assume that considering minority arguments might result in divergent processing that operates at a non-conscious level.

In sum, we argue that automatic associations of consensus cues affect the persuasive outcome - either at an implicit level or by indirectly affecting explicit evaluative judgments (Figure 1). How automatic associations can affect explicit judgments will be outlined next.

4.2 Explicit minority and majority influence

We assume that more systematic processing minority and majority communication can be measured with explicit self reports - like propositional processes in the APE model and systematic processing in the HSM. In line with the APE model we assume that the most common case of propositional thinking is approval of the automatic affective reaction. When motivation and opportunity are sufficiently high to elaborate further, automatic evaluations are compared with inferences about the information. For example, the association "majority = correct = positive" could be questioned when propositions like "majorities also supported genocides" come into play. Such a consideration would create cognitive inconsistency (Festinger, 1957), which could be reconciled by rejecting the association on the basis of strong arguments. The amount of propositions that are taken into account is affected by the amount of time new propositions are considered, which in turn can depend on (a) current processing goals that define whether the actual level of confidence in the judgment is sufficient or not (Bohner et al., 1995), (b) context effects, e.g. how clearly the information is presented, and (c) available processing capacity. Hence, changes in the considered set of propositions result in changes in explicit evaluative judgments. The content of propositions can - like automatic associations - depend on processing goals and context of presentation.

For example, when accuracy motivation is high, the automatic reaction to the majority label could be positive (see above). Because accuracy-motivated individuals are likely to consider a large range of propositions, they might bring to mind instances where the majority heuristic was misleading. When arguments are strong, this might attenuate the heuristic value of consensus information for accuracy-motivated individuals (see attenuation hypothesis Bohner et al., 1995) - resulting in rejection of the automatic affective reaction - and guide their attention toward other information in the persuasive setting. Thus, when processed with the goal of accuracy, attitudes should be determined by argument quality. However, when arguments are ambiguous, participants with high accuracy motivation presumably accepted the positive automatic reaction toward the majority as a valid source for correct attitudes (Bohner et al., 2008, accuracy conditions), and moderately agreed with the majority. Importantly, if the goal to affiliate or to maintain a positive self-concept is active, the set of considered propositions may differ according to their relevance for the current motive.

The motive to affiliate with others, too, will affect the considered set of propositions that are aggregated in an evaluative judgment or explicit attitude. In general, individuals will strive to identify and adopt attitudes and arguments that are socially accepted. Participants with a highly activated affiliation motive (Bohner et al., 2008, affiliation conditions) accepted the majority's position - irrespective of argument quality. In our terms, they presumably based their judgment predominantly on the positive automatic evaluation of the majority cue as a large source of social support. As motivation to discount majority arguments was presumably low, search for more thoughts was ended relatively early, not bringing to mind conflicting propositions. In contrast, minority positions were scrutinized for valid arguments. As being associated with a minority is usually seen as opposed to the goal to affiliate (see Mugny, 1982), minority arguments have to be really convincing to be adopted.

A study by Erb et al. (2002) illustrates how the need for a positive self-concept can shape propositional processes in minority and majority influence. The authors found more systematic processing of majority messages than minority messages when participants' prior attitudes were moderate; however, when participants' prior attitudes were opposed to the message's position, minority messages were considered more extensively than majority messages. When prior attitudes oppose persuasive arguments, the motivation to maintain a positive self and to reject the arguments is likely to be high. Thus, as it serves the current motivational state, participants will consider a selection of propositions that can easily be discounted and dismissed - resulting in regained consistency between considered thoughts. Here, consensus information can corroborate inferences that the information given is invalid. The aspect of minorities' being deviant and incorrect is highlighted. Consequently, searching for the flaws in minorities' argumentation may appear more fruitful than scrutinizing majorities' messages - higher levels of systematic thinking are thus more likely for opposing minority views (Erb et al., 2002, p. 1180). However, when arguments are strong, and thus validated to be correct, the proposition that the minority is probably incorrect has to be rejected, to re-establish consistency among propositions. Moreover, an additional proposition might be generated like 'a correct minority is brighter than the majority and brave', which should contribute to the positive evaluation of strong arguments. On the other hand, when arguments are weak, source status implies a simple new proposition that can resolve inconsistency between recipients' own attitudes and views communicated by minorities: Arguments dysfunctional to maintain a positive self-concept can be rejected on the basis that the source is probably incorrect anyway.

Attitude change through effortful thinking following minority and majority communication emerges not only via consideration of different sets of thoughts and motivated rejection of certain parts of the active set of thoughts, it can also be due to changes in the strategy to reconcile contradicting propositions into a consistent judgment (see Gawronski & Bodenhausen, 2006a, p. 701). For instance, by giving example to solve tasks in an unconventional manner, minority sources will highlight the possibility to think outside the box. Although this point should generally transfer to majorities, minorities seem to trigger a processing style that may be characterized as creative or divergent (see above). Thus, contradicting propositions may be more easily reconciled when a person is thinking in a more creative or open way (for theoretical frameworks of processing styles see e.g. Förster & Dannenberg, 2010). Thinking more creatively may well be grounded in automatic processes. On the basis of automatic divergent associations (Dickel, 2011; Galinsky & Moskowitz, 2000; Sassenberg & Moskowitz, 2005) creative thoughts might be more accessible. Also, if group status is manipulated between participants, the existence of more than one alternative group beside a minority could be inferred by the participants, setting a higher norm of general divergence. This reasoning is less likely for (large) majorities (see also Naumer, 1996). Strategies to reconcile contradicting propositions can, again, be shaped by motives and context.

How automatic associations can affect explicit judgments beyond mere approval or disapproval of their evaluative implications will be considered in our assumptions on the interplay of automatic and systematic processing of minority or majority communication.

4.3 Interplay of automatic and systematic processing in minority and majority influence

From the perspective of the APE-model changes in associative structure and/or pattern activation can influence propositional thinking when the automatic association is considered a valid or invalid basis to form an evaluative summary (case 1). Conversely, change in propositions can mediate associative processes by bringing propositions to mind that activate automatic associative reactions (case 4). These cases appear to be conceptualized in the APE model as additive influences with varying weights on associations and propositions. For example, in the evaluative conditioning study described above (Field, 2006), where children liked cartoon characters more after they had been presented together with ice-cream (than with Brussels sprouts), the APE model would assume a change in associative structure of the character's representation. Corresponding change on explicit measures would be due to the approval of the associative implication (Gawronski & Bodenhausen, 2006a).

By contrast, we assume that automatic associations can trigger assimilating and contrasting biases in propositional thinking. Consensus information and dominant features of the message will automatically activate certain aspects of the concepts. Which aspects will be activated depends on the context of presentation and on the perceiver's motivational state. For example, a majority cue could activate the concept 'correct' or 'safe' when an accuracy goal prevails. Based on these active concepts effortful thinking will bring to mind inferences about source implications and the topic. Thus, once a majority cue has been evaluated positively (e.g. due to the perceiver's motivational state), the perceiver will be more likely to generate thoughts that will support the majority's arguments. Hence, the valence of thoughts will be assimilated to the initial automatic affective reaction. We assume that an assimilating bias in effortful thinking will occur only when message arguments are open to interpretation to some extent. If, however, message arguments violate the implications of initial associative reactions to the source, these initial reactions will be actively rejected, and the result will be a contrasting bias in effortful thinking (see Bohner et al., 2008).

4.4 New predictions

Implicit attitudes toward consensus information and toward the message topic change according to motivational states and context factors. When accuracy motivation prevails, high consensus usually activates positive (goal-serving) associations of correctness, whereas low consensus activates negative associations of incorrectness. When affiliation motivation prevails, minority and majority stimuli will activate different aspects of the concept: Belonging to a majority will usually satisfy the need to be connected more effectively than being associated with a minority. When the motivation to maintain a positive self-concept prevails, consensus information can be functional to discount or corroborate a perceiver's own views, which will trigger appropriate automatic associations. Depending on the information given in the context, different associations can be activated.

Explicit attitudes toward consensus information and toward the message topic also change according to motivational states and context factors. When accuracy motivation prevails, evaluative judgments will usually be based on argument quality. When arguments are unclear, however, individuals can rely on consensus information as indicating the level of support for the message position. Thus, arguments will be assimilated to (automatic) source evaluation. If arguments clearly violate such initial evaluations, more effortful judgments of the issue will be contrasted to them. Correlations between implicit and explicit change will increase when assimilating bias occurs, and decrease when contrasting bias occurs. When affiliation motivation prevails, perceivers will bring to mind or highlight thoughts that are functional for social affiliation. When the motivation to maintain a positive self-concept prevails, consensus information can be functional to discount or corroborate the perceiver's own views, which will trigger appropriate thoughts. Depending on the information given in the context, different thoughts will be brought to mind.

The amount of listed thoughts is a function of motivation strength and opportunity to process the information of interest. The larger the gap between perceivers' actual and desired confidence in their own judgment, the greater will be the perceivers' effort to scrutinize given information and to generate thoughts (see sufficiency threshold, e.g. Bohner et al., 1995).

The content of both thought listings and automatic associations is influenced by more divergent processing following minority than majority communication. Whether this is due to different levels of arousal or the activation of different mindsets should be investigated further. Instruments that assess the novelty of concepts (Vinokur & Burnstein, 1974) or self-generated arguments (Bohner & Schwarz, 1993) can be applied to address this question.

4.5 Discussion

We acknowledge that, to date, much of our analysis is speculative and many of our conclusions are based on plausible inferences rather than on empirical findings. Thus, the predictions outlined above have to undergo extensive testing. However, we hope to have demonstrated the exciting opportunities of integrating theorizing on automatic associations into the study of minority and majority influence.

Going beyond the APE model and the HSM, we have outlined in detail how automatic associations may bias systematic thinking. This is specified for the case of consensus effects on persuasion. Although the APE model mentions that motivational states affect propositional thinking (Gawronski & Bodenhausen, 2006a, p. 711) and automatic associations (p. 700), they do not explain in detail how motivational states affect attitude change. We assume that motivational states affect both implicit and explicit attitudes by making goal appropriate associations and/or propositions more accessible. Moreover, we allow for and predict assimilating and contrasting bias in the interplay of automatic and systematic processing.

Different from the APE model and the HSM, we do not assume two distinct processes but rather a continuum of implicitness versus explicitness in the processing of consensus and message information.

5. Conclusion

In conclusion, we argue that - as persuasion research has cross-fertilized research on minority and majority influence - new methodological and theoretical paradigms in attitude research have the potential to generate new insights into minority and majority influence processes. Applying implicit measures of attitude to majority and minority influence can enhance our understanding of which cognitive processes are affected by consensus information. In particular, the use of response-time based paradigms may enhance our understanding of the extent to which consensus information and messages aspects may be processed automatically. The assumption of a continuum of explicitness may help us to generate and test new hypotheses about consensus effects. More generally, the concept of gradually changing explicitness of evaluations (instead of dichotomous implicit versus explicit evaluations) could provide a noteworthy extension for attitude change theories.

6. References

Abrams, D., Wetherell, M., Cochrane, S., Hogg, M. A., & Turner, J. C. (1990). Knowing what to think by knowing who you are: Self-categorization and the nature of norm formation, conformity and group polarization. *British Journal of Social Psychology, 29,* 97–119.

Alvaro, E. M. & Crano, W. D. (1997). Indirect minority influence: Evidence for leniency in source evaluation and counterargumentation. *Journal of Personality and Social Psychology, 72,* 949–964.

Allport, G. W. (1935). Attitudes. In C. Murchinson (Ed.), *A Handbook of Social Psychology* (pp. 798–844). Worcester, MA, US: Clark University Press.

Asch, S. E. (1952). Social Psychology. Englewood Cliffs, NJ, US: Prentice Hall.

Asch, S. E. (1956). Studies of independence and submission to group pressure: I. A minority of one against a unanimous majority. *Psychological Monographs*, 70(9, Whole No. 417).

Baker, S. M., & Petty, R. E. (1994). Majority and minority influence: Source-position imbalance as a determinant of message scrutiny. *Journal of Personality and Social Psychology, 67*, 5–19.

Barden, J., Maddux, W. W., Petty, R. E., & Brewer,M. B. (2004). Contextual moderation of racial bias: The impact of social roles on controlled and automatically activated attitudes. *Journal of Personality and Social Psychology, 87,* 5–22.

Bargh, J. A. (2007). Social psychology and the unconscious: The automaticity of higher mental processes. New York, NY, US: Psychology Press.

Bem, D. J. (1972). Self-perception theory. *Advances in Experimental Social Psychology, 6,* 1–62.

Bond, R. & Smith, P. B. (1996). Culture and conformity: A meta-analysis of studies using Asch's (1952b, 1956) line judgment task. *Psychological Bulletin, 119*, 111–137.

Bohner, G., & Dickel, N. (2011). Attitudes and attitude change. *Annual Review of Psychology, 62*. 391–417.

Bohner, G., Dykema-Engblade, A., Tindale, R. S., & Meisenhelder, H. (2008). Framing of minority and majority source information in persuasion: When and how "consensus implies correctness". *Social Psychology,* 108–116.

Bohner, G., Erb, H.-P., Reinhard, M.-A., & Frank, E. (1996). Distinctiveness across topics in minority and majority influence: An attributional analysis and preliminary data. *British Journal of Social Psychology, 35*, 27–46.

Bohner, G., Frank, E., & Erb, H.-P. (1998). Heuristic processing of distinctiveness information in minority and majority influence. *European Journal of Social Psychology, 5,* 855–860.

Bohner, G., Moskowitz, G. B., & Chaiken, S. (1995). The interplay of heuristic and systematic processing of social information. *European Review of Social Psychology, 6,* 33–68.

Bohner G., Ruder,M., & Erb, H.-P. (2002). When expertise backfires: Contrast and assimilation effects in persuasion. *British Journal of Social Psychology, 41,* 495–519.

Bohner, G., & Schwarz, N. (1993). Mood states influence the production of persuasive arguments. *Communication Research, 20*, 696–722.

Chaiken, S. (1987). The heuristic model of persuasion. In M. P. Zanna, J. M. Olson, & C. P. Herman (Eds.), *Social Influence: The Ontario Symposium* (Vol. 5, pp. 3–39). Hillsdale, NJ: Erlbaum.

Chaiken, S., Liberman, A., & Eagly, A. H. (1989). Heuristic and systematic information processing within and beyond the persuasion context. In J. S. Uleman & J. A. Bargh (Eds.), *Unintended thought* pp. 212–252). New York: Guilford.

Chaiken, S., & Maheswaran, D. (1994). Heuristic processing can bias systematic processing: Effects of source credibility, argument ambiguity, and task importance on attitude judgment. *Journal of Personality and Social Psychology, 66,* 460–473.

Conrey, F. R., Sherman, J.W., Gawronski, B., Hugenberg, K., & Groom, C.J. (2005). Separating multiple processes in implicit social cognition: the quad model of implicit task performance. *Journal of Personality and Social Psychology, 89,* 469–487.

Conrey, F. R., & Smith, E. R. (2007). Attitude representation: attitudes as patterns in a distributed, connectionist representational system. *Social Cognition, 25,* 718–735

Cialdini, R. B., & Goldstein, N. J. (2004). Social Influence: Compliance and Conformity. In S. T. Fiske, D. L. Schacter, & C. Zahn-Waxler (Eds.), Annual Review of Psychology (Vol. 55). Annual Reviews, Inc., pp. 591-621.

Cialdini, R.B., & Trost, M.R. (1998). Social influence: Social norms, conformity, and compliance. In D. Gilbert, S. Fiske, & G. Lindzey (Eds.) The handbook of social psychology, (4th edition) vol. 2, pp. 151-192. New York: McGraw-Hill.

Crano, W. D., & Alvaro, E. M. (1998). The context/comparison model of social influence: Mechanisms, structure, and linkages that underlie indirect attitude change. In W. Stroebe & M. Hewstone (Eds.), *European Review of Social Psychology* (Vol. 8, pp. 175–202). Chinchester, UK: Wiley & Sons Ltd.

Crano, W.D., & Hannula-Bral, K.A. (1994). Context/categorization model of social influence: Minority and majority influence in the formation of a novel response norm. *Journal of Experimental Social Psychology, 30*, 247–276.

Crutchfield, R. S. (1955). Conformity and character. *American Psychologist, 10*, 191–198.

David, B., & Turner, J. C. (1999). Studies in self-categorization and minority conversion: The ingroup minority in intragroup and intergroup contexts. *British Journal of Social Psychology, 38*, 115–134.

De Houwer, J. (2009). The propositional approach to associative learning as an alternative for association formation models. Learning & Behavior, 37, 1–20.

De Houwer, J., Teige-Mocigemba, S., Spruyt, A., & Moors, A. (2009). Implicit measures: a normative analysis and review. *Psychological Bulletin, 135*, 347–368

Dickel, N. (2011). Implicit minority and majority influence. Talk presented at the *Transfer of Knowledge Conference, ESCON2*, at Sligo, Ireland, 24.–28. Aug. 2011.

Doms, M. & van Avermaet, E. (1980). Majority influence, minority influence and conversion behavior: a replication. *Journal of Experimental Social Psychology, 16*, 283–292.

Erb, H.-P. & Bohner, G. (2001). Mere consensus effects in minority and majority influence. In: C. K. W. De Dreu & N. K. De Vries (Eds.), *Group consensus and minority influence: Implications for innovation* (pp.40–59). Oxford, UK: Blackwell publishers.

Erb, H.-P., & Bohner, G. (2010). Consensus as the key: Towards parsimony in explaining minority and majority influence. In R. Martin & M. Hewstone (Eds.), *Minority influence and innovation: Antecedents, processes and consequences* (pp. 79–103). Hove, UK: Psychology Press.

Erb, H.-P., Bohner, G., Hewstone, M., Wert, L., & Reinhard, M.-A. (2006). Large minorities and small majorities: Interactive effects of inferred and explicit consensus on attitudes. *Basic and Applied Social Psychology, 28*, 221–231.

Erb, H.-P., Bohner, G., Schmälzle, K. & Rank, S. (1998). Beyond conflict and discrepancy. *Personality and Social Psychology Bulletin, 24*, 620–633.

Erb, H.-P., Bohner, G., Rank, S., & Einwiller, S. (2002) role of prior attitudes

Erb, H.-P., Büscher, M., Bohner, G., & Rank, S. (2005). Starke und schwache Argumente als Teile derselben Botschaft: Die "Mixed-Message Methode" zur Erfassung des kognitiven Aufwands bei der Verarbeitung persuasiver Kommunikation. *Zeitschrift für Sozialpsychologie, 36*, 61–75.

Erb, H.-P., Hilton, D. J., Bohner, G., & Krings, L. (2009). The minority position – A risk-seeking choice. unpublished manuscript.

Erb, H.-P., Pierro, A., Mannetti, L., Spiegel, S., & Kruglanski, A. W. (2007). Biased processing of persuasive information: on the functional equivalence of cues and message arguments. *European Journal of Social Psychology, 37*, 1057–1075.

Fazio, R. H. (2007). Attitudes as object-evaluation associations of varying strength. *Social Cognition, 25*, 603–637.

Fazio, R. H., Jackson , J. R., Dunton, B. C., & Williams, C. J. (1995). Variability in automatic activation as an unobtrusive measure of racial attitudes: a bona fide pipeline? *Journal of Personality and Social Psychology, 69*, 1013–1027.

Ferguson, M. J., & Bargh, J. A. (2004). Liking is for doing: The effects of goal pursuit on automatic evaluation. *Journal of Personality and Social Psychology, 87,* 557–572.

Festinger, L. (1957). *A theory of cognitive dissonance.* Evanston, IL: Row Peterson.

Festinger, L., & Carlsmith, J. M. (1959). Cognitive consequences of forced compliance. *Journal of Abnormal and Social Psychology, 58,* 203–210.

Field, A. P. (2005). Is the meta-analysis of correlation coefficients accurate when population effect sizes vary? *Psychological Methods,* 10 (4), 444–467.

Fiske, S. T. and Taylor, S. E. (1991). *Social cognition* (2nd ed.). New York: McGraw Hill.

Foroni, F., & Mayr, U. (2005). The power of a story: New, automatic associations from a single reading of a short scenario. *Psychonomic Bulletin & Review, 12,* 139–144.

Förster, J. & Dannenberg, L. (2010). GLOMO sys : A Systems Account of Global versus Local Processing. *Psychological Inquiry, target article, 21,* 175–197.

Friese, M., Hofmann, W., & Wänke, M. (2008). When impulses take over: Moderated predictive validity of explicit and implicit attitude measures in predicting food choice and consumption behaviour. *British Journal of Social Psychology, 47,* 397–419.

Galinsky, A. D. & Moskowitz, G. B. (2002). Counterfactuals as behavioral primes: Priming the simulation heuristic and consideration of alternatives. *Journal of Experimental Social Psychology, 36,* 384–409.

Gawronski, B., & Bodenhausen, G. V. (2006a). Associative and propositional processes in evaluation: An integrative review of implicit and explicit attitude change. *Psychological Bulletin, 132,* 692–731.

Gawronski, B., & Bodenhausen, G. V. (2006b). Associative and propositional processes in evaluation: Conceptual, empirical, and meta-theoretical issues. Reply to Albarracín, Hart, and McCulloch (2006), Kruglanski and Dechesne (2006), and Petty and Briñol (2006). *Psychological Bulletin, 132,* 745–750.

Gawronski, B., & Payne, B. K. (Eds.). (2010). *Handbook of implicit social cognition: Measurement, theory, and applications*. New York: Guilford Press.

Gilbert, D. T., & Hixon, J. G. (1991). The trouble of thinking: Activation and application of stereotypic beliefs. *Journal of Personality and Social Psychology, 60,* 509–517.

Greenwald, A. G., McGhee, D. E., & Schwartz, J. K. L. (1998). Measuring individual differences in implicit cognition: The Implicit Association Test. *Journal of Personality and Social Psychology, 74,* 1464–1480.

Hodges, B. H., & Geyer, A. (2006). A nonconformist account of the Asch experiments: Values, pragmatics, and moral dilemmas. *Personality and Social Psychology Review, 10,* 2–19.

Hofmann, W., Friese, M., & Strack, F. (2009). Impulse and self-control from a dual-systems perspective. *Perspectives on Psychological Science, 4,* 162–176.

Hofmann, W., Gawronski, B., Gschwendner, T., Le, H., & Schmitt, M. (2005). A meta-analysis on the correlation between the Implicit Association Test and explicit self-report measures. *Personality and Social Psychology Bulletin, 31,* 1369–1385.

Imhoff, R., & Erb, H.-P. (2009). What motivates nonconformity? Uniqueness seeking blocks majority influence. *Personality and Social Psychology Bulletin, 35,* 309–320.

Jones, E., & Sigall, H. (1971). The Bogus Pipeline: A new paradigm for measuring affect and attitude. *Psychological Bulletin, 76,* 349–364.

Kelley, H. H. (1967). Attribution theory in social psychology. In D. Levine (Ed.), *Nebraska symposium on motivation* (pp. 192–238), Lincoln: University of Nebraska Press.

Kelley, H. H. (1973). The process of causal attribution. *American Psychologist, 28,* 107–128.

Kruglanski, A. W., & Dechesne, M. (2006). Are associative and propositional processes qualitatively distinct? Comment on Gawronski and Bodenhausen (2006). *Psychological Bulletin, 132,* 736–739.

Kruglanski, A. W. & Mackie, D. M. (1990). Majority and minority influence: A judgmental process analysis. In: W. Stroebe & M. Hewstone (Eds.), *European Review of Social Psychology* (pp. 229-161). Wiley & Sons Ltd.

Kruglanski, A.W. & Thompson, E.P. (1999). Persuasion by a single route: A view from the unimodel. *Psychological Inquiry, 10,* 83–109.

Latané, B., & L' Herrou, T. (1996). Spatial clustering in the conformity game: Dynamic social impact in electronic games. *Journal of Personality and Social Psychology, 70,* 1218–1230.

Latané, B. & Wolf, S. (1981). The social impact of majorities and minorities. *Psychological Review, 88,* 438–453.

Likert, R. (1932). A Technique for the Measurement of Attitudes. *Archives of Psychology, 140,* 1–55.

Maass, A., & Clark, R. D. III (1983). Internalization versus compliance: Differential processes underlying minority influence and conformity. *European Journal of Social Psychology, 13,* 197–215.

Maass, A., & Clark, R. D. III (1984). Hidden impact of minorities: Fifteen years of minority influence research. *Psychological Bulletin, 95,* 428–450.

Mackie, D. M. (1987). Systematic and nonsystematic processing of majority and minority persuasive communications. *Journal of Personality and Social Psychology, 53,* 41–52.

Martin, R., & Hewstone, M. (2001). Afterthoughts on after-images: A review of the literature using the afterimage paradigm in majority and minority influence. In C. De Drew & N. De Vires (Eds.), *Group innovation: Fundamental and applied perspectives* (pp. 15–39). Oxford: Blackwell.

Milgram, S., Bickman, L., Berkowitz, L. (1969). Note on the drawing power of crowds of different size. *Journal of Personality and Social Psychology, 13,* 79–2.

Miller, N., & Pederson, W. C. (1999). Assessing process distinctiveness. *Psychological Inquiry, 10,* 150–156.

Mitchell, C. J., De Houwer, J., & Lovibond, P. F. (2009). The propositional nature of human associative learning. *Behavioral and Brain Sciences, 32,* 183–198.

Monroe, B. M., & Read, S. J. (2008). A general connectionist model of attitude structure and change: The ACS (Attitudes as Constraint Satisfaction) model. *Psychological Review, 115,* 733–759.

Moors, A., & De Houwer, J. (2006). Automaticity: theoretical and conceptual analysis. *Psychological Bulletin, 132,* 297–326.

Moscovici, S. (1980). Toward a theory of conversion behavior. In L. Berkowitz (Ed.), *Advances in experimental social psychology* (Vol. 13, pp. 209–239). New York: Academic Press.

Moscovici, S., Lage, E., & Naffrechoux , M. (1969). Influence of a consistent minority on the response of a majority in a color perception task. *Sociometry, 32,* 365–380.

Moscovici, S. & Personnaz, B. (1980). Studies on social influence V. Minority influence and conversion behavior in a perceptual task. *Journal of Experimental Social Psychology, 16,* 270–282.

Mucchi-Faina, A., Pacilli, M. G., & Pagliaro, S. (2011). Automatic reactions to the labels "minority" and "majority" are asymmetrical: Implications for minority and majority influence. *Social Influence, 6,* 181–196.

Mugny, G. (1982). *The power of minorities.* London: Academic Press.

Naumer, B. (1996). Auswirkungen wahrgenommener Festgelegtheit eines Entscheidungsprozesses auf die Diverenz des Denkens [How perceived determination of decisions affects divergent thinking]. Unpublished manuscript.

Nemeth, C. J. (1986). Differential contributions of majority and minority influence. *Psychological Review, 93,* 23–32.

Nemeth, C., & Kwan, J. (1985). Originality of word associations as a function of majority vs. minority influence. *Social Psychology Quarterly, 48,* 277–282.

Nemeth, C., Mayseless, O., Sherman, J., & Brown, Y. (1990). Exposure to dissent and recall of information. *Journal of Personality and Social Psychology, 58,* 429–437.

Nemeth, C., & Wachtler, J. (1983). Creative problem solving as a result of majority *vs* minority influence. *European Journal of Social Psychology, 13,* 45–55.

Petty, R.E., Briñol, P., & DeMarree, K.G. (2007). The Meta-Cognitive Model (MCM) of attitudes: Implications for attitude measurement, change, and strength. *Social Cognition, 25*(5), 657–686.

Petty, R. E. & Cacioppo, J. T. (1986). The elaboration likelihood model of persuasion. In L. Berkowitz (Ed.), *Advances in experimental social psychology* (Vol. 19, pp. 123–205), New York: Academic Press.

Petty, R. E., Haugtvedt, C. P., & Smith, S. M. (1995). Message elaboration as a determinant of attitude strength. In R. E. Petty & J. A. Krosnick (Eds.), Attitude strength: Antecedents and consequences. Hillsdale, NJ: Lawrence Erlbaum Associates.

Petty, R. E., & Wegener, D. T. (1998). Attitude change: Multiple roles for persuasion variables. In D. Gilbert, S. Fiske, & G. Lindzey (Eds.), The handbook of social psychology (4th ed., pp. 323–390). New York: McGraw-Hill.

Rothermund, K., & Wentura, D. (2004). Underlying processes in the Implicit Association Test: Dissociating salience from associations. *Journal of Experimental Psychology: General, 133,* 139–165.

Sassenberg, K. & Moskowitz, G. B. (2005). Don't stereotype, think different! Overcoming automatic stereotype activation by mindset priming. *Journal of Experimental Social Psychology, 41,* 506–514.

Schwarz, N., & Bohner, G. (2001). The construction of attitudes. In A. Tesser & N. Schwarz (Eds.), Blackwell handbook of social psychology, Vol. 1: Intraindividual processes (pp. 436–457). Oxford, UK: Blackwell.

Smith, E. R. (1996). What do connectionism and social psychology offer each other? *Journal of Personality and Social Psychology , 70,* 893–912.

Snyder, C. R., & Fromkin, H. L. (1977). Abnormality as a positive characteristic: The development and validation of a scale measuring need for uniqueness. *Journal of Abnormal Psychology, 86,* 518–527.

Strack, F., & Deutsch, R. (2004). Reflective and impulsive determinants of social behavior. *Personality and Social Psychology Review, 3,* 220–247.

Thoben, D. F. & Erb, H.-P. (2010). Wie es euch gefällt: Sozialer Einfluss durch Mehrheiten und Minderheiten. *In-Mind Magazine, 1(2).*

Tanford, S. E. & Penrod, S. (1984). Social influence model: A formal integration of research on majority and minority influence processes. *Psychological Bulletin, 95,* 189–225.

Vinokur, A., & Burnstein, E. (1974). Effects of partially shared persuasive arguments on group-induced shifts: A group-problem-solving approach. *Journal of Personality and Social Psychology, 29*(3), 305–315.

Wood, W., Lundgren, S., Oullette, J. A., Busceme, S., & Blackstone, T. (1994). A meta-analytic review of social influence processes. *Psychological Bulletin, 115,* 323–345.

14

Conformity, Obedience, Disobedience: The Power of the Situation

Piero Bocchiaro and Adriano Zamperini
Department of Philosophy, Sociology, Education and Applied Psychology, University of Padua, Italy

1. Introduction

From the beginning social psychology has concerned itself, from different perspectives, with processes of social influence, producing an imposing amount of research. Given this vastity and heterogeneity, it is opportune to restrict the sphere of these studies, to understand better their specific nature. Social influence can be assessed in all situations where there are two "social entities" (two people, two groups, a person and a group), where one is the source of influence and the other the target; both interact through an "object" which can be an opinion or a behaviour. The purpose of these studies is to reveal whether the reactions of people faced with a certain social object can change in terms of the relationship engaged in and how, in the present chapter, to what the phenomena of conformism and obedience are connected.

Conformism can be defined as the change in thinking, feeling or acting following pressure, real or imaginary, exercised by the group (Moghaddam, 1998). Obedience is instead that modification that is manifested carrying out the instructions issued by figures given authority. The two phenomena are connected (often conformism is a mental direction more easily inclined towards obedience) and both imply the themes of independence and submission. For sure living in a society we develop a sense of dependence on others as regards the way of understanding and acting in social reality. We can sometimes reach an authentic shared consensus, other times no. There are situations in which we cannot freely express our ideas, and this activates our resources in order to affirm ourselves and our values. Instead others can resign themselves and become submissive, even coming to the point of aligning themselves with their oppressor. Analyzing similar situations enables us to distinguish the presence or the forming of binding forces in the social environment, just like the forces that individual people put into action to resist coercion.

Conformism and obedience are not necessarily negative phenomena. The list of their positive aspects is decidedly long. In fact, without conformism and obedience social life would be governed by chaos. We could not circulate in the streets nor even hold a civil conversation. However in the present chapter we shall concern ourselves mainly with their negative consequences. Starting from the analysis of what is the basis of conformism and obedience: the formation of social norms.

2. Conformism

A social norm is generally an accepted way of thinking, feeling or acting, emphasized and expected by members of a particular community or social group since it is considered the right thing (Turner, 1991). A norm is the standard of reference for judging what is correct and appropriate to do in specific situations, providing people with criteria of validity and reducing their sense of uncertainty. Therefore norms exercise their own influence on people in terms of how to perceive social reality (the function of understanding) and how to behave inside social reality (axiological function).

First research on interaction in small groups has demonstrated that when called to express judgment, people tend to develop a certain agreement. For Sherif (1936) this agreement is the equivalent of the formation of social norms. In one of his classic studies he used an optical illusion called "autokinetic effect": in a completely dark room, fixing on a luminous point the sensation is created, though immobile, that it begins to move irregularly. The participants in Sherif's experiment, placed in this ambiguous situation and assigned with the task of estimating the width of movement of the luminous stimulant, manifested a progressive tendency to establish a common rule, producing a convergence in their judgment. A mutual adaptation that may be interpreted as the internalization of a social norm, a framework of common reference that establishes judgment and reduces uncertainty.

Something analogous is present in the work of Leon Festinger (1950), where conformity is seen as pressure towards the uniformity that the group exercises on its members. A uniformity that, excluding deviants, favours the cohesion of the group. But probably the most brilliant demonstration of pressure towards conformism is retraced in the pioneer studies of Solomon Asch (1951).

2.1 Independence and submission to judgment

The experimental context provided by Asch (1956) was simple: a length comparison task was proposed for the participants. They were placed in front of two white cardboards: on the left one there was a single line (the sample line) and on the right one were three other lines. They had to indicate which of the three lines was the same length as the sample line. Once all participants had formulated their judgment the two cardboards were replaced by another two, again with a sample line and three lines to compare. The sequence foresaw 12 evaluations. The difference between the line and the other two different lines was so marked that it was unmistakably visible.

The experiment proceeded regularly for the first two trials. Being quite simple judgments, the response was the same for all participants. But during the third trial and in subsequent ones some changes occurred: the members of the group, except for one (usually situated in the last but one place in the row), were in reality accomplices in the experiment and had the task of providing the seven judgments clearly contrary to the perceptive evidence. The group involved in the experiment was thus composed of two types of participant: a majority of people aware of the characteristics and of the results of the experiment and a minority (just one participant) unaware of anything. As was immediately intuitable, the real "experimental subject" (the "critical subject", according to terminology used by Asch) had to confront a highly problematic condition. On the one hand the task appeared very simple, as it was easily perceptible which of the three lines was the same length as the sample; on the other hand the situation was disorientated since the accomplices claimed to have completely different perceptions from those suggested by the senses.

Since he had to express his own opinion after theirs, the critical subject suffered the pressure of the majority and therefore was faced with a dilemma: would he have to express without wavering what he really saw, thus showing his own disagreement with respect to the rest of the group, or provide the same response given by the others, conforming in this way to general opinion?

Results proved that, while in a control group errors had been very few, in the experimental groups the wrong evaluations expressed by the majority had influenced about a third of the judgments expressed by the critical subjects (33.2% of total responses). If it was also true that independence had prevailed among the critical subjects (the percentage of exact responses was 66.8%), what is striking is the high percentage of participants who submitted to the clearly wrong opinion of the majority in a substantially insignificant task. If 6 of the critical subjects maintained a firm position, altogether 25 people out of 31 involved claimed they perceived what for sure they could not have seen.

It is also interesting to consider the behaviour shown by the critical subjects. None of them neglected the responses of the others and all demonstrated that they had been struck by the fact that a unanimity of judgment had not been reached in this simple perceptive test. The immediate reaction of most of the critical subjects was perplexity, unease, confusion. Some of them, after two or three trials in which disagreement was registered, attempted to stop the experiment to ask the experimenter to repeat the instructions, while others tried to speak with their neighbours to find out why they had given such unexpected responses. If at the beginning of the series of discordances the critical subjects thought that dissent was by chance, with the continuation of the trials they were forced to confront another unequivocal fact: their perception was different from that of the others. Also many of them attributed the cause of the disagreement not so much to the others, but rather to themselves. All of this shocked Asch who expected that very soon the game would be up and the experiment would come to nothing. What happened instead was the opposite: in the face of such a clearly mistaken opinion, the critical subjects did not call into question the judgments of the majority but tried to defend their own position or be even safer, even going so far as to approach the two cardboards with the lines to see better and, finally, to doubt their own perceptive capacity.

One comment reported at the end of the experiment, by one of the critical subjects is exemplary: "I didn't think I was mistaken, but reason told me I was wrong because it was impossible that so many people could be wrong and that only I was right". Even the few that never conform to the responses of the majority confessed that they had experienced a profound sense of unease and a painful uncertainty. Among these few those who resisted did it to hold on to the trust in themselves, through exercising internal coherence in their judgments. Among those who instead aligned themselves to the opinions of the majority, besides those no longer trusting their own visual capacity, many claimed they had felt the need not to be excluded from the group ("I didn't want to appear stupid"), giving less importance to any concern relative to what they had effectively perceived.

In these experiments the numerical rapport between the two sides takes centre stage. In fact when the sides are one to one (one accomplice and one critical subject) conformism is almost zero; after all we are in a situation of the type "your word against mine". The breaking point comes when the rapport becomes one (critical subject) to three (accomplices); a higher proportion does not increase significantly the entity of conformity. When however a person who thinks like the critical subject is inserted in the group despite a substantial confirmed majority in an opposing position, conformity falls visibly. Another dissenting individual breaks up the unanimity and shows that it is possible to have different opinions, creating at the same time a psychological tension in whoever has to manifest an opinion. It is interesting to note that in such a predicament very few of the critical subjects interviewed fully appreciated the role played by the deviant judge; although admitting that his presence was one of support, they did not seem to realize that he had been the determining factor in allowing them independence of judgment. When however the accomplice of the experimenter was instructed to be the only one to give the wrong response, the participants in the experiment ridiculed him.

2.2 The explanation of conformism

To understand the phenomenon of conformism a distinction was advanced between "informational influence" and "normative influence" (Deutsch & Gerard, 1955).

The first, consisting in taking positions expressed by others to resolve doubts deriving from ambiguous situations, is utilized to integrate sketchy skills and so gain greater security in facing up to life's chores. In such a case the group offers its members informational influence.

The second form of influence, pertaining to affiliation (the assumption of the norms of the group as an expression of the link between individuals), manifests itself in situations where a person intends to communicate to others a positive image of himself, or wants to avoid embarrassment and sanctions, like exclusion from the group.

Both these processes of sharing norms and knowledge assume importance for the people, and the prevalence in exercising one or the other varies according to the situation. In fact they produce their psychological effects at different levels. In this way two essential forms of conformism originate: acquiescence, when the person externally agrees with the group to avoid argument, although disagreeing, and internalization, when the person conforms because he is trustful of the responses given by the others and so is convinced of their goodwill (Kelman, 1958).

In the experiment conducted by Sherif on the autokinetic effect, the group exercised informative influence which induced a process of internalization. The individual judgments converge towards uniform regulation decided at group level without excessive difficulty, since there is no chance of objectifying the perception of luminous movement, being an optical illusion. As with many other real ambiguous or dangerous situations people authentically accept the influence exercised by the group they belong to.

In Asch's experiment, although both are present, the normative influence turns out to be more important than the informational one. This derives from the fact that public responses suffer more from the judgment of the group with respect to those given in private, generating in deviants a feeling of shame (Scheff, 1988). In addition this study has shown above all the type of conformism known as acquiescence, since the participants regain independence of judgment, once separated from group pressure. In this case you can speak of false conformism.

Naturally, acquiescence and internalization are not phenomena that exclude each other, rather they are understood to be polarities of a continuum. To do something because circumstances force us to do so can in fact induce a change of behaviour compared with what you are doing, as shown by the theory of cognitive dissonance (Festinger, 1957).

The "Asch effect", to follow the norms of the group even when they are so clearly against the data of reality, has raised several questions. Besides explanations linked to group processes (informational and normative influence), some authors (for example, Berry 1967; Frager, 1970) have also analyzed the rapport between conformism and socialization. In fact different societies tend to encourage behaviour of independence rather than submission, and viceversa. Otherwise to attach great importance to conformism compared with norms fixed by unknown people. At the same time, every society is characterized by the presence of various sub-cultures, which can orientate its members differently with respect to the dominant culture. For example, homosexuals often conform to the norms of the group they belong to but turn out to be non-conformist compared with the remaining society of heterosexuals.

Reference to homosexuals enables us to remember how, next to the influence of the majority, precisely in the studies of Asch, there is also an influence of the minority (Moscovici, 1976). Assigning a central role to social conflict, the minority, as for example illustrated by the history of the homosexual movement, have shown that it is possible to induce a change in the majority.

3. Obedience

If for the studies of Asch we can speak of a conformism in words the research conducted by Stanley Milgram (1974) on obedience describes instead how conformity comes to involve conduct. Obedience is a particular form of conformity: it manifests itself when the "majority" is not a quantitative dimension but qualitative. At the bottom of this there is a difference of status: the one who exercises a power superior to others operates a direct explicit pressure on them, who adapt to his will.

3.1 Immoral orders and dilemmas of conscience

"We will pay you $4.00 for one hour of your time. People needed for a study of memory". With this announcement published in a local newspaper participants were recruited to the first of a series of experiments which signalled the story of social psychology (Milgram, 1974).

Those who had responded to the announcement were invited to a laboratory to carry out actions which became more and more in contrast with their moral conscience. What interested the experimenters was to understand to what point the participants would obey to orders and when or how they would rebel. To make the prearranged situation credible a particular strategy was used: staging an experiment which had as its fictitious objective the study of processes of memory and learning; two participants were assigned the roles of teacher and learner. The experimenter informed both that it was an investigation aimed at investigating the effects of punishment on learning. The learner was taken into a room, made to sit, with hands tied in such a way as to make it evident that freedom of movement would be removed, while an electrode was applied on one pulse. The task of the learner consisted in learning a series of word associations, but for each error of memory apparently an electric shock was received increasing in intensity each time.

In reality the real "experimental subject" was not the learner but rather the teacher who, after helping to accommodate the former, was placed in another room before a false electricity generator contrived with a series of modulators of intensity ranging from 15 to 450 volts, rising on a scale by 15 volts with 30 lever switches. The instrument indicated, with special labels, the sequence from "light shock" to "dangerous shock". The teacher had the task of subjecting the learner to the word memory test: when the latter responded correctly the rule was that the test passed to the subsequent series of words, while when a mistake was made an electric shock was administered starting from the lowest level and proceeding as required upwards. As an accomplice of the experimenter, the false guinea pig did not receive any torture but the teacher was convinced that real damage was being inflicted.

The objective of the experimenter was that of observing to what point the teacher would agree to inflict violence on a person who manifested the will to defend himself, interrupting the test and unable to do it as he was tied up. The contrast between moral conscience and received orders was primed so that when the learner, pretending, manifested his discomfort: around 75 volts the first groans could be heard clearly, at 120 volts there was strong invective, at 150 volts the request that the experiment be suspended, finally, when the shocks were now reaching 285 volts excruciating gasps. How did the teachers behave? The results were surprising. Although manifesting tension and protesting energetically, 65% of the participants continued to punish the learner to the last beat. The groans and imploring of the victim were insufficient to make them desist from carrying out the orders of the experimenter.

What has just been described illustrates the standard condition of the experiment and the general results obtained but, to understand the problems faced better, it is opportune to analyze the different experimental modifications introduced to identify which conditions influence the behaviour of obedience. Milgram conducted several variations on his baseline study and found that obedience was maximized when participants merely assisted someone else giving the electric shocks (92.5%) and when they first observed a peer complying with the experimenter until the end (68.75%) (Milgram, 1974).

From these variations of situational stimuli, an important element regards the closeness of teacher and learner: the data show that there is an inversely proportional rapport between the tendency to inflict electric shocks and the proximity of the victim. As can be seen from table 1, Milgram arranged four different experimental conditions; if we observe how many participants arrived at the extreme point, corresponding to the most dangerous shocks, we note that the percentage of obedient participants follow the course of the levels of proximity. In fact the closer the teacher gets to the learner, until they touch, the less the phenomenon of obedience to the orders of the experimenter is registered. It can be affirmed that closeness of the victim, on the perceptive plane, increases the link between action and consequence, raising personal responsibility for the suffering inflicted. The principal morals that guide the action thus seem to be subject to the laws of proximity and distance. To act with ferocity towards a nearby or faraway victim certainly does not change the moral quality of the action; in spite of this intervention in the spatial rapport profoundly affects the disposition towards obedience. Therefore every element that reduces the proximity between action and victim inhibits the voice of conscience and makes the execution of the violent task easier.

	REMOTE	**VOICE FEEDBACK**	**PROXIMITY**	**TOUCH PROXIMITY**
EXTREME POINT OF OBEDIENCE (Shocks XXX) (435-450 volts)	The victim is not visible or audible	The victim is not visible and only his groans can be heard	The victim is in the same room as the person administering the electric shocks	The victim receives the shocks only if his arm is pushed by the teacher on a metal plate
% Participants	65.0%	62.5%	40.0%	30.0%

Table 1. Rapport between the proximity "teacher-learner" and level of obedience in Milgram's studies.

Even when the experimenter behaves incorrectly, reaching preliminary agreement less with respect to the moment of interruption of the experiment, most of the teachers respected their decisions of authority. Already evident is that the substance of the order is not so important as its origin; in fact, in the situation where roles are manipulated it turned out that any man placed in the role of the experimenter was unable to obtain obedience and when the part of the learner was recited by the experimenter, the moment the latter asked that the experiment be suspended, all participants stopped, disregarding the orders given by any man, while 65% of teachers continued when the commands were given by another experimenter: the orders of a source without authority had no power.

3.2 The explanation of destructive obedience

The explanation adopted by Milgram (1974) to understand the results of his research is founded on the concept of *agentic state*. A person inserted in an authoritarian system passes from an autonomous state to an agent state since he no longer feels free to act and considers himself as an agent who must satisfy the requirements of others, accepting the definition of the situation provided by authority. Thus a subject finds himself in an agentic state when he is willing to regulate his conduct according to directives coming from a person of higher status. In this condition the individual is no longer considered responsible for his own actions but is defined as an instrument to carry out the orders of others (Zamperini, 2003).

The root of behaviour of obedience is however singled out by Milgram outside the experimental context, calling socialization into question: the role of the family structure, school, institutions as agents that promote teaching of rules of obedience. And science does not escape similar considerations: the figure of the scientist, cloaked in prestige and superiority thanks to social legitimization, induces respect and acceptance.

The experimental model of Milgram is known also by the term "Eichmann experiment", since the condition in which participants are found evokes something analogous in the activity of this nazi bureaucrat, who from one side of a desk, absorbed in the work to be carried out, organized the expedition of trains loaded with Jews, destined for the extermination camps. Without drawing any equivalence between the participants in these experiments and those marked with collective atrocities these studies have, in any case, provided important indications in order to understand human behaviour in extreme situations like the Holocaust (for a critical review, Miller, 2004). The power of the situation in transforming ordinary people into torturers ready to commit acts of violence has also been analyzed by Kelman and Hamilton (1989). The authors give the name "binding forces" to all those elements of a situation that psychologically bind an individual to the definition of the reality provided by authority. The power of these forces is emphasized by the presence of numerous factors: the pressure of a group of equals, being watched, finding oneself involved in an ambiguous or new situation, the existence of a chain of command (like the military hierarchy), the grave consequences in case of disobedience. The massacres of civilians perpetrated by soldiers, as in the slaughter of My Lai during the Vietnam war, represent a tragic manifestation of similar forces.

The rapport of power between the dominant and the subordinate is shown effectively by a famous simulation: the imprisonment study of Philip Zimbardo (for a detailed summary, Zimbardo, 2007). In the simulated prison set up in the rooms of Stanford University, whoever wore the guard's uniform became aggressive while those who wore that of the prisoner took on an apathetic manner. This condition would have induced a psychological feeling of de-individualization, since the uniforms caused anonymity and loss of awareness of oneself. This seems to show that social roles may have a powerful effect on our behaviour. The guards are invested with authority and expect obedience. The expectation of role of the prisoners is obedience. In the study it does not just turn out that the latter obey the former but that all of them obey their social role (Zamperini, 2004).

3.3 Administrative obedience

In Milgram's study we are in the presence of conduct which (apparently) causes physical suffering, but we know that there are forms of violence and oppression that produce less visible damage and perhaps, just for this reason, are more insidious and worrying. The problem was confronted in a series of experiments on administrative obedience conducted in the eighties at Utrecht University, in Holland (Meeus & Raaijmakers, 1995).

The participants were asked to administer an enrolment test to an unemployed person and, to enable the scientist to collect data for personal research, completely unrelated to the selection process, they had to create a degree of psychological tension so as to cause a very poor performance. In this way the unemployed person lost any chance of obtaining the job he had applied for.

Comparing results obtained using the violence administered with those of Milgram, it turned out that in the first condition a greater level of obedience was achieved with respect to the second. It is the type of violence that enables us to understand this difference: physical violence (Milgram's experiments) is more direct and therefore more difficult to apply compared with the more indirect psychological-administrative violence. It was also shown that the participants were able to oppose authority: when they had to sign beforehand a declaration that made them legally responsible to the unemployed person, there was a significant reduction in the degree of obedience.

The explanation for the results are collocated in the theoretical perspective of Milgram, calling into question the status of agent and thus the psychological change inherent in the responsibility perceived in the participants. The experimenter is a representative of social institutions, authorized to act in a certain way and in a certain direction, while the unemployed person is perceived as a neutral and insignificant individual. For this reason the participants feel no emotional involvement with the victim and let themselves be guided by an institution considered legitimate.

4. Ethical issues and the (limited) validity of scenario studies

As we have seen from the above analysis, it seems difficult for people not to obey in the presence of an authority figure perceived as legitimate. Although social psychologists know much about this pervasive phenomenon – particularly with regard to the role of situational influences –, they would have known even more if ethics committees within universities or research institutions, established to protect the rights of human subjects, had not discouraged them from extending Milgram's research because of the stress experienced by participants. In the end, stricter ethical standards placed studies using procedures similar to Milgram's out of bounds – the last methodological replication was made in Austria, in the eighties, by Grete Schurz (Schurz, 1985).

Diana Baumrind was one of Milgram's most severe critics. In a famous article published in the *American Psychologist*, Baumrind (1964) argued that the extreme stress and emotional conflict described by Milgram could have easily modified the participants' self-image and/or their ability to trust authority figures in the future. Perhaps only an intense corrective interpersonal experience could have helped the subject to recover after such a distressing event. Without it, Baumrind expected a sensitive individual to remain hurt and anxious for some time, and a cynical subject to become even more alienated and distrustful. Similar critics and concerns for the welfare of subjects who served in the Milgram's experiment were expressed in the following years by several other scholars (Kaufmann, 1967; Mixon, 1972).

In his defense, Milgram (1964) claimed that the stress experienced by participants dissipated quickly and was not injurious – when, a year after the research program was completed, a medical examiner interviewed 40 experimental subjects, no evidence was found of any traumatic reactions. Also, follow-up data indicated that many participants not only felt gratified to have taken part in that study but said they viewed their participation as an opportunity to learn something important about themselves and wanted to be in further experimental research.

Milgram's arguments were not enough to put an end to the controversy. From that point on, social researchers interested in exploring the mechanisms of obedience have relied upon their creativity to set up experimental paradigms able to minimize participants' emotional strain. Electric shocks were then replaced with verbal insults (Bocchiaro & Zimbardo, 2010; Meeus & Raaijmakers, 1986), the real victim with a puppy (Sheridan & King, 1972) or with a (female) virtual human (Slater et al., 2006), and the intimidating laboratory settings with more familiar, real world ones (Bickman, 1974; Hofling et al., 1966).

Recently, a partial replication of Milgram's experiment was conducted in the United States by Jerry Burger (2009). Burger received approval from his university ethics committee by modifying several of the experimental protocols in order to reduce the emotional discomfort experienced by participants. First, through several screenings (tests and interviews), he rejected people who might have negative reactions to participating in the study. Second, participants were given a milder sample shock (15 volts) rather than in the Milgram study (45 volts). Third, and most important, Burger stopped the procedure at 150 volts, when the learner-confederate protested for the first time and clearly said he wanted out because of the excessive pain. The 150-volt solution was based on previous analyses showing that 79% of Milgram's subjects (Exp. 5; see Milgram, 1974) who had followed the experimenter's orders at this level went on until the last shock. As noted by Burger, knowing people's reactions to the 150-volt point allows one to estimate what they would do if allowed to continue, without exposing them to the extreme tension exhibited by Milgram's participants.

What did Burger find 45 years after Milgram? Despite the important historical and cultural changes that have occurred over four decades, the power of authority figures to claim people's allegiance and obedience remains very strong: 70% of participants obeyed until the end. Milgram, at the same point in his most comparable condition, had found 82.5%, but such a difference does not come close to statistical significance — in comparing these percentages, it is crucial to consider also that Burger had implemented a few procedural changes that should have made it easier to disobey.

Results obtained by Burger are not surprising: correlational analyses conducted by Blass (1999) on 24 studies spanning a period of 22 years (from 1963 to 1985) clearly indicate that the rates of obedience show no systematic change over time. These findings, taken together, provide indirect evidence against the "enlightenment effects" thesis proposed by social psychologist Kenneth Gergen (1973). According to Gergen, "sophistication as to psychological principles liberates one from their behavioral implications" (1973, p. 313). If Gergen is right, participants in the more recent studies would have been more familiar with Milgram's work and thereby become enlightened about the demands of authority; as a consequence, the later studies should have found lower rates of obedience than the earlier ones. A more direct test of the "enlightenment effects" thesis was provided by a study in which participants were asked to serve as experimenters and oversee a "teacher" who had to teach a verbal-learning task to a "learner" by using increasing shocks as punishment on each mistake (Shelton, 1982). As the shock levels escalated, the teacher, who unbeknownst to the experimenter-participant was a confederate, "expressed uneasiness, then became quite anxious, angry, on the verge of tears; cursed, complained of stomach pains, asked for a glass of water, and pleaded with the experimenter to stop the session ..." (p. 31). Although participants had first been given a synopsis of the obedience experiment – in Gergen's words, they had been "enlightened" –, 92% of them continued to command the teacher to keep increasing the voltage to the maximum level. As noted by Blass (1999):

> ...contrary to what is implied by Gergen's "enlightenment effects" notion, knowledge does not or cannot always lead to action. Being enlightened about the unexpected power of authority may help a person to stay away from an authority-dominated situation, but once he or she is already in such a situation, knowledge of the drastic degree of obedience that authorities are capable of eliciting does not necessarily help to free the individual from the grip of the forces operating in that concrete situation; that is, to defy the authority in charge. (p. 971)

The aforementioned stringent ethical standards, besides hindering research on obedience, have indirectly delayed the systematic investigation of the socially positive aspects of the interaction individual-unjust authority, notably disobedience and whistle-blowing – we will talk about them in the next paragraph–, investigation that would seem to be essential for understanding some preconditions of social/political revolutions. Our knowledge about "rebellious" individuals is gradually increasing, but there are still no clear cut answers to basic questions: do disobedient people/whistleblowers have special values or personality traits? Or why do they choose to defy unjust authority/to report the misconduct to higher authorities?

In order to resolve the ethical controversy and find answers to these important questions, some social scientists feel that scenario studies are a viable methodology (King, 1997; Sims & Keenan, 1998). Basically, in scenario studies participants are presented with a detailed description of a given situation, asked to reflect carefully on it and, finally, to predict their behaviour. It is a research method that can be appropriate and useful when respondents are asked to predict their own behaviour under situations that have been experienced frequently. Predictions in these cases will likely be correct because based on people's personal histories. On the contrary, complex and unfamiliar circumstances have a flavor that is hard to grasp by simply imagining them; as a logical result, respondents are especially inaccurate in guessing what they would do. Also, as correctly noted by Miceli and colleagues (2008), would people accurately report their behaviour, or would they report what they believe most others will view favorably? Or would they give the researcher the responses they believe would support his/her hypotheses rather than their "real" feelings?

Before the study was conducted, Milgram (1963) had provided 14 psychology graduate students with a detailed description of his experimental paradigm on obedience, then asked them to predict the behaviour of one hundred hypothetical Americans of various ages and occupations who were placed in that situation. Students predicted that about 1% of the subjects would continue to obey to the end. The same question was posed informally to a group of experts, professors of psychology and psychiatry, and again the prediction was that virtually all participants would refuse to go on at a certain point of the procedure. As you remember, in Milgram's baseline condition 65% of participants turned out to be fully obedient to the authority. Similarly, Bocchiaro and colleagues (2011) found a striking difference between estimated and observed data. Their experimental paradigm allowed participants to deal with an unreasonable, unethical request by the experimenter-authority with options of obeying, disobeying, or blowing the whistle. In the scenario study, only 3.6% of total respondents (138 undergraduate students) indicated they would obey; by contrast, most believed they would be either disobedient, 31.9%, or whistleblowers, 64.5%. Data from the laboratory presented a very different picture: 76.5% of participants (a separate sample of 149 undergraduate students) obeyed the experimenter, 14.1% disobeyed, and 9.4% challenged the alleged unethical nature of the experiment by reporting the misconduct of the experimenter to higher authorities.

Far from launching a generic attack on scenario studies, we want to point out again that it is feasible for social scientists to use this research method when they want to explore human behaviour in situations that are familiar to respondents. Otherwise, it is more appropriate to use or develop research paradigms that (a) allow for the analysis of spontaneous reactions to events that are real in the participants' eyes and that (b) protect their psychological and emotional well-being. The 150-volt solution proposed by Burger is a valid contribution in this direction. In the next paragraph we will see a few more.

5. Resisting to social pressures: Disobedient people and whistleblowers

It is worth noting that, independent of the procedure used, all studies on obedience invariably report a percentage of participants that defy the authority (Hofling et al., 1966; Meeus & Raaijmakers, 1986; Sheridan & King, 1972; Slater et al., 2006). This defiant decision, at least in Milgram-style experiments, appears most likely at the critical point when the victim's first requests to terminate the study (Gilbert, 1981; Packer, 2008). Other subsequent analyses, this time performed on Milgram's "Bridgeport" condition (his second laboratory site in an office suite in Bridgeport, Connecticut), reveal that the earlier in the procedure subjects begin to oppose the experimenter (by questioning or objecting to his demands), the more likely they are to end up defiant (Modigliani & Rochat, 1995). "Thus it appears that the timing of a participant's first firm opposition is important in shaping final outcomes. Firm, early opposition seems to be a sufficient condition for successful defiance, and, not surprisingly, total lack of such firm opposition is a sufficient condition for ending up obedient" (Rochat et al., 2000, p. 171).

Monin and colleagues (2008) demonstrated that *moral rebels* – "individuals who take a principled stand against the status quo, who refuse to comply, stay silent, or simply go along when this would require that they compromise their values" (pp. 76-77) – often do not receive the respect they deserve. In a series of studies, such rebel behaviour turned out to elicit resentment and rejection in those participants who had not taken this brave course of action, implicitly perceived as an indictment of their own misconduct. As a further, indirect proof of the validity of these results, the authors report comments made at debriefing by Milgram's obedient participants on those who had disobeyed (1965, Study 2): they were "ridiculous" (p. 132), they "lost all control of themselves" (p. 132), and "they came here for an experiment, and I think they should have stuck with it" (p. 132).

More recently, Bocchiaro and Zimbardo (2010), through a research paradigm modeled after that of the Utrecht studies (Meeus & Raaijmakers, 1986), tried to cast some light on the psychological factors involved in fostering disobedience. In this study, the participant, called "coach", was asked to assist a "performer"(confederate) in solving a sequence of syllogisms. The task for the performer was to find the logical conclusions, for the coach to give critical feedback in case of mistake. Critical feedback consisted of a graded series of negative comments and rude remarks. For example, a mild criticism was "You are going bad…", a moderate feedback was "You are really ridiculous!", and an extremely negative feedback was "You are really the most stupid person I have ever seen!". The performer solved only 4 of the 19 syllogisms, mostly at the beginning. His emotive reactions were also predetermined and their intensity increased as critical feedback turned more hostile.

The results of this exploratory study revealed that 70% of participants (Italian undergraduate students) disobeyed the unjust authority at the victim's first request to be released (the confederate pretended to suffer a lot and shouted that he wanted to leave) – such a high level of disobedience was mainly due to the combination of condition "proximity of teacher to learner" with "remote authority". The study also showed similarities between obedient and disobedient participants: the two groups were equivalent in terms of personality traits, stress reactions to the experimental setting, and verbal dissent (form and frequency) towards authority. Among the disobedient participants, post-experimental interviews revealed their decision to be impulsive, and believed to be the most obvious for anyone to make in that situation. Moreover, disobedience turned out to be typically motivated by emergent empathy for the victim-confederate ("I felt pity for him") and, to a lesser extent, by moral/ethical considerations ("I stopped because it didn't seem fair to me to go on in those conditions. I wouldn't have had a clear conscience").

In another study (Bocchiaro et al., 2011), conducted in the basement of the VU University of Amsterdam, participants were asked by the experimenter-authority to write and sign a brief statement to convince their fellow students and friends to participate in an experiment on sensory deprivation to be done at the VU University. The experiment appeared immediately unethical: in a similar one, allegedly carried out in Rome (allegedly, as no experiment had actually been done), subjects had panicked, experienced visual and auditory hallucinations, and described the experience as a frightening one. Two participants had even asked the researchers to stop because of their strong symptoms.

Besides the possibility to disobey the experimenter's request to write the statement in support of the sensory deprivation experiment, participants had the opportunity to report his misconduct by putting a form in the "research committee" box. As mentioned in the previous paragraph, 76.5% of participants obeyed, 14.1% disobeyed, and 9.4% blew the whistle.

When considered retrospectively, the decision to disobey seemed fairly obvious to participants: 81% of disobedient subjects stated it had been "easy" for them to act that way, mainly because of their perception of the obviously unethical aspects of the sensory deprivation experiment. Such a perception of "easiness" was also linked with a firm resolution not to involve other people. The dominant feeling, at the end, was one of "pride" (52.4%), and of "relief" (28.6%).

Obeying was considered an easy path as well. Authority of the experimenter (34.2%), importance of scientific research (17.5%), and money (16.7%) were the factors that, in that order, contributed most in making such a decision. In sharp contrast, it was mainly the wish to protect their own friends (52.4%) and the ethically unacceptable sensory deprivation experiment (14.3%) that triggered participants' disobedience.

When asked about the thoughts that went through their mind before choosing what to do, many disobedient participants (42.9%) thought about how "not fair" the sensory deprivation experiment was ("It is unethical… it goes against my principles"). As regards their feelings, a clear sense of uneasiness was experienced by 47.6% of disobedient participants ("I felt under pressure, morally oppressed", "I got a strange feeling in my gut").

The pattern of responses given by obedient participants proved to be more articulated: some of them (18.4%) were confused about what to do ("Would it be weird to stop?", "Shall I get up and leave?"), others (14.9%) concentrated on their friends ("I thought to warn my fellow students before they would receive that message", "What are they going to do with the friends I wrote down?"), and some others (6.1%) were preoccupied with the task ("My thoughts went to the message… how to write a good and short piece"). Almost one third of obedient participants (30.7%) experienced conflicting feelings before deciding to comply ("On the one side I did want to help the experimenter, but on the other I did not want to involve my friends"), whereas 23.7% explicitly claimed to have felt "uneasy" ("I did get a nasty feeling", "I was uneasy because I had the idea that it was not ethically correct"). This same feeling of uneasiness accompanied the act of writing the statement for the experimenter by 30.7%. However, this figure grew to 48.2% when the categories "uneasy", "guilty", and "forced, used" were combined.

Subjects were also specifically asked whether they had realized that, in writing the statement, they were lying. Only 47.4% of respondents said "yes." Even so, they continued for one of the following reasons: "People who would receive the message still have the freedom to choose what to do" (25.9%), "authority of the experimenter" (14.8%), "already committed to the task" (14.8%), value of "science" (9.3%), and the "possibility to adapt the message" (9.3%). All the remaining answers were included in the category "other". Those who had said "I did not realize I was lying" actually resorted to a mechanism of denial. They stated that they just left out crucial information, adapted the message, withheld information - but actually they did not.

In general, disobedient participants stated they were not worried about possible negative effects arising from their behavior ("no money" was the worst consequence for 28.6% of those who disobeyed). Surprisingly, the same lack of consequential concern was true of many obedient participants: most of them were not concerned because "people who would receive the message still have the freedom to choose what to do" (38.8%), because "these people can be warned in advance" (28.8%), or because "the last word is up to the Research Committee" (10.%).

Finally, disobedient participants were asked why, although they refused to comply, they refrained from going further to denounce the authority misconduct by reporting it to the higher authorities. Many of them (42.9%) answered that, by opposing the experimenter, they had already done their duty ("I thought it did not apply to me"). Others (19%) made reference to the experimenter ("I would have felt guilty", "The mail box looked like it could be opened by the experimenter"), whereas 14.3% refrained from blowing the whistle because in any case the Research Committee would monitor the experiment ("The Research Committee was informed, so…").

What about the whistleblowers? Before going into details of their post-experimental responses, it is probably useful to present here the whistle-blowing phenomenon. Whistleblower is a general term applied to anyone who discloses illegal, immoral or illegitimate practices under the control of his/her employer to persons or organizations that may be able to effect remedial action (Near & Miceli, 1985). Although protected by a number of laws (at least in some countries), the act of reporting internal wrongdoing is clearly demanding for people: a prospective whistleblower, in fact, is typically concerned about ostracism, harassment, blame, demotion, discharge. Moreover, there is no warranty that the unlawful practices will be corrected, especially when the correction is costly, damages the reputation of the company or institution, or when there is a culture of complicity from top down in the company or system of control.

Miethe (1999) noted that the act of blowing the whistle is often followed by bankruptcy, depression, and alcoholism, whereas Alford (2001) found that somewhere between half and two-thirds of the whistleblowers lose their jobs — they rarely get them back and most will never work in that field because of informal blacklists spread across sister organizations. But usually they are not fired outright. "The organization's goal is to disconnect the act of whistleblowing from the act of retaliation, which is why so much legislation to protect the whistleblower is practically irrelevant. The usual practice is to demoralize and humiliate the whistleblower, putting him or her under so much psychological stress that it becomes difficult to do a good job. If the whistleblower is under enough stress, he or she is likely to make a bad decision, justifying disciplinary actions." (Alford, 2001, pp. 31-32).

Retaliation seems then a key element in the whistleblowing phenomenon. It can be work-related or social — the first being tangible and formal whereas the second more informal and undocumented in employment records — and it is inversely associated with the whistleblower's power and credibility (Near & Miceli, 1987). However, "where the organization depends heavily on the wrongdoer or the wrongdoing itself, even a whistle-blower with high status may not have sufficient relative power to escape retaliation" (Miceli et al., 2008, p. 104).

Having said all that, it is not surprising that only a small minority of people is willing to perform such an extraordinary act. The value of this percentage will depend on situational factors (seriousness and type of wrongdoing, characteristics of the organization, wrongdoer power) more than on personality traits (see Miceli et al., 2008). Regarding this latter point, research reveals that whistleblowers are not different in terms of personality traits or personal values from those who chose not to report the observed wrongdoing (Near & Miceli, 1996). This lack of difference may sound somewhat strange at first, as one might expect a whistleblower being more altruistic, courageous, empathetic than the rest of the people. It is not like this. Of course, there must be personal variables that distinguish between "categories" of individuals, but the psychological tests so far used by psychologists are probably not so subtle to pick up such difference.

Let us go back to data. In the post-experimental interviews collected by Bocchiaro and colleagues (2011), 78.6% of whistleblowers stated it had been an easy decision, followed by a feeling of "pride" (42.9%), and of "relief" (35.7%). Whistleblowers declared that they were not worried about possible effects arising from their behavior, and that their decision was almost entirely a matter of principle of fairness and justice. When asked about the thoughts that went through their mind before choosing what to do, whistleblowers were mainly focused (57.1%) on the moral "rightness" of the decision they were about to make ("I thought I would do something good by sending the form"). As regards their feelings, a clear sense of uneasiness was experienced by 57.1% of them ("I was scared, my hands started to shake", "I felt used").

It is important to note that no statistically significant differences were found among whistleblowers, obedient, and disobedient participants in any of the personality factors measured. Also, no significant differences were found in any of these groups in relation to religious affiliation, religious involvement, or gender.

6. Conclusion

We opened this chapter by noting that conformism and obedience are essential elements in maintaining social order. However, as clearly demonstrated by Solomon Asch and Stanley Milgram in the controlled setting of a laboratory, the desire to conform and obey can lead ordinary people into even mistrust their own experiences or inflict serious harm on others. The implicit message is that, in certain contexts, apparently simple situational factors are more powerful than personality traits in shaping human behaviour.

The good news is that these same situational factors can be manipulated to stimulate people to act in a positive way. In other words, virtually anyone, independently of his/her personality structure, can overcome social pressures toward conformity and obedience. Although we expect many social psychologists to agree with us, our statement may appear provocative or even absurd to those who think that behaviours stem from a specific constellation of personality: for them, we assume, rebels must be more courageous than others or must have been nurtured properly, in a supportive environment, by parents or teachers. This reasoning is surely plausible, but at present there is insufficient evidence to support it. To us, it seems much more reasonable to argue that nonconformers, disobedients, and whistleblowers are ordinary people whose action is extraordinary, and that some of them, if not many, are unlikely to engage in another disobedient act given that the first one was situationally-specific.

It is essential to understand the forces that catalyse people from passive bystanders to active responders able to challenge immorality and injustice. To do that, we call for studies that, while protecting the welfare and dignity of individuals, explore the foundation of defiance both in the person and in the situation. On the one hand, social researchers should make use of more refined psychological measures to capture even the most subtle difference between categories of people; on the other, they should systematically manipulate a set of variables to develop in the participants a sense of personal responsibility, morality, and pressure necessary for disobeying and blowing the whistle. Also, it would be important to manipulate the power held by the authority figure and observe whether, and to which extent, different typologies of power shape the participants' behavior.

If conformism and obedience are basic elements in our culture, nonconformity, disobedience, and whistle-blowing are vital for its progress.

7. References

Alford, C. F. (2001). *Whistleblowers: Broken Lives and Organizational Power*, Cornell University Press, Ithaca (NY).

Asch, S. (1951). Effects of Group Pressure Upon the Modification and Distortion of Judgment, In: *Groups, Leadership and Men*, H. Guetzkow (Ed.), 177-190, Carnagie Press, Pittsburgh (PA).

Asch, S. (1956). Studies of Independence and Conformity: 1. A Minority of One Against a Unanimous Majority. *Psychological Monographs*, Vol. 70, No. 416, pp. 1-70.

Baumrind, D. (1964). Some Thoughts on Ethics of Research: After Reading Milgram's "Behavioral Study of Obedience." *American Psychologist,* Vol. 19, No. 6, pp. 421–423.

Berry, J. W. (1967). Independence and Conformity in Subsistence-Level Societies. *Journal of Personality and Social Psychology*, Vol. 7, No. 4, pp. 415-418.

Bickman, L. (1974). The Social Power of a Uniform. *Journal of Applied Social Psychology,* Vol. 4, No. 1, pp. 47-61.

Blass, T. (1999). The Milgram Paradigm After 35 Years: Some Things We Now Know About Obedience to Authority. *Journal of Applied Social Psychology,* Vol. 29, No. 5, pp. 955-978.

Bocchiaro, P., & Zimbardo, P. G. (2010). Defying Unjust Authority: An Exploratory Study. *Current Psychology,* Vol. 29, No. 2, pp. 155-170.

Bocchiaro, P., Zimbardo, P. G., & Van Lange, P. A. M. (2011). *To Defy or Not to Defy: Unpacking Disobedience and Whistle-blowing as Extraordinary Forms of Resistance to Authority.* Unpublished manuscript, VU University of Amsterdam, Amsterdam, The Netherlands.

Burger, J. M. (2009). Replicating Milgram: Would People Still Obey Today? *American Psychologist,* Vol. 64, No. 1, pp. 1–11.

Deutsch, M. & Gerard, H. B. (1955). A Study of Normative and Informational Social Influence. *Journal of Abnormal and Social Psychology,* Vol. 51, No. 3, pp. 629-36.

Festinger, L. (1950). Informal Social Communication. *Psychological Review,* Vol. 57, No. 5, pp. 271-282.

Festinger, L. (1957). *A Theory of Cognitive Dissonance,* Stanford University Press, Stanford (CA).

Frager, R. (1970). Conformity and Anti-Conformity in Japan. *Journal of Personality and Social Psychology*, Vol. 15, No. 3, pp. 203-210.

Gergen, K. J. (1973). Social Psychology as History. *Journal of Personality and Social Psychology,* Vol. 26, No. 2, pp. 309-320.

Gilbert, S. J. (1981). Another Look at the Milgram Obedience Studies: The Role of the Gradated Series of Shocks. *Personality and Social Psychology Bulletin,* Vol. 7, No. 4, pp. 690-695.

Hofling, C. K., Brotzman, E., Dalrymple, S., Graves, N., & Pierce, C. (1966). An Experimental Study of Nurse-Physician Relations. *The Journal of Nervous and Mental Disease,* Vol. 143, No. 2, pp. 171-180.

Kaufmann, H. (1967). The Price of Obedience and the Price of Knowledge. *American Psychologist,* Vol. 22, No. 4, 321–322.

Kelman, H. C. (1958). Compliance, Identification, and Internalization: Three Processes of Attitude Change. *Journal of Conflict Resolution,* Vol. 2, No. 1, pp. 51-60.

Kelman, H. C., & Hamilton, V. L. (1989). *Crimes of Obedience: Toward a Social Psychology of Authority and Responsibility,* Yale University Press, New Haven (CT).

King, G., III. (1997). The Effects of Interpersonal Closeness and Issue Seriousness on Blowing the Whistle. *Journal of Business Communication,* Vol. 34, No. 4, pp. 419-436.

Meeus, W. H. J., & Raaijmakers, Q. A. W. (1986). Administrative Obedience: Carrying Out Orders to Use Psychological-Administrative Violence. *European Journal of Social Psychology,* Vol. 16, No. 4, pp. 311-324.

Meeus, W. H. J. & Raaijmakers, Q. A. W. (1995). Obedience in Modern Society: The Utrecht Studies. *Journal of Social Issues,* Vol. 51, No. 3, pp. 155-75.

Miceli, M. P., Near, J. P., & Dworkin, T. M. (2008). *Whistle-Blowing in Organizations,* Routledge, New York.

Miethe, T. D. (1999). *Whistleblowing at Work: Tough Choices in Exposing Fraud, Waste, and Abuse on the Job,* Westview Press, Boulder (CO).

Milgram, S. (1963). Behavioral Study of Obedience. *Journal of Abnormal and Social Psychology,* Vol. 67, No. 4, pp. 371–378.

Milgram, S. (1964). Issues in the Study of Obedience: A Reply to Baumrind. *American Psychologist,* Vol. 19, No. 11, pp. 848-852.

Milgram, S. (1965). Some Conditions of Obedience and Disobedience to Authority. *Human Relations,* Vol. 18, No. 1, pp. 57–76.

Milgram, S. (1974). *Obedience to Authority: An Experimental View,* Harper & Row, New York.

Miller, A. G. (2004). What Can the Milgram Obedience Experiments Tell Us about the Holocaust?: Generalizing from the Social Psychology Laboratory, In: *The Social Psychology of Good and Evil,* A. G. Miller (Ed.), 193-239, The Guilford Press, New York.

Mixon, D. (1972). Instead of Deception. *Journal for the Theory of Social Behavior,* Vol. 2, No. 2, pp. 145–177.

Modigliani, A., & Rochat, F. (1995). The Role of Interaction Sequences and the Timing of Resistance in Shaping Obedience and Defiance to Authority. *Journal of Social Issues,* Vol. 51, No. 3, pp. 107-123.

Moghaddam, F. M. (1998). *Social Psychology. Exploring Universals Across Cultures*, W. H. Freeman and Company, New York.

Monin, B., Sawyer, P. J., & Marquez, M. J. (2008). The Rejection of Moral Rebels: Resenting Those Who Do the Right Thing. *Journal of Personality and Social Psychology*, Vol. 95, No. 1, pp. 76-93.

Moscovici, S. (1976). *Social Influence and Social Change*, Academic Press, New York.

Near, J. P., & Miceli, M. P. (1985). Organizational Dissidence: The Case of Whistle-Blowing. *Journal of Business Ethics*, Vol. 4. No. 1, pp. 1-16.

Near, J. P., & Miceli, M. P. (1987). Whistle-Blowers in Organizations: Dissidents or Reformers?, In: *Research in Organizational Behavior*, B. M. Staw and L. L. Cummings (Eds.), 321-368, JAI Press, Greenwich, CT.

Near, J. P., & Miceli, M. P. (1996). Whistle-Blowing: Myth and Reality. *Journal of Management*, Vol. 22, No. 3, pp. 507-526.

Packer, D. J. (2008). Identifying Systematic Disobedience in Milgram's Obedience Experiments: A Meta-Analytic Review. *Perspectives on Psychological Science*, Vol. 3, No. 4, pp. 301-304.

Rochat, F., Maggioni, O., & Modigliani, A. (2000). The Dynamics of Obeying and Opposing Authority: A Mathematical Model, In: *Obedience to Authority: Current Perspectives on the Milgram Paradigm*, T. Blass (Ed.), 161-192, Lawrence Erlbaum Publishers, Mahwah (NJ).

Scheff, T. J. (1988). Shame and Conformity: The Defence-Emotion System. *American Sociological Review*, Vol. 53, No. 3, pp. 395-406.

Schurz, G. (1985). Experimentelle überprüfung des zusammenhangs zwischen persönlichkeitsmerkmalen und der bereitschaft zum destruktiven gehorsam gegenüber autoritäten [Experimental Examination of the Relationships Between Personality Characteristics and the Readiness For Destructive Obedience Toward Authority]. *Zeitschrift für Experimentelle und Angewandte Psychologie*, Vol. 32, No. 1, pp. 160–177.

Shelton, G. A. (1982). *The Generalization of Understanding to Behavior: The Role of Perspective in Enlightenment*. Unpublished doctoral dissertation, University of British Columbia, Vancouver, Canada.

Sheridan, C. L., & King, R. G. (1972). Obedience to Authority With an Authentic Victim, *Proceedings of the 80th annual convention of the American Psychological Association*, pp. 165-166, Honolulu, Hawaii, USA, September 1-8, 1972.

Sherif, M. (1936). *The Psychology of Social Norms*, Harper, New York.

Sims, R. L., & Keenan, J. P. (1998). Predictors of External Whistleblowing: Organizational and Intrapersonal Variables. *Journal of Business Ethics*, Vol. 17, No. 4, pp. 411-421.

Slater, M., Antley, A., Davison, A., Swapp, D., Guger, C., Barker, C., Pistrang, N., Sanchez-Vives, M. V. (2006). A Virtual Reprise of the Stanley Milgram Obedience Experiments. *PLoS ONE, 1:* e39.

Turner, J. C. (1991). *Social Influence*, Open University Press, Buckingham.

Zamperini, A. (2003). Obbedienza distruttiva e crisi dell'azione [Destructive Obedience and Action Crisis], In: S. Milgram, *Obedience to Authorithy: An Experimental View*, 9-42, Einaudi, Torino, (Introductory essay to the Italian translation).
Zamperini, A. (2004). *Prigioni della mente. Relazioni di oppressione e resistenza [Mind Prisons. Rapports of Oppression and Resistance]*, Einaudi, Torino.
Zimbardo, P. (2007). *The Lucifer Effect*, Random House, New York.

15

Selected Social Psychological Phenomena's Effect on Educational Team Decision Making

Laurie McGary Klose and Jon S. Lasser
Texas State University-San Marcos
USA

1. Introduction

School psychologists practice in complex eco-systemic contexts that present unique challenges and opportunities to impact the education and mental health of children (Borgelt & Conoley, 1999; Curtis & Stollar, 2002; Lusterman, 1992). Social psychology explores human cognition, behavior, and emotion in the context of social interactions (Bernstein & Nash, 2002). This chapter examines the influence of several social psychological phenomena on school psychologists' participation in group decision-making, and presents case examples to illustrate these descriptions. Finally, recommendations for school psychology practice are given to minimize potential negative effects of group decision-making phenomena.

The practice of psychology in the schools presents challenges that are specific to working with teams, systems, and groups. School psychologists must frequently navigate systems' boundaries, conflicting values and beliefs, and multiple roles. Some of these roles include evaluator, counselor, mediator, administrator, consultant, advocate and educator. Each of these roles brings complex issues of privacy, confidentiality, informed consent, and multiple relationships when working with students, parents, teachers, administrators, and other school personnel. School psychology can be conceptualized through an eco-systemic framework that presents schools operating as interrelated systems. Each of these systems contains complex interactions between many individuals including parents, teachers, administrators, service professionals and children. These individuals and systems interact and engage in decision making that determine the educational programming for children in the schools. Therefore, understanding group decision-making necessitates an understanding of social influence.

Although social psychology research has been applied broadly to the practice of school psychology (Medway & Cafferty, 1992, 1999), the specific implications for ethics have not yet been addressed. The need to address the ethical decision-making of school psychologists through an understanding of social psychological phenomena is significant because such decisions occur in social contexts. Because ethical decisions are typically made based upon how they will impact others, the application of various social psychological phenomena to ethical decision-making can serve as an appropriate and useful tool. Failing to recognize the influence of social psychological phenomena on group decision making can result in unintended consequences that can give rise to ethical concerns. What follows are overviews of selected social psychological phenomena that have implications for group decision making and potential ethical concerns, a case example for illustration, and recommendations for best practice.

2. The foot-in-the-door phenomenon

The foot-in-the-door phenomenon, also known as sequential-request compliance, predicts that, having complied with a small or initial request, respondents are more likely to comply later with a larger request (Kaufmann-Bryant & Mullen, 1995). For example, after consenting to allow a sales person to enter a home and deliver a demonstration, the homeowner may be more likely to purchase the product being demonstrated. This may result from inferences one might make about compliance with the initial request (e.g., I must be the kind of person that complies with requests because I complied with the last request this person made). Implications of this phenomenon can have significant applications for school psychologists and educational decision makers.

Four decades of support indicate the foot-in-the-door phenomenon clear, yet qualified, base of empirical support. Beginning with the first study related to phone and then in person interviews about household products, (Freedman & Fraser, 1966) more than 100 foot-in-the-door phenomenon experiments have been published (Burger, 1999). Burger's (1999) systematic review and meta-analysis of foot-in-the-phenomenon research carefully delineated the contextual factors that influence compliance. While an extensive discussion of these factors goes beyond the scope of this chapter, a summary of research findings include labeling the participant who agreed to the first request as helpful before making the second request, proximity of the second request to the first and from the same person making the second request that made the first, and making the second request similar to the first. Readers interested in more detailed discussions of the foot-in-the-door phenomenon are referred to more extensive reviews (e.g., Burger, 1999; Dillard, Hunter, & Burgoon, 1984).

Perhaps the impact of foot-in-the-door is most logically considered in the context of informed consent. Informed consent for services is paramount in school psychology. Informed consent is a process rather than an occurrence. "Blanket consent" (in which an individual consents to any and all services that the school psychologist wishes to perform) is inappropriate (Jacob & Hartshorne, 2003). As a result, the school psychologist may engage in sequential requests for each specific type of service that is to be provided. Typically, school psychologists employ a process-oriented approach to informed consent (Pope & Vasquez, 1991), where the school psychologist and parent/guardian revisit issues related to consent issues as proposed services change over time and circumstance. Sometimes, consent is sought for small requests (permission to consult with the child's teacher) and subsequent requests are for more significant services (permission to engage in ongoing counseling with a child). Another common situation for school psychologists occurs when they seek permission to conduct an evaluation of a student suspected of having a disability and then later participates in discussions regarding parental consent for placement in special education services. In this natural course of events, opportunities for the foot-in-the-door type influence should be avoided. The following case example and discussion illustrate the significance of the potential impact of foot-in-the-door phenomenon in school psychology practice with regard to sequential requests for consent. The case example is not an actual case but reflects an amalgamation of many situations that could occur in school based practice. All names are fictional and do not represent actual people.

3. Case example

Bailey Jenkins, the school psychologist, has asked Susan and Dale for their consent to conduct an evaluation to determine if their daughter is a student with a learning disability. Bailey has emphasized that she is seeking consent for evaluation only, and that consenting to the evaluation does not indicate that the parents are agreeing to placement in special education. Susan and Dale agree that there is little risk in giving their consent for the assessment. Bailey shares with the parents that the results of the evaluation indicate that their daughter, Jennifer, meets the eligibility criteria for special education services as a student with Specific Learning Disability in basic reading. Susan and Dale inform Jennifer's teacher and the principal that they will not agree to Jennifer receiving special education services. The principal suggests that Bailey speak to the parents to gain consent as she was able to obtain consent for the evaluation.

This case example illustrates a situation where Bailey, the school psychologist, may unwittingly pressure Jennifer's parents toward consent to placement in special education. Although the primary motivation driving Bailey's attempts to gain the parents' consent may be her belief that the recommendations are in the best interest of the child, the consent for the smaller request for evaluation may influence the parent's willingness to agree to the larger request for placement in special education. This could result in Jennifer's parents making a decision that they might not have made in the absence of the foot-in-the-door phenomenon, thus exercising influence rather than allowing the parents to make an informed decision in the absence of influence.

When a school psychologist has a clear understanding of the foot-in-the-door phenomenon and its implications, she would be cognizant of the issues that arise when the same person asks for consecutive consents. The impact of the foot-in-the-door phenomenon can be minimized if the school psychologist maintains a role of "informer" rather than "persuader". The school psychologist can engage in ethical best practice by providing the parents all the information that they need to arrive at an informed decision and reiterating that their consent for the evaluation should not influence their decisions about consent for services.

Lasser and Klose (2007) suggest the following steps to minimize the impact of foot-in-the-door on decision making in school settings: "a proactive, family empowering approach that utilizes awareness of social psychological principles could involve: discussing with the parents about the importance of making decisions with which they are comfortable; framing parental consent for placement in special education as an option or choice rather than a request for compliance; educating the Individual Educational Plan team to minimize exploitation of the foot-in-the-door phenomenon."

4. Conformity

An important aspect of school psychological services is the participation in meetings with other education professionals in an effort to identify and analyze academic, behavioral, and social problems of students and develop interventions for identified problems. In fact, some aspects of school psychological services must be conducted in group settings according to legal requirements (e.g., IDEIA, 2004 the current federal law that governs special education and related services) that specify required participants (e.g., parents, evaluation personnel, etc.). As a result, an understanding of social psychological phenomena on group decision making is an important component of school psychological services.

Groups can have tremendous social power over individuals and, in some cases, exert pressure on the individual to go against his/her better judgment (Turner, 1995). Conformity has been well studied in numerous social psychology experiments. One of the most well-known of these studies was conducted by Solomon Asch (1952). This study involved the manipulation of subjects' responses to the length of vertical lines. Almost 75% of the subjects conformed at least once in the experiments by giving a response that was consistent with researcher confederates but objectively untrue. Thus, the motivation to conform was more salient than the motivation to be accurate.

Additional studies examined the impact of conformity on decision making processes. By conforming to the opinions of others rather than stating an individual, divergent opinion a group member may minimize stress by avoiding arguing, not appearing to be different or difficult or having to devise a reasonable argument for an unpopular position. People make judgments about those who agree with them and see those who agree as more intelligent and more likeable (Braver et al., 1977). In addition, when one is aware of the opinion of others in advance, one is more likely to conform when expressing his/her individual opinion (Tetlock et al., 1989). Conformity influence has been show to occur even in situations where individuals feel a high degree of personal importance and/or personal consequences for the group decisions being made (Brief et al., 1991; Brockner et al., 1981).

In contrast, the circumstances that are established for the group decision making process can alter the effect of conformity on individual and group decision making. Chen, Shechter and Chaiken (1996) found that when the group circumstance was established to value "getting along", individuals were more likely to show a conformity effect than when the group decision making circumstance was defined as finding the "truth." In another study, when an individual was called upon to explain or defend his or her view that was divergent from the rest of the group, that individual was more likely to change his/her opinion by conforming with the opinion of the group (Cialdini et al, 1976).

The application of conformity to group decision making in schools is frequently observed when school personnel collaborate to present a "united front" to parents. The case of Jennifer can be expanded to demonstrate this case.

> Since Jennifer's parents have expressed that they are not in favor of special education placement, the principal suggests that school staff involved in Jennifer's educational program meet for a "staffing" (a meeting *prior* to the official meeting that typically does not include the parents) to ensure that they are all in agreement with the recommendation that Jennifer be placed in special education. The principal feels that if the school staff iron out any differences or concerns, they can present a "united front" and Jennifer's parents will be more likely to agree with the recommendation.

Unofficial meetings conducted by school personnel that occur prior to an official meeting with a parent, frequently referred to as "staffings", occur routinely and can include important processes related to a child's educational program. For example, the staffing can be used to explore alternatives, problem solve, and identify resources, which may be confusing or inappropriate to discuss with parents. However, when educators work to present a united front to parents, they may unwittingly produce results such as those seen in the Asch experiments. When a parent participates in a meeting and hears the same recommendation made by the teacher, the principal, the school psychologist and the counselor, the motivation to conform may influence the parent to agree with the recommendation, even if the recommendation does not represent the parent's individual preference. Therefore, the pressure to conform may undermine the parent's right to act autonomously on behalf of his/her child. If school personnel do not share the information that the pre-meeting staffing occurred, the educators may be (wittingly or unwittingly) engaging in deception (such as in Asch's experiments) to achieve a desired outcome. Such deception creates ethical problems for educational professionals and can result in negative outcomes for the student.

To minimize conformity, school psychologists should encourage team decision making processes that promote truly meaningful discussion among members. Meaningful discussion that values input from all members cannot occur if categorical, predetermined decisions have already been made in advance of the meeting. As mentioned previously, there are aspects of pre-meetings that may be appropriate, but teams should avoid making important decisions about a child's educational program until all parties are present. By doing this, conformity effects can be minimized. Lasser and Klose (2007, p. 492) suggest that educational planning teams could "formally adopt an approach that honors dissent, promotes a dialectical process, and encourages individual thought." This approach must be valued and followed by all team members. In addition, it is important that educators follow up with parents following meetings to evaluate their perceptions of their participation in the process. If parents report feeling conformity pressures, the decision making process should be re-evaluated. Finally, if school psychologists learn that parents have felt conformity pressures, they should follow-up to ensure that decisions were made out of conviction rather than social pressure.

5. Authority and obedience

Stanley Milgram's (1963, 1965, 1974) experiments involving administering electric shocks in obedience to authority figures constitute some of the most profound research involving the social psychological constructs of authority and obedience. As a result of the negative effects on subjects and confederates in Milgram's research new standards were developed regarding the treatment of research participants (e.g., Baumrind, 1964 and Ableson, Frey, & Gregg, 2004) and, consequently, Milgram's studies have not been replicated. However, similar studies have also shown obedience to authority, such as in the area of nursing (Hofling et al., 1966) and studies similar to the Milgram experiments in countries other than the United States (e.g., Kilham & Mann, 1974; Meeus & Raaijmakers, 1995). In addition, the Stanford Prison Experiment (Haney, Banks, & Zimbardo, 1973) demonstrated the importance of social roles in authority and obedience.

Because students and their parents may perceive school personnel as authority figures, care must be taken to ensure that decisions are not made under the influence of obedience to authority and are instead based on careful consideration of information. However, as the continued expansion of Jennifer's case illustrates, authority and obedience dynamics can come into play not only between parents and school staff, but also within school system hierarchies.

> When the principal presented her ideas about the pre-meeting staffing to present a united front to Jennifer's parents, Bailey, the school psychologist and Mr. Suarez, Jennifer's classroom teacher, expressed concerns. The principal informed Bailey and Mr. Suarez that participating in the staffing was mandatory and not participating would be considered insubordination and be reflected in their annual performance reviews.

The school principal's leadership role includes the supervision and evaluation of all school personnel. As a result, there are many circumstances in which deference to this authority might be expected and appropriate. However, when making important decisions regarding the educational programming for an individual student, especially one who is being considered for special education, is not one of these instances. In this type of instance, a multi-disciplinary team should make a decision that is based on data and thoughtfully considers information from all team participants. Further, failure to make sound decisions in an effort to comply with the command of authority figures potentially violates ethical and legal standards.

The problem posed in the case example is common and challenging. Bailey and Mr.Suarez's non-compliance with the principal's plans could lead to a poor performance evaluation and possibly dismissal. However, the educational decision making team has an obligation to the child to engage in an appropriate and data-based decision making process regarding the child's educational program.

In addition to the situation described in the case example, educators need to take steps to manage the impact of authority influence in group decision making. Lasser and Klose (2007, p. 493) make the following recommendations:

> "First, team members could be designated specific roles and responsibilities that could functionally reduce any given member's authority over the group. For example, the principal could be assigned the role of parent liaison, the school psychologist the role of note taker, the general education teacher the role of data presenter. By diffusing the responsibility and functions across team members, the team may effectively transfer some authority associated with one individual across the team. Another improvement to the general education problem solving teams that could potentially deemphasize authority could be the development of a team mission statement and ground rules that explicitly emphasize shared governance and democratic process. Such a statement could be posted on the conference room wall where the meetings are held and/or reviewed before each meeting. Efforts to undermine such a process would be difficult to reconcile in the face of a public commitment to free thought and speech."

Another technique to minimize power differentials and lessen the impact of authority influence is the practice of "one-downsmanship" (Caplan & Caplan, 1993). This allows decision making team members to collaborate in a decision making process that emphasizes an egalitarian approach.

6. Fear appeals

Most of the research on the impact of fear appeals is related to advertising campaigns. However, some empirical data is available that examines the impact of fear appeals on personal decision making (Smith & Lazarus, 1993; Lerner & Keltner 2000). When fear appeals are employed, individuals tend to make decisions that they perceive will avoid unpleasant outcomes rather than effectively solve problems. This can result in denial of responsibility for the decision (Keller & Block, 1996) and avoidance of making a decision (Dubachek, 2005). However, fear appeals may also be used to highlight specific aspects of a particular situation (Frijda, 1986). For example, advertisements may predict or imply dire consequences for not using the product being shown. In summary, fear appeals may be used to emphasize the seriousness of a particular situation, however, fear appeals may also negatively impact the group decision-making process.

While additional research is needed into the impact of fear appeals on group decision making, available information can be applied to the context of educational decision-making. For example, a suggestion that a certain decision will result in negative outcomes for a child is likely to influence a parent's decision making process.

When the disadvantages of a course of action are emphasized to influence outcomes with the intent of arousing anxiety, the fear appeal phenomenon is at work (Manstead, 1995). While it is true that educational decision making groups should consider potential positive and negative outcomes when evaluating alternatives, a fear appeal occurs when communication between group members is specifically designed to instill anxiety in specific group members. Parents may be particularly vulnerable to fear appeals in the context of making educational decisions regarding their child. Parents may have negative school experiences that make participating in any educational decision making an anxiety provoking experience. Jennifer's case example is further detailed to examine the impact of fear appeals.

> When Jennifer's parents attend the team meeting where Jennifer's evaluation results are discussed and plans are going to be made, they enter the room with trepidation. Jennifer's father had difficulty learning to read and as a result was retained in third grade and this led to a great deal of subsequent difficulties in school. During the course of the meeting, in addition to the recommendation for Jennifer to be placed in special education, the teacher mentions that if Jennifer is not placed in special education, she is likely to be retained as her performance is not on grade level.

In this situation, the teacher uses the unpleasant outcome of grade retention in an attempt to influence Jennifer's parents in giving their consent for special education placement. Roger's (1983) protection motivation theory proposes that fear appeals have the most influence on behavior when the individuals see the problem as a serious problem, the individuals are vulnerable to the problem and the individuals can do something about the problem. In the case example, Jennifer's parents are concerned about her difficulties in school and presumably feel that this a significant problem in that these difficulties could influence her academic progress in later years. Jennifer is certainly vulnerable to the negative consequences that can be associated with retention in a grade. Jennifer's parents are being told that they can do something about the problem and avoid the negative outcome of grade retention by agreeing to placement in special education. Consequently, Jennifer's parents may be influenced to consent to special education services, in spite of their original objections. Lasser and Klose (2007, p. 496)page) suggest that "the school psychologist has a responsibility to explain the impact of fear appeals to administrators and other educational professionals to ensure that school personnel do not exploit the fears and anxieties of parents."

7. Informational influence

Informational influence occurs when a member of a group influences the decisions of a group by presenting him/her self as an undisputed expert (Turner, 1995). Members of the group are influenced because the expert is viewed as having the most valid and most important contribution to the group. As a result, the group may be more likely to make a decision that is recommended by the expert, rather than arrived at by the entire group. Members of a group are influenced to agree with the information presented by the expert in order to appear attractive/intelligent to the rest of the group and thereby obtain social approval. This type of influence increases as the uncertainty of individual group members increases.

Burnstein and Vinokur (1973, 1975) demonstrated shifts in group decisions based on informational persuasions and when compared to the influence of conformity, informational influence has been shown to yield "more frequent and stronger shifts" in groups' decision outcomes (Kaplan & Miller, 1987, p. 306). Other studies have examined other variables such as the type of issue discussed by a group (e.g., intellectual vs. judgmental) (Laughlin & Earley, 1982) and the types of decision rules needed for action (e.g., unanimous vs. majority) (Miller, 1985). Kaplan and Miller (1987) demonstrated that intellectual decisions under a unanimous decision rule were most susceptible to informational influence.

In an educational group decision making team meeting, each member brings information and areas of expertise. These areas can overlap as all team members are involved in the education of a particular child being discussed. The multidisciplinary team is involved in developing the educational plan for a student because each member of the team contributes valuable information toward the development of the plan. Jennifer's case example continues with an illustration of informational influence.

> The first meeting of the decision making team involved with Jennifer's educational program did not result in a final decision as to how to progress. Jennifer's parents decided to consult a private educational psychologist for a second opinion regarding Jennifer's learning needs and profile. Dr. Frankle attended the second team meeting and presented his findings. He reported that his assessment did not indicate that Jennifer was a child with a learning disability and he cited his years in private practice and the number of his clients as evidence of his authority to make such a claim. Further, Dr. Frankle recommended that a specific reading program be utilized in the regular classroom to maximize Jennifer's probability of success in reading.

Jennifer's parents have a right to seek a second opinion regarding their daughter and to invite others to participate in decision making teams. However, school psychologists should be cognizant of the ways in which Dr. Frankle's status could potentially override other team members' contributions, whether intentionally or unintentionally. Consequently, the school psychologist should make efforts to ensure that Dr. Frankle's influence is not given more weight than other team members.

Encouraging and validating each group members contribution is an important way to minimize informational influence. If the group appears to be experiencing informational influence, the school psychologist can use group facilitation skills to ensure that each member is able to contribute.

Parents may be vulnerable to more subtle forms of informational influence in that they may feel that they have less to offer in an educational decision making because the school personnel are the experts in education, and this uncertainty may result in an increase of vulnerability to informational influence (Turner, 1995). As a result, parents may agree in an effort to appear socially acceptable and cooperative instead of asserting their own expertise related to their child. By being aware of this phenomenon, the school psychologist can encourage parents by soliciting contributions and framing information so that other team members understand the relevance of the parent information.

8. Recommendations

The case example illustrated how a variety of social psychological phenomena can potentially influence the outcomes of important educational decisions. Lasser and Klose (2007, 497-8page) offer the following recommendations to minimize the unwanted consequences of impact of these social psychological phenomena on educational group decision making:

1. Maintain "dual citizenship" as a member of decision-making groups and as an outsider that is "meta the group." In doing so, school psychologists can actively participate as team members but have the added advantage of stepping outside of the group to better observe and understand its processes. While this may be challenging, it is certainly not unusual for school psychologists to work in multiple roles that transcend systems. Just as a social constructivist can step back to critique a system in which he/she lives, so can the school psychologist simultaneously work in a system and cognitively remove himself/herself to monitor the process.
2. Promote independent thought among team members. This effort could be supported by solicitation of individual input prior to group meetings. Ultimately, this serves children and adolescents because decisions are made in consideration of them rather than as a response to social pressures.
3. Teach teachers and administrators about the impact of social psychological phenomena to reduce the use of inappropriate behaviors (e.g., fear appeals).
4. Work collaboratively to decrease perceived power differentials. Any effort to reduce perceptions that team members must obey authority figures will promote meaningful involvement from all team members. This can be accomplished through Caplan and Caplan's (1993) *one-downsmanship*, which emphasizes the coordinate status of personnel, deemphasizes hierarchical relationships, and actively counters deference.
5. When social psychological phenomena are interfering with sound decision-making, bring the concern to the attention of the group. Teams can identify the problem and take steps to correct it.

9. Conclusion

While social psychological phenomena will always be a part of school psychologists' work, the problems associated with these factors need not be problematic or pervasive. With greater awareness and proactive approaches, school psychologists may be better able to improve the functioning of educational decision-making groups and better understand the social world of schools. Future research should include investigations of the extent to which practicing school psychologists are aware of the social psychological phenomena occurring in their daily practice. This research could utilize questions about vignettes that describe the various phenomena. In addition, the level of knowledge regarding social psychological phenomena in general should be assessed. Perhaps revisions of entry level qualification exams should be revised to include this content. An important extensive of research in this domain is the evaluation of parents perceptions of the impact of social psychological phenomena their own decision making regarding their own child. Data from these types of studies would provide important information for trainers of school psychologists to use in the preparation of future practitioners.

10. References

Ableson, R.P, Frey, K.P., & Gregg, A.P. (2004). Experiments with people: Revelations from social psychology. Mahwah, NJ: Lawrence Erlbaum.

American Psychological Association (2002). Ethical Principles of Psychologists and Code of Conduct. *American Psychologist, 57,* 1060-1073.

American Educational Research Association, American Psychological Association, & National Council on Measurement in Education (1999). *Standards for educational and psychological testing (2nd ed.).* Washington, DC: American Educational Research Association.

Asch, S.E. (1952). *Social Psychology.* Englewood Cliffs, NJ: Prentice Hall.

Baumrind, D. (1964). Some thoughts on ethics of research: After reading Milgram's 'Behavioral Study of Obedience.' *American Psychologist, 19,* 421-423.

Bernstein, D.A., & Nash, P.W. (2002). *Essentials of Psychology (2nd ed.).* Boston: Houghton Mifflin.

Borgelt, C.E., & Conoley, J.C. (1999). Psychology in the schools: Systems intervention case examples. In C.R. Reynolds & T.B. Gutkin (Eds.), *The handbook of school psychology* (1056-1076). New York: John Wiley & Sons.

Braver, S. L., Linder, D. E., Corwin, T.T. & Cialdini, R.B. (1977). Some conditions that affect admissions of attitude change. *Journal of Experimental Social Psychology, 13,* 565-576.

Brief, A.P., Dukerich, J.M., & Doran, L.I. (1991). Resolving ethical dilemmas in management: Experimental investigations of values, accountability and choice. *Journal of Applied Social Psychology, 21,* 380-396.

Brockner, J., Rubin, J.Z., & Lang, E. (1981). Face-saving and entrapment. *Journal of Experimental Social Psychology, 17,* 68-79.

Burger, J.M. (1999). The foot-in-the-door compliance procedure: A multiple-process analysis and review. *Personality and Social Psychology Review, 3,* 303-325.

Burnstein, E., & Vinokur, A. (1973). Testing two classes of theories about group-induced shifts in individual choice. *Journal of Experimental Social Psychology, 9,* 123-137.

Burnstein, E., & Vinokur, A. (1975). What a person thinks upon learning he has chosen differently from others: Nice evidence for the persuasive arguments explanation of choice shifts. *Journal of Experimental Social Psychology, 11,* 412-426.

Caplan, G., & Caplan, R.B. (1993). Mental health consultation and collaboration. Prospect Heights, IL: Waveland Press.

Chen, S., Shechter, D., & Chaiken, S. (1996). Getting at the truth or getting along: Accuracy-versus impression-motivated heuristic and systematic processing. *Journal of Personality and Social Psychology, 71,* 262-275.

Cialdini, R.B., Levy, A., Herman, C.P., Kozlowski, I.T., & Petty, R.E. (1976). Elastic shifts of opinion: Determinants of direction and durability. *Journal of Personality and Social Psychology, 34,* 663-672.

Curtis, M.J., & Stollar, S.A. (2002). Best practices in system-level change. In A. Thomas & J. Grimes (Eds.), *Best practices in school psychology IV* (pp. 223-234). Bethesda, MD: NASP.

Dillard, J.P., Hunter, J.E., & Burgoon, M. (1984). Sequential-request persuasive strategies: Meta-analysis of foot-in-the-door and door-in-the-face. *Human Communication Research, 10,* 461-488.

Dubachek, A. (2005). Coping: A multidimensional, hierarchical framework of responses to stressful consumption episodes. *Journal of Consumer Research, 32,* 130-146.

Freedman, J.L., & Fraser, S.C. (1966). Compliance without pressure: The foot-in-the door technique. *Journal of Personality and Social Psychology, 4,* 195-202.

Frijda, N. H. (1986). *The emotions.* Cambridge, UK: Cambridge University Press.

Gottlieb, M.C. (1995). Ethical dilemmas in change of format and live supervision. In R.H. Mikesell, D. Lusterman, & S.H. McDaniel (Eds.). Integrating family therapy: Handbook of Family Psychology and Systems Therapy (pp. 561-570). Washington, D.C.: American Psychological Association. Reprinted in D. Bersoff (Ed.) (1995). Ethical Conflicts in Psychology. Washington, D.C: American Psychological Association.

Haney, C., Banks, C., & Zimbardo, P. (1973). Interpersonal dynamic in a simulated prison. *International journal of criminology and penology, 1,* 69-97.

Hofling, C.K., Brotzman, E., Dalrymple, S., Graves, N., & Pierce, C.M. (1966). An experimental study in nurse-physician relationships. *The Journal of nervous and mental disease, 143,* 171-180.

Individuals with Disabilities Education Improvement Act (IDEIA) of 2004. 20 U.S.C. § 1401 (c)(5)(F).

Jacob, S., & Hartshorne, T. (2003). *Ethics and law for school psychologists* (4th ed.). New York: John Wiley & Sons, Inc.

Kaplan, M.F., & Miller, C.E. (1987). Group decision making and normative versus informational influence: Effects of type of issue and assigned decision rule. *Journal of Personality and Social Psychology, 53,* 306-313.

Kaufman-Bryant, B. & Mullen, B. (1995). Foot-in-the-door. In A.S.R. Manstead & M. Hewstone (Eds.), *The Blackwell encyclopedia of social psychology* (250). Oxford: Blackwell Publishers.

Keller, P. A. & Block, L. G. (1996). Increasing the persuasiveness of fear appeals: The effect of arousal and elaboration. *Journal of Consumer Research, 22,* 448-459.

Kilham, W., & Mann, L. (1974). Level of destructive obedience as a function of transmitter and executant roles in the Milgram obedience paradigm. *Journal of Personality and Social Psychology, 29,* 696-702.

Lasser, J. & Klose, L.M. (2007). School psychologists' ethical decision-making: Implications from selected social psychological phenomena. *School Psychology Review, 36,* 1-18.

Laughlin, P.R., & Earley, P.C. (1982). Social combination models, persuasive arguments theory, social comparisons theory, and choice shift. *Journal of Personality and Social Psychology, 42,* 273-280.

Lerner, J., & Keltner, D. (2000). Beyond valence: Toward a model of emotion-specific influences on judgment and choice. *Cognition and Emotion, 14,* 473-493.

Lusterman, D-D. (1992). Ecosystemic treatment of family-school problems: A private practice perspective. In M.J. Fine & C. Carlson (Eds.), *Handbook of family-school interventions: A systems perspective* (363-373). Boston: Allyn & Bacon.

Manstead, A.S.R. (1995). Fear appeals. In A.S.R. Manstead & M. Hewstone (Eds.), *The Blackwell encyclopedia of social psychology* (249-250). Oxford: Blackwell Publishers.

Medway, F.J., & Cafferty, T.P. (1992). School psychology: A social psychological perspective. Hillsdale, NJ: Erlbaum.

Medway, F.J., & Cafferty, T.P. (1999). Contributions of social psychology to school psychology. In C.R. Reynolds & T.B. Gutkin (Eds.), *The handbook of school psychology* (194-222). New York: John Wiley & Sons.

Meeus, W.H.J., & Raaijmakers, Q.A.W. (1995). Obedience in modern society: The Utrecht Studies. *Journal of Social Issues, 51,* 155-175.

Milgram, S. (1963). Behavioral study of obedience. Journal of Abnormal and Social Psychology, Vol. 67, pp. 371-378.

Milgram, S. (1965). Some conditions of obedience and disobedience to authority. *Human Relations, 18,* 57-76.

Milgram, S. (1974). *Obedience to Authority*. London: Tavistock.

Miller, C.E. (1985). Group decision making under majority and unanimity decision rules. *Journal of Applied Social Psychology, 7,* 38-56.

National Association of School Psychologists (2010). *Principles for Professional Ethics.* Bethesda, MD: Author.

Pope, K.S. & Vasquez, M.J.T. (1991) Ethics in psychotherapy and counseling. San Francisco: Josey- Bass.

Rogers, R.W. (1983). Cognitive and physiological processes in fear appeals and attitude change: A revised theory of protection motivation. In J.T. Cacioppo & R.E. Petty (Eds.), *Social Psychophysiology: A sourcebook* (pp.153-76). New York: Guilford Press.

Smith, C. A. & Lazarus, R. S. (1993). Appraisal components, core relational themes and the emotions. *Cognition and Emotion, 4,* 233-269.

Tetlock, P.E., Skitka, L., & Boettger, R. (1989). Social and cognitive strategies for coping with accountability: Conformity, complexity, and bolstering. *Journal of Personality and Social Psychology, 57,* 632-640.

16

The Social Value of Persons: Theory and Applications

Nicole Dubois[1] and Jean-Léon Beauvois[2]
[1]*University of Lorraine (University Nancy2)*
[2]*University of Nice-Sophia Antipolis*
France

1. Introduction

When people talk about an object in their environment, they have recourse not to scientific language, but to evaluative language. This evaluative language allows them to say what one does, can do or must do with that object (i.e., its functional or social value). For instance, when Mrs Smith talks about an orchid that someone has given her, she says, *It's so delicate and refined! Its flowers come in fantastic shapes and yet it's really easy to grow.* When she talks about the meat she is cooking for dinner, she says, *It's tender, juicy, and smells good.* Statements like these make sense, but not *scientific* sense. These words are not the words of a botanist or a physiologist. This is a language used to say what one does, can do or must do with a flower or a cut of meat, something that is never expressed in descriptive or scientific language. A botanist might say, for example, that an orchid has three colorful sepals and three petals, that two of the petals are underdeveloped, that the third, on the contrary, is highly developed and forms the labellum, and so on. A physiologist might say that muscle is made up of thousands of cylindrical cells called muscle fibers, that each fiber is enveloped and separated from the others by a thin layer of connective tissue - the endomysium -, and so on. Curiously, though, when Mrs Smith talks about her friends or neighbors, many social psychologists opine that the words she uses to describe those friends and neighbors are more like the descriptive or scientific words of the botanist or physiologist than the evaluative words she uses to talk about meat or flowers.

1.1 Memories of the 1950s

This curious phenomenon has a long history. In his famous book on interpersonal relations, Heider (1958) stated that (1) naive psychology should be a key topic of psychosocial research, and that (2) people resemble professional scientists in their daily lives. More specifically, when attempting to understand either other people or themselves, they operate as intuitive scientists. The theorists of the causal attribution will attempt to exemplify this postulate which poses man as a scientist. Heider's view rested on a continuist epistemology, in that he assumed that a continuity exists between the commonsense way of thinking and scientific reasoning, the only difference being that scientists devote more resources to meeting their knowledge goals. These ideas were very much of their day, for in the 1950s, theorists felt it was important to reinstate human rationality in the social sciences, after decades of psychoanalysis and psychology of affects and motivations. However, such was their overpowering influence on social psychology throughout the second half of the twentieth century that we can legitimately ask whether they did not do more harm than good. These ideas led social psychologists to forget that human beings essentially are evaluative creatures (Kluckhohn, 1954). And yet, it can be argued that the approach that people have to objects (animate or inanimate) traditionally called "objects of knowledge" prevents them from knowing what those objects are from a descriptive point of view. Instead, it allows them to decide what one can or should do with them (*Can I get involved in this project with him?*) or what one can make them do (*Can I persuade this pupil to embark on a lengthy course of study?*). In other words, it allows them to evaluate the objects (Beauvois & Dubois, 2000, 2009). Thus, instead of being "objects of knowledge", objects are actually "objects of evaluation" to people. This conception rests on a different, noncontinuist epistemology, wherein science can only flourish if it breaks away from common sense (Bachelard, 1938, 1953). The fact of seeing the science everywhere in the thought and in the judgment is linked to a dichotomous conception according to which the science opposes to the error, maybe to the madness. A noncontinuist position moves forward that the science is only one of the possible modes of knowledge of the objects which do not have all the rationality of the science. Common sense is certainly not irrational, but its rationality is different from that of science. Common sense cannot be judged on the criterion of truth value, but it can be judged on the criterion of social acceptability. The common sense's statements must be acceptable (versus unacceptable) by people rather than be true (versus false). This is the case when we use naive psychology and, in particular, personality traits to understand the people with whom we have dealings. In this conception, traits are regarded as genuine concepts, but concepts that are not descriptive (or scientific) but that are directly, genuinely evaluative.

The purpose of this chapter is to outline a set of theoretical formulations and some studies that rely on an *evaluative conception* of intuitive psychology (Beauvois, 1976, 2011; Beauvois & Dubois, 2000, 2008, 2009; Dubois, 2006; Dubois & Beauvois, 2011) and, more specifically, of the intuitive psychology of personality traits. While this conception differs from most current theories, it can be likened to the formulations of researchers who differentiate between a paradigmatic manner of thinking and a narrative one (Zuckier, 1986).

1.2 Psychological realism: Traits and implicit personality theories

The continuist claim that the concepts handled by the naive, or intuitive, psychologist are descriptive or quasi-scientific has been referred to as *psychological realism* (Beauvois & Dépret, 2008). In psychological realism, the use of traits is regarded as a realist approach to a *person's psychological nature* and these traits are assumed to be intrinsic properties of the person, the *homo sapiens sapiens,* about whom the intuitive psychologist is talking. This idea is based on a more basic hypothesis (the lexical hypothesis; see Mollaret & Mignon, 2006) that traits are efficient tools for decoding the psychological reality. Obviously, psychological realism does not presuppose that the intuitive psychologist never makes mistakes. As such, psychological realism is less concerned with the functioning of an individual than with the nature of the concepts he/she uses, in particular personality and personality traits. Because traits, as quasi-scientific constructs, cannot be "seen" directly, they have to be apprehended via their visible behavioral manifestations. Accordingly, many models of social cognition (and, in particular, person memory; Srull & Wyer, 1989) stipulate that knowing about a person's psychological nature means being able to encode his/her behaviors as traits.

We use the term *TB behaviors* to designate the behaviors of a target person associated with a trait in memory (see Beauvois & Dubois, 2000). The well-known example of "pointing out a mistake made in one's favor" is a TB that allows us to attribute the *honest* trait to a target person. For convenience's sake, we consider that TB behaviors reflect knowledge that can be viewed as descriptive at the operational level.

In intuitive psychology, one important line of research concerns the dimensions underlying the psychological descriptions made by people in terms of traits. These dimensions are seen as the *implicit personality theories* of the intuitive psychologist (Beauvois, 1982; Bruner & Tagiuri, 1954; Rosenberg & Sedlak, 1972; Schneider, 1973). When people are asked to describe either themselves or others using personality traits, their psychological descriptions are generally framed by a very limited number of dimensions, either one (Kim & Rosenberg, 1980), two (Rosenberg & Sedlak, 1972) or five (Passini & Norman, 1966). Explanations for the theoretical foundations of these dimensions are often anchored in psychological realism, in that the dimensions are seen as referring to a psychological reality[1]. They are assumed to correspond to the structure of human personality, and the perceiver, as a quasi-scientific intuitive psychologist, therefore seeks to answer the question *How can I characterize this person according to the basic dimensions of human personality?* (Abele & Wojciszke, 2007; Judd, James-Hawkins, Yzerbyt, & Kashima, 2007; Suitner & Maass, 2008). Obviously, perceivers rapidly deduce the *evaluative implications* of the psychological realities they discover (Srull & Wyer, 1989). Moreover, psychological information is often processed precisely with the aim of arriving at these evaluative implications. However, the evaluations are reached on the basis of a presumed psychological reality by people who are explicitly or implicitly seen as potential intuitive scientists, even if they may, like all scientists, sometimes make mistakes. These errors do not invalidate the idea that the dimensions are genuine psychological dimensions that arise from people's actual nature.

By contrast, in the evaluative conception, dimensions are thought of as fundamentally social, and belonging to the registers of social values.

1.3 The evaluative approach: Traits are criteria of social value but not descriptive constructs

The evaluative approach rests on two major arguments:

---

[1] This can be problematic when these dimensions are used in studies of stereotypes. The latter prompt the elaboration of a supposedly universal model: the Stereotype Content Model (see Echebarria Echabe, in this book). These presuppositions are problematic insofar as the truth value of stereotypes is often questioned in the psychosocial literature. The foundations of psychological realism can nevertheless be preserved by arguing that if the truth value of a stereotype is questionable, it is because that stereotype is the product of errors of judgment, which can be explained by social necessities. We may, for instance, think that the Chinese are smaller than the Indonesians. This is doubtless an error, but the fact remains that the size of a person is an authentic individual variable which allows us to express true or false judgments. After all, psychological realism does not imply that intuitive psychologists are accurate in all their judgments.

- An empirical argument: the main personality traits, the central most frequently used traits (Asch, 1946), are known to be strongly evaluative and only weakly descriptive in meaning (Labourin & Lecourvoisier, 1986). We have also known for a long time that the dimensions of implicit personality theories are clearly evaluative: they set "good traits", such as *intelligence* and *competence*, against "bad traits", such as *stupidity* and *laziness* (for a brief review, see Cambon, 2006). This opposition between good and bad traits rests on a social point of view (people who behave intelligently are more highly paid than people who behave stupidly because the former are more socially useful than the latter). The defenders of psychological realism therefore have to answer the following puzzling question: Why are humans (*Homo sapiens sapiens*) the only creatures in nature whose intrinsic properties vary linearly with social utility or value?
- A cognitive and epistemological argument: an analysis of the cognitive construction of the meaning of personality traits (Beauvois, 1976, 1984; Beauvois & Dubois, 2000) reveals that the social value of people's behaviors[2] (e.g., the social value of the behaviors of a student said to be *intelligent* or *honest*) is not a secondary, post hoc inference (*intelligent* => intelligent behaviors => individual's social value), but rather is inherent to the meaning of the traits in the first place (*intelligence* = a set of behavioral social values). A set of behavioral social values is the sole basis for the emergence of a personality trait. Most traits are constructed not to grasp an *invisible* individual characteristic, but to express the *observed* behavioral social value. This process is doubtful from an epistemological point of view. The mere connection between a behavior (or performance) and a personality-trait implies that the numerous variables (in particular situational variables) which, according to the determinist point of view, affect this behavior (or performance) are forgotten. Only the social value of behavior is retained and is "psychologized" through the use of an assumed *causal* trait (see Beauvois & Dubois, 2000, for a formal description of this process).

In other words, when a pupil is said to be *intelligent*, the *intelligence* trait tells us nothing other than: this pupil has displayed a behavior (or performance) characterized by a certain kind of social value. Good (or poor) behavior (or performance) is thus translated into traits. These traits convey the person's social value without any descriptive or scientific (determinist) basis. In the above example, the value is named *intelligence*. Thus, personality traits *intelligent, competent, helpful* vs. *weak, stupid, selfish* are merely paraphrases of the social value of the behaviors or performances of the person concerned (Beauvois, 2011). This is the reason why traits tell us what we can or should do with people (the purpose of any evaluative activity), but say nothing about the *individual variables* that affected this behavior or performance.

We use the term *OB behaviors* (see Beauvois & Dubois, 1992, 2000) to designate the behaviors that others can or should display towards a person known either by a trait or by a set of behaviors endowed with some social value that is expressed by that trait. For instance, for *honest, you can give him confidential information* or *you can lend him your office keys*. By definition, OB behaviors reflect an evaluative knowledge. If the evaluative conception is correct, traits in psychological descriptions should directly activate OB behaviors in memory, as well as TB behaviors.

---

[2] It should be noted that the word *value* implies both positive and negative values (e.g., to successfully / unsuccessfully resolve a problem).

In short, the evaluative conception merely assumes that, through evaluative practices, everyone learns to use the language of personality traits and hence, implicit personality theories with the purpose of grasping and expressing, in psychological terms, the main aspects of the social value of people's behaviors both the positive value (e.g., *intelligent*) and the negative value (e.g., *stupid*).

In the following three sections, we discuss a variety of empirical studies whose findings provide strong support for the evaluative approach in psychological description (for a more comprehensive review, see Beauvois & Dubois, 2000, 2008, 2009). Section 2 deals with studies showing that OB behaviors are at least as important as TB behaviors in intuitive psychology (we use everyday psychological language to talk about what we do, can do and must do with people). Section 3 looks at studies showing that the evaluative conception allows us to account for the meaning of the dimensions at work in psychological description (the main factors extracted from psychological descriptions correspond to the main dimensions of people's social value). Section 4 describes studies exploring the relevance of the evaluative conception in organizational contexts (recruitement, leadership, salaries).

2. TBs and OBs in naive psychology: We use everyday psychological language to talk about what we do, can do or must do with people

2.1 Semantic decision

It was important at the beginning of this trend of research to show that OBs provide a system for encoding personological information that is just as efficient as the TB system.

To this end, Beauvois and Dubois (1992, Study 1) conducted an experiment whereby a list of 33 positive and negative traits was read out to a group of students who had to write down a behavior they considered to be characteristic of a person defined by each of those traits in turn (TB list). A second group had to write down a behavior that people might or should have towards that person (OB list). In a second phase, different students were shown the most frequent behaviors associated with each of the 33 traits on the TB or OBs lists. Then they were asked to select those they considered to be *the most representative of each trait*. They were also asked to rate their confidence after each choice on a 100-point scale. Results are given in Table 1 for positive and negative traits: the frequency hierarchies are virtually identical, as are the confidence curves for TBs and OBs. Similar results were obtained by Mignon and Mollaret (2002).

	Rank 1	Rank 2	Rank 3	Rank 4	Rank 5
TB frequency*	68	54	43	38	31
OB frequency*	62	49	45	38	34
TB confidence**	41.2	39.6	37.6	33	33.4
OB confidence**	40.9	39.7	36.9	35.5	33.4

* Rank 1= Mean frequency of choice (on all traits) for the top-ranking behaviors. Rank 2 = mean frequency of choice (on all traits) of the behaviors ranked second, etc.
** Rank 1= Means on a 0-100 rating-scale (on all traits) for the top-ranking behaviors. Rank 2 = means (on all traits) of the behaviors ranked second, etc.

Table 1a. OB and TB hierarchies and confidence for positive traits in Beauvois and Dubois (1992, Study 1)

	Rank 1	Rank 2	Rank 3	Rank 4	Rank 5
TB frequency*	62	54	45	41	30
OB frequency*	63	52	48	44	38
TB confidence **	40.1	38.85	38.3	36.5	36.9
OB confidence**	36.8	34.8	34.1	33.7	33.5

* Rank 1= Mean frequency of choice (on all traits) for the top-ranking behaviors. Rank 2 = mean frequency of choice (on all traits) of the behaviors ranked second, etc.
** Rank 1= Means on a 0-100 rating-scale (on all traits) for the top-ranking behaviors. Rank 2 = means (on all traits) of the behaviors ranked second, etc.

Table 1b. OBs and TBs hierarchies and confidence for negative traits in Beauvois and Dubois (1992, Study 1)

In the two tables, no comparison of frequencies (X^2) nor means (t test) inside the same rank reached the threshold of significance (.05). So, these results show that the OB register is no more ambiguous than the TB register[3]. They exclude the idea that the OB register is more idiosyncratic than the TB register. They seem hardly compatible with the idea that OBs are post hoc inferences made on the basis of TBs. One could, for example, claim that it is because I have stored *honest => hands in wallets to the police* (TB) in memory that I can infer that an honest person is *someone to whom I can lend money* (OB).

Beauvois and Dubois (1992, Study 2) used a semantic decision task precisely to reject this idea as far as main traits are concerned. Subjects were asked to indicate as quickly as possible whether or not a particular OB or TB behavior was characteristic of a trait that had just been presented. Traits were either strongly evaluative (traits whose evaluative component outweighed the descriptive component: e.g., *honest*, *dynamic*) or weakly evaluative (traits whose descriptive component outweighted the evaluative component: e.g., *shy* or *talkative*). The twenty OB and TB were chosen so that twelve of them (6 OBs and 6 TBs with comprable association frequencies) exemplify the given trait, six of them (3 OBs and 3 TBs) exemplify another trait and two of them (one OB and one TB) exemplify an antonym of the given trait. Reaction times were recorded. The significant behavior x traits interaction: $F(1,17)= 13.30$, $p<.002$ indicated that, for positive and negative responses alike, the OBs were judged as rapidly as TBs on strongly evaluative traits (1328ms vs. 1307 ms). On the other hand, they were judged more slowly on weakly evaluative traits (1647 ms vs. 1308 ms)[4]. These results allow us to contend that when highly evaluative traits are at stake (the most central traits), OBs are indeed stored and granted a status in long-term memory that is at least equivalent to that of TBs. In a subsequent semantic decision experiment, Beauvois, Dubois, and Tarquinio (1994) assigned half the subjects to a "social context" condition, where TBs and OBs were placed in a social setting that was relevant to the trait in question

[3] The small difference between the two confidence curves for the negative traits is easily explained. Students were probably reluctant to attribute confidence to a decision that implied that they might act towards others in a negative way. For example, *It is necessary to know how to shut him (her) up* for *chatterbox*. Or *It is necessary to put him (her) in his place* for *conceited*

[4] These studies and the studies of Beauvois, Dubois, Mira and Monteil, 1996, presented immediately after, were performed about twenty years ago. At this time, the publishers only demanded mean values, results with significance levels. As we have not the data files, we regret not beeing able to provide other statistical indicators than those given in the published papers.

(*at a party*, he enjoys talking to everyone). Interestingly, in this condition, and always for the most evaluative traits, reaction times were *shorter* for OBs than for TBs, whereas no such difference was found in the "no social context" condition (i.e., the same condition as in Study 2 of Beauvois & Dubois, 1992). Again, these results are in line with the idea that the OBs for more central traits are activated without having to call upon TBs beforehand, in particular when there is a social context.

2.2 Person memory

Beauvois, Dubois, Mira, and Monteil (1996; see also Milhabet, 2004) described three studies exploring the person memory paradigm. Students listened to lists of behaviors comprising filler items, OBs and TBs said to characterize a single person. Four OBs and four TBs were provided in Studies 1 and 2, and six OBs and six TBs in Study 3. In all three studies, half the OBs and half the TBs were representative of a single trait that was either strongly evaluative (*honest*, *dynamic*, etc.), or weakly evaluative (*shy*, *passionate*, etc.) These traits varied from one experiment to another. In all three studies (see Table 2), the same significant behavior x trait interaction was observed: in study 1: $F(1,216)= 53.03$, $p<.0001$, with simple effects all $p <.01$; in study 2: $F(1,191)= 36.07$, $p<.0001$ with simple effects all $p <.001$; in study 3: $F(1,114)= 61.27$, $p<.0001$ with simple effects all $p <.001$.

	Study 1		**Study 2**		**Study 3**	
	OB behaviors	TB behaviors	OB behaviors	TB behaviors	OB behaviors	TB behaviors
Most evaluative traits	2.76	2.37	2.54	1.92	2.68	1.59
Least evaluative traits	1.96	3.10	1.86	2.68	1.74	2.29

Table 2. Means for OBs and TBs recalled in Beauvois, Dubois, Mira, and Monteil (1996)

For highly evaluative traits, subjects remembered more OBs than TBs, and vice versa for less evaluative traits. Results suggested that OBs are endowed with a memory structuring power that exceeds that of TBs. In the third experiment, the virtual social relation between target and participant was manipulated. The subjects were students, while the target was said to be either "a person", "a student" or "a teacher". The interaction was strongest, and accounted for a greater proportion of variance, when the target was one of the student's professors (i.e., power relationship) than when the target was a student or a person. Again, as in Beauvois, Dubois and Tarquinio's study (2004), the structuring power of the OBs was strongest when a social context was induced.

2.3 Implications

The above-described studies validate three implications of the evaluative conception. As far as the more central traits are concerned:

a. the evaluative component is mobilized just as much as the descriptive component in the intuitive use of traits. In other words, OBs constitute a means of encoding the knowledge provided by the traits and are called upon either in conjunction with TBs or as an alternative to them;
b. evaluative knowledge is not the product of inferences drawn from descriptive knowledge. In other words, from an operational standpoint, OBs are part of the meaning of a trait and do not presuppose TBs;
c. the evaluative component of traits becomes more accessible and is more frequently used when the social context is made salient.

Others studies (see Beauvois & Dubois, 2000) have yielded further empirical evidence of the validity of the evaluative conception of trait meaning. In particular, they have shown that OBs and TBs have different effects on first impressions (zero-acquaintance paradigm): OBs are more effective than TBs as far as interpersonal differentiation (evaluation) is concerned, while TBs are better than OBs at allowing intraindividual analysis of targets (description). It has also been shown that OBs are just as good recall cues as TBs in person memory and that OBs define a universe that is a good approximation of implicit personality theories established on the basis of the traits themselves. Moreover, people whose job involves judging other people for the purposes of determining which actions to take towards them (e.g., social workers) exhibit a sociocognitive functioning which relies more on the evaluative component of intuitive psychology than on the descriptive one.

The choice of the word "evaluative" to refer to a register of knowledge may seem surprising. In the psychosocial literature, it is always associated with the affective or emotional register, which is why the evaluative process has attracted so little attention from social cognition theorists. This is the consequence of the dichotomous thinking that we mentioned above. Evaluation can rarely be considered as a scientific activity. It cannot therefore be considered as a competence of the intelligent thinking. Thus, evaluation is of the emotional register. And yet it seems clear that OBs give rise to genuine knowledge (from this point of view, they have the same status as TBs), namely the knowledge of what we can or should do with people. Of course, this knowledge is sometimes inferred from another, possibly more descriptive kind of knowledge (TBs). But for traits that are very common in psychological descriptions, namely the most central ones, which are more evaluative than descriptive in nature, the evaluation is supplied directly as knowledge of what we can or should do with people, that is, knowledge of their social value (Beauvois, 2011). People's social value cannot be a mere individual fact. Human resources managers cannot refer to their affective reactions to fix salaries or grant promotions. Nor can professors bank on their emotions when marking their students' work. Both can very exceptionally only justify their evaluation by the science. Now, their decisions must be understandable. Social evaluative knowledge, we said it, must be endowed with social acceptance. Obviously, the managers' and professors' decisions can still be disputed, but any contestation must be based on a piece of acceptable evaluative knowledge. We can see how the prevalent idea in social psychology that evaluation is derived from an emotional register has caused social psychologists to neglect an important aspect of the knowledge conveyed by naive psychology.

3. The evaluative conception and the two-factor model: The main factors extracted from psychological descriptions are the main dimensions of people's social value

We have said that when people are asked to describe either themselves or others using personality traits, the psychological descriptions they produce are generally framed by one, two or five main factors (or dimensions). The two-dimensions approach is the most stimulating one today (see Special Issue, *European Journal of Social Psychology*, 2008; see also Echebarria Echabe, in this book). The first dimension pertains to the quality of the target person's interpersonal relationships (e.g., *warm, helpful, honest* vs. *cold, irritable, selfish*), while the second refers to the energy and resources that the target person invests in his/her activities (e.g., *intelligent, ambitious, active* vs. *lazy, weak, careless*). These two dimensions have been given various names which, from a theoretical standpoint, may seem arbitrary: value vs. dynamism (Osgood, 1962), social good-bad vs. intellectual good-bad (Rosenberg & Sedlak, 1972), other-profitability vs. self-profitability (Peeters, 1992), morality vs. competence (Wojciszke, 1994, 2005), warmth vs. competence (Fiske, Cuddy, & Glick, 2007), communion vs. agency (Abele & Wojciszke, 2007), etc. Except for a few variations, however, these two dimensions always contain the same traits, at least as far as the positive pole is concerned.

According to psychological realism, these two dimensions are clearly derived from genuine psychological knowledge of what people are (i.e., from the standpoint of a virtually scientific or quasi-scientific descriptive psychology). They refer to a psychological reality in the form of psychological information that is extracted by the perceiver and/or derived from the dimensions of human personality.

This view is challenged by the advocates of the evaluative conception. They assume that both types of information are derived not from truly psychological knowledge of people, but rather from a social evaluation of people that is directly supplied by interchangeable traits (i.e., *intelligent, capable, clever, gifted*). In addition to the above arguments, there is an important historical argument: the two dimensions were identified by industrial psychologists studying the *occupational value* of men and women in the workplace (see De Montmollin, 1972; Tiffin & McCormick, 1965). These two dimensions therefore emerged from people's knowledge of two basic aspects of the social value of employees in organizations. In this context, but also in a more general way, the value of a person is generally apprehended through the observation of poor or good behaviors, judgments or performances. As we demonstrated earlier, poor or good behaviors (or performances, or judgments) are then given labels (assumed causal traits). Implicit personality theories, which are essentially semantic or conceptual in nature (Shweder & D'Andrade, 1979) are then activated, giving rise to descriptions that go far beyond what has actually been observed (*intelligent* and *competent* activate *ambitious, ambitious* activates *dynamic; helpful* activates *nice, nice* activates *sociable, sociable* activates *honest*, and so on.) This evaluative view led Beauvois (1995) to propose new names for the two dimensions and to emphasize their evaluative nature by presenting them from an evaluator's viewpoint: social desirability for the former, social utility for the latter.

Their definitions are set out below. First, however, we describe three sets of studies which have yielded strong evidence supporting this evaluative view.

3.1 Social desirability and social utility of professionals. Is a factory manager more competent than a hospital manager?

Cambon (2004) borrowed Ricardo's and Smith's opposition (echoed by Marx) between production (production of goods for the market) and maintenance (taking care of the producers) within a social structure. In several studies, he studied the psychological descriptions of different professionals known only by their occupation (e.g., a factory manager in the production sector vs. a hospital manager in the maintenance sector). These descriptions were made in terms of positive or negative traits indicating social desirability or social utility. Every description was analyzed using a utility index and a desirability index *(*number of positive adjectives minus number of negative adjectives*)*. In studies where gender stereotypes and professional status were manipulated or controlled, Cambon observed that professionals working in the production sector were seen as more useful than desirable, whereas professionals working in the maintenance sector were often described as more desirable than useful (see Table 3 for the data of Study 4 in which the gender of the targets was controlled).

	Production	Maintenance
Social utility	1.06	0.31
Social desirability	0.10	0.63

Table 3. Mean desirability index and mean utility index for psychological descriptions of professionals working in production versus maintenance sectors (subjects: economics students) in Cambon (2004, study 4)

These data were submitted to a 2 (professional sector: production vs. maintenance) x 2 (traits: social utility vs. social desirability) ANOVA. This analysis yielded the predicted interaction, $F(1,49)= 28,56$; $p <.001$. Such results are not easy to explain from the psychological realism perspective (who can say that the director of a hospital is less "competent" than the director of a factory?) On the contrary, they are typical of our evaluative approach and justify our quasi-economic idea of social utility. Adam Smith said that when a worker is hired, (economic) value is created, while when a domestic is hired, (economic) value is consumed. Economists have indeed often claimed that production activities are more typical of (economic) value than maintenance activities. We can understand why production professionals are more highly rated on the most "economic" dimension (i.e., the social utility dimension). This certainly does not mean that they are, from a purely "psychological" point of view, more competent, more dynamic than maintenance professionals, who are supposedly nicer and more honest. Rather, it simply means that, because they occupy different economic positions, they are not judged on the same social values. Since we do not use the same traits to express different values, production and maintenance professionals are described using different personality traits. Intuitive psychologists have no access to invisible psychological realities. They talk about what they see or think they are seeing in a social structure or in a given context. The words they use are embedded in that social structure or context. Consequently, intuitive psychologists always talk about a target and about the value of that target within the social structure or context.

3.2 A human psychological reality is not a prerequisite for the emergence of either dimension: Are some pet rabbits more competent than others?

The evaluative approach assumes that social desirability and social utility do not have a human psychological reality as empirical reference. Rather, they operate independently of any kind of empirical or even conceivable human psychological reality. The notion of "human psychological reality" is specific to psychological realism: a human psychological reality is any human object that can be thought of and studied via a descriptive scientific or quasi-scientific psychology. The advocates of the "man as scientist" axiom or of psychological realism will necessarily agree with this definition. They will contend that the two dimensions of social judgment are linked to two human psychological realities (two registers of personality-traits). We, however, take the view that they are two basic aspects of people's social value: the value of people in interpersonal contexts and the value of people in activity (work) contexts. It has been asserted (cf. Dubois & Beauvois, 2011) that these two dimensions exist independently of an empirical and even a conceivable human psychological reality, and are activated through implicit personality theories, solely via the retrieval of the described object's social value. This is why the subjects in Dubois and Beauvois' experiment (2011, Study 2) were told to pick personality traits from a list to describe not people but pet rabbits, after they had been given two pieces of information about the mere social value of those rabbits, namely price ([in]expensive) and love ([un]loved). No other information was given. The traits provided for the "description" were located at the positive and negative poles of either the social desirability dimension (*likeable, pleasant, warm* vs. *aggressive, irritable, cold*) or the social utility dimension (*active, intelligent, dynamic* vs. *stupid, lazy, weak*). Two principal component analyses were performed (PCA).

a. The first PCA (see Table 4) revealed two factors accounting for 50% of the variance. We considered only the first two factors because we wanted to verify that they were in accordance with those brought out in the literature. In addition, we observed an important drop in the explained variance between the second factor (15.85%) and the third factor (10.58%). These two factors were identical to those usually found in psychological description studies. The first factor (accounting for 35.02% of the variance) set high social-desirability traits (*likeable, pleasant, warm*) against low social-desirability traits (*aggressive, irritable, cold*). The second factor (accounting for 15.85% of the variance) set high social-utility traits (*dynamic, intelligent, active*) against low social-utility traits (*lazy, spineless, stupid, weak*).
b. A second PCA was then performed with *price* and *love* (see Table 4). The introduction of these two variables did not change the factor structure. The PCA also revealed two first factors accounting for more than 50% of the variance (35.78% for the first factor and 18.06% for the second factor)[5]. Taken together, these results confirmed the evaluative nature of the factors).

Love was associated with social desirability, price with social utility. The fact that the two classic dimensions of social judgment were obtained in conditions where no descriptive information was available but only information about the rabbits' social value (love: social desirability, and price: social utility) led us to question the descriptive basis of person description. We think that these results validate our claim that person description simply

[5] The third factor was accounting for 11.04% of the variance.

amounts to situating individuals on the two basic dimensions of social value rather than on the two dimensions of a true psychology of *Homo sapiens sapiens* (psychological realism), a true psychology which thus remains uncharted waters. These dimensions only tell us about the social value of individuals.

	First PCA without Price and Love		Second PCA with Price and Love	
	Factor1	Factor2	Factor1	Factor2
Likeable	.876	-.116	.884	.281
Pleasant	.871	-.112	.843	.285
Warm	.838	-.129	.795	.188
Aggressive	*-.843*	0	-.833	-.263
Irritable	*-.780*	.225	-.813	0
Cold	*-484*	.361	-.615	0
Dynamic	0	*-.751*	.492	-.597
Intelligent	.114	*-.537*	.188	-.553
Active	0	*-.532*	178	-.497
Lazy	0	.624	-.321	.625
Stupid	-.137	.616	-.387	.567
Weak	-.139	.443	-.190	.538
Spineless	-475	.621	-.475	.479
Love			.778	.341
Price			-.287	-.427

Table 4. Factor matrix for the two PCA (without and with love and price) in Dubois and Beauvois (2011, study 2)

3.3 Social value of people and social value of everyday objects: From a person to a car

Recent studies (Cambon, 2007; Schiffler, Dubois, & Mollaret, 2010) have shown that the bidimensional evaluation of people bears some similarity to the bidimensional evaluation of everyday objects, such as watches, tables and cars. Readers who recall Osgood's writings will not be surprised (Osgood, Suci, & Tanenbaum, 1957): with his theory of semantic mediation, Osgood would certainly not have been a proponent of psychological realism[6]. When Schiffler et al. (2010) ran a PCA on descriptions of everyday objects, they came up with two dimensions. On the first one, *attractive, nice,* and *amusing* were contrasted with *horrible, ugly* and *square*. On the second one, *luxury, extremely expensive* and *chic* were set against *cheap, bottom of the range* and *poor quality*. The first dimension was named "agreeableness" and the second "market value". Results were similar to those obtained with pet rabbits. We can therefore legitimately wonder whether evaluative processes are

[6] Remember that the component of the connotative meaning is nothing other that a kind of memories of anterior responses towards objects.

characterized by a fundamental duality, in that, at least in our societies, these processes distinguish between pleasure derived from contact with an object and the economic value of that object. If this is indeed the case, the social desirabilty and social utility of human beings correspond to the agreeableness and market value of objects. This fundamental duality obviously only fits in with the evaluative conception put forward in this chapter.

Schiffler et al. conducted an experiment to confirm this fundamental duality. Subjects first had to make a decision concerning photos of target individuals' faces. This decision was manipulated through instructions steering them towards the social desirability of these targets (*choose the person who has most friends)*, or their social utility (*choose the person who has the highest salary*). In the second phase of the experiment, the same subjects had to choose the most typical adjectives for 12 objects (armchair, car, pen, etc.). Adjectives were selected on the basis of the above-mentioned PCA. They were either descriptive or evaluative (either high in agreeableness: *amusing, ugly,* or high in market value: *luxurious, downmarket*). Phases 1 and 2 were presented as pertaining to two distinct experiments (priming paradigm). Schiffler et al. expected decisions about target individuals in the first phase to prime the choice of adjectives in the second phase. More specifically, they predicted that the social desirability instruction would drive the choice of agreeableness and that social utility instruction would drive the choice of market value. Results are given in Table 5.

The 2 (kind of priming: social desirability vs. social utility) x 2 (kind of adjectives: agreeableness vs. market value) ANOVA performed on the data (see Table 5) showed a significant interaction effect, $F(1,47) = 14.38$ $p < .001$, $\eta^2 = .234$. Results confirmed expectations: the social desirability of people primed the agreeableness of objects ($F(1,47) = 11.14$ $p < .002$, $\eta^2 = .192$), whereas the social utility of people primed market value ($F(1,47) = 4.15$ $p < .05$, $\eta^2 = .081$). These results can be perfectly explained by the evaluative conception, but not by a strictly realist conception. When individuals look at an object, they see it from an evaluative point of view which is not an implication of the object's nature. This evaluative point of view can be acquired through a previous evaluative experience with another kind of object. Furthermore, evaluative experiences would appear to be shaped by two types of relationship with an object, confirming the idea of a fundamental evaluative duality.

Kind of adjectives	Kind of priming	
	Social desirability	Social utility
Agreeableness	0.62 (0.15)	0.51 (0.16)
Market value	0.41 (0.23)	0.64 (0.18)

The chosen adjectives were coded 1; the not chosen adjectives were coded 0. The scores given in the table correspond to the average difference between the chosen adjectives and the not chosen adjectives pertaining to the considered dimension.

Table 5. Saliency indexes (means and standard deviations) as a function of kind of priming and kind of adjectives in Shiffler, Dubois and Mollaret (2010)

However, even if social desirability and social utility are homologous with agreeableness and market value, we cannot bank on their strict equivalence. The fundamental evaluative duality takes diverse forms according to the type of object. The social desirabilty of human beings, for instance, seems to have at least two components, namely morality (*honest, sincere*) and sociability (*helpful, warm*). While sociability can be seen as the "human" shape of agreeableness, there seems to be no relevant equivalent of morality for a watch or a rabbit. This is why we can surmise that this fundamental duality results from people's evaluative experience, particularly through evaluative practices, which is then generalized to the evaluation of nonhuman objects.

3.4 Social utility is associated with social differentiation

Other research that is typical of the evaluative conception can be summed up in a single proposition: "*worthful* people" are seen as being socially useful rather than socially desirable. It has been shown that "*worthful* people" make normative judgments (see Dubois, 2003 and Beauvois & Dubois, 2009 for the concept of social judgment norms). For example, "*worthful* people" have been found to be more internal, more self-sufficient and more optimistic than others. Several studies have shown that the more normative people are in their judgments, the more they are considered and consider themselves to be socially useful. In these studies, subjects were given questionnaires filled out by a person showing himself/herself to be either normative or counternormative in his/her answers. They were then asked to describe, usually with adjectives[7], the person that was supposed to have filled out the questionnaire. Results showed that the internal targets were seen as more socially useful than the external ones (Cambon, Djouari, & Beauvois, 2006; Dubois & Beauvois, 2005). The self-sufficient targets were also seen as more socially useful that the non-self-sufficient targets (Dubois, 2005; Dubois & Beauvois, 2005), and the optimistic targets were likewise seen as more socially useful than the nonoptimistic or pessimistic targets (Le Barbenchon & Milhabert, 2005; Milhabet, 2011). This link between normativeness and social utility persists in self-descriptions. Cambon et al. asked students to fill out an internality questionnaire, then describe themselves using adjectives. They observed an almost linear relationship between the internality of these students and the social utility they assigned themselves.

This body of research is interesting because it shows that "psychological description", regarded as an evaluative —and as such attributing social utility or social desirability—, is a way of communicating a person's social value when this value is assessed on other criteria. The above-mentioned normativeness of judgment is not the only criterion of people's social value. Other criteria are linked to social structure, in particular the positions occupied by individuals within that structure as well as the profits associated with those positions. We have good reason to think that psychological descriptions vary with these criteria, as we saw with Cambon (2004)'s results. These criteria are discussed below in the organizational context.

We conclude this section with a hypothesis derived from previous research. Significant social differences have been shown to give rise to differences in social utility, but less so in social desirability (professionals working in the production sector are seen as more socially useful but not more socially desirable than professionals working in the maintenance sector; normative individuals are seen as more socially useful but not more socially desirable than counternormative individuals). We can therefore deduce that while social utility is used to corroborate some important *social* differences, social desirability is used to compensate for a lack of social valorization. Social desirability is thus used by people who are not socially valued as a means of self-promotion, in other words, to earn a judgment that is not too pejorative: *I am certainly not dynamic and ambitious* (understood: like *worthful* individuals), *but*

[7] More rarely by means of rating scales.

I am honest and helpful (see Kervyn, Yzerbyt & Judd, 2011; Yzerbyt, Kervyn, & Judd, 2008, for compensation effects).

4. Social desirability and social utility in organizational contexts: Social utility corresponds to people's economic value

This section is divided into two parts. Part 1 deals with the role of social utility in the organizational context. Part 2 discusses the relevance of breaking social utility down into three components, each with a different status in an organization and, more generally, in society.

4.1 Social utility in recruitment

4.1.1 Recruitment or cooptation?

In a study by Dubois and Aubert (2010, Study 1), executives in charge of a team and who had considerable experience in assessment were told to put themselves in the position of recruiting a target peer described in terms of socially useful or socially desirable adjectives. As predicted (see Table 6, study 1), the socially useful target candidate (*active, intelligent, organized,* etc.) was judged by the vast majority to be more recruitable than the socially desirable target candidate (*agreeable, honest, helpful,* etc.): $F(1,70)= 80.42$, $p<.001$, $\eta^2= .535$.

In a second study, Dubois and Aubert compared a recruitment condition to a co-optation condition. In this last condition, students were asked to coopt a target person to go on vacation. This target person was described using the same socially useful or socially desirable adjectives as those used in the recruitment condition. The 2(condition: recruitment vs. co-optation) x 2 (target: socially useful vs. socially desirable) between-subjects ANOVA performed on the data (see Table 6, study 2) showed a significant interaction effect, $F(1,396)= 1552.445$, $p<.001$, $\eta^2= .797$). Whereas a similar result to that of Study 1 was observed in the recruitment condition (the socially useful target was the one most frequently recruited), an opposite result was found in the friend cooptation situation (the socially desirable target was this time the most frequently coopted).

The results of these two studies led to a simple idea that we have already touched on, namely, that social utility is a relevant selection criterion as far as economic value is concerned (i.e., in organizations and the workplace), but social desirabilty is a relevant selection criterion as far as interpersonal relations are concerned.

	Socially useful target	Socially desirable target
Study 1 recruitment condition 88 executives	6.11 (*1.14)*	3.39 (*1.42)*
Study 2 recruitement condition 200 students	79.24 (*11.66)*	35.95 (*10.02)*
Study 2 co-optation condition 200 students	43.55 (*11.22)*	81.60 (*8.01)*

Table 6. Selection of a socially useful vs. socially desirable target person (means and standard deviations) in Dubois and Aubert (2010, Study 1 and Study 2)

4.1.2 Recruitment for a job in production or a job in maintenance?

The above results nevertheless raise an important question. We have already seen (Cambon, 2004) that while social utility is the main value in production, this is not the case in maintenance. Dubois and Aubert's studies therefore needed to be replicated in the light of these two sectors. To this end, Dubois (2010a, Study 4) looked at ordinary employees' ratings of a target applicant's chances of being hired when the applicant was said to be either socially useful (*active, intelligent, organized, efficient, hardworking*) or socially desirable (*agreeable, honest, open-minded, helpful, likeable*). Vacant positions were a high- or low-ranking position in either the production sector or the maintenance sector of the economy (head of an automobile company for the high-status production job, milling machine operator for the low-status production job, artistic director at an opera house for the high-status maintenance job, and sports coach at a summer camp for the low-status maintenance job). A 2(types of trait descriptions: socially useful vs. socially desirable) x 2 (job sectors:production vs. maintenance) x 2 (job statuses: high vs. low)) between-subjects ANOVA performed on the data (see Table 7) showed a significant types of traits x job sectors interaction effect, $F(1,53) = 19.42$, $p < .001$, $\eta^2 = .113$. The breakdown of this interaction indicated firstly that the type-of-trait effect was only found for the production jobs ($F(1,53) = 36.03$, $p < .001$, $\eta^2 = .191$): when presented as socially useful, both applicants applying for a production job were rated as more likely to be hired ($M = 3.64$) than when they were presented as socially desirable ($M = 2.42$). For the maintenance jobs, whether presented as socially useful ($M = 3.30$) or socially desirable ($M = 3.35$), the applicant's chances of being recruited were the same ($F(1,53) = .06$, ns). The fact that the second-order interaction was nonsignificant (F(1,53) = .70, ns) showed that the job-rank variable did not affect the type-of-trait by job-sector interaction. Such results clearly showed that social utility was the dominant value when the production sector was involved (whether for a job as the head of an automobile company or as a milling machine operator). There was no such finding for applicants seeking a position in the maintenance sector (whether as an artistic director or a sports coach).

Applicant's profile	Job economic sector			
	Production		Maintenance	
	High-status	Low-status	High-Sstatus	Low-status
Socially useful	3.70 (*0.86*)	3.57 (*0.81*)	3.20 (0.83)	3.40 (1.05)
Socially desirable	2.35 (*0.75*)	2.50 (*1.05*)	3.35 (0.88)	3.35 (0.99)

Table 7. Mean scores and standard deviations for the target applicant's chances of being hired by job economic sector, status and profile of the target in Dubois (2010a, Study 4)

4.2 Three components of social utility[8]

When we look at the actual meaning of the words, we find that the traits located at the positive poles of the two dimensions are not at all similar. *Honesty* and *helpfulness*, for instance, (two traits traditionally found at the positive pole of the first dimension) do not belong to the same register of meaning. Similarly, *ambition* and *competence* (two traits found

[8] The studies which follow are very recent. They have been presented at scientific meetings, but have not yet been published.

at the positive pole of the second dimension) belong to two different registers, as far as their simple meaning is concerned. These same semantic problems are observed when we consider the negative poles. Why would a *shy* person (trait located at the negative pole of the second dimension) not be *competent* (trait located at the positive pole of this same second dimension)? Similarly, why would a *liar* (located at the negative pole of the first dimension) not be *warm* (located at the positive pole of this same first dimension)? This observation has led researchers to introduce a distinction between morality and sociability within the first dimension (Brambilla, Rusconi, Sacchi, & Cherubini, 2011). French researchers have proposed several differentiations within the second factor which have recently turned out to be very productive. While certain traits belonging to the second dimension (which we call "social utility" but many name "competence") directly evoke ideas of competence or incompetence (*intelligent* and *capable* at the positive pole, and *stupid* and *out of his/her depth* at the negative pole), other traits (e.g., *courageous* at the positive pole, and *shy* at the negative pole) have nothing to do with (in)competence. This is why the second factor has been broken down into the following three components.

1. effort (in an activity; i.e., *persevering*). Description of someone who is hardworking, extremely conscientious and always sees his or her work through to the end, even if it is difficult;
2. competence (in an activity; i.e., *capable*) Description of someone who has considerable abilities, masters techniques well and knows how to resolve problems;
3. ease (in an activity; i.e., *competitive*). Description of someone who is ambitious, feels at ease with the competition and is never temperamental.

We evoke just two studies here. Dubois (2010b) asked subjects to read the three above descriptions through carefully. The latter were said to be descriptions of three employees. The experimenter then informed the subjects of these employees' status: one was said factory manager, another was said foreman and the third, manual worker. Subjects had to match descriptions and status. In another group, instead of statuses, Dubois gave the salaries of these employees: one earned €6,000 a month, another earned €3,000, and the third €1,500. Similarly, subjects had to match descriptions and salaries. The results (Tables 8a and 8b) support the predictions in a very significant way for the statuses (for « factory manager » : $X_{(2)}{}^2= 29.4$, $p< .001$, for « foreman » : $X_{(2)}{}^2= 22.4$, $p< .001$, for « manual worker » : $X_{(2)}{}^2= 35$, $p<.001$) and in an only marginally way for salaries, although the salaries associated with the three components were in the expected direction (for "€6,000": $X_{(2)}{}^2= 2.4$, ns, for « €3,000" : $X_{(2)}{}^2= 4.2$, ns, and for "€1,500": $X_{(2)}{}^2= 5,4$, $p <.07$).

These results suggest that the highest status was associated with the "at ease in the activity" portrait and the lowest status was associated with the "effort" portrait and, to a lesser extent that the lowest salary was associated with the "effort" portrait.

These results prompted the author to wonder whether the observed hierarchy of the three components of social utility was specific to one particular organizational culture. A study by Mollaret and Miraucourt (n.d) has now provided an answer to that question. These researchers asked servicemen, public-sector workers and the employees of a large private company to say how much money (7-point rating scale) 75 traits would fetch a member of the organization to which they belonged. The traits were representative either of effort, competence, or ease. The researchers were thus able to calculate how much money the three components were worth in each organization. Ease was found to be the dominant value in the private sector, but not in the other two organizational models under scrutiny. Interestingly, when they asked people encountered in their own homes or in the street, to say what the same 75 traits might bring someone in a general way (without referring to any particular organization), they reproduced the results for the private sector. The results are set out in Table 9.

status	At ease in the activity	Competence	Effort
Factory manager	80%	10%	10%
Foreman	20%	73.33%	6.67%
Manual worker	0%	16.67%	83.33%

Table 8a. Status associated with the three components of social utility in Dubois (2010b)

Salaries	At ease in the activity	Competence	Effort
€6,000	46.67%	26.67%	26.67%
€3,000	30%	50%	20%
€1,500	23.33%	23.33%	53.37%

Table 8b. Salaries associated with the three components of social utility in Dubois (2010b)

	Ease (E)	Competence (C)	Effort (Ef)
Employees of a private company	5.72 (0.54)	4.86 (1.11)	4.78 (0.95)
Servicemen	4.87 (0.62)	4.87 (0.85)	5.38 (0.78)
Public-sector workers	4.71 (0.89)	5.28 (0.82)	4.65 (0.77)
Random sample	5.48 (0.65)	4.80 (1.33)	4.60 (1.28)

Table 9. Mean economic value (and standard deviations) for adjectives associated with ease, competence and effort worth in three organizational models and in a random sample in Mollaret and Miraucourt (n.d)

"Ease" seemed to be the preferred value in private companies ($F(2, 44)= 16.91$, $p <.001$; $\eta^2 = .43$). The analysis of contrasts showed that subjects choosed significantly more "Ease" than "Competence" and "Effort" (undifferentiated). "Competence" seemed to be the most chosen value by public-sector workers ($F(2, 44)= 6.65$, $p < .01$; $\eta^2 = .23$). The analysis of contrasts showed that subjects choosed significantly more "Competence" than "Ease" and "Effort" (undifferentiated). "Effort" seemed the value prized by servicemen ($F(2, 44)= 5.61$, $p < .01$; $\eta^2 = .20$). The analysis of contrasts showed that subjects choosed significantly more "Effort" than "Ease" and "Competence" (undifferentiated). As we might have expected on the basis of an analysis of ideological processes in our society, the general public seemed to be imbued with the private-sector model ($F(2, 44)= 9.67$, $p <.001$; $\eta^2 = .30$). The analysis of contrasts showed that subjects choosed significantly more "Ease" than "Competence" and "Effort" (undifferentiated).

The research described in this section confirms the idea that social utility is the most relevant dimension in business organizations in the production sector and that it comes in the shape of a hierarchy indicating people's market value in these organizations. Ease is at the top of this hierarchy, with the highest status, and effort at the bottom, with the lowest status. To the best of our knowledge, social desirabilty has yet to give rise to studies that would allow us to organize morality and sociability in a similar hierarchy.

Taken together, these findings can help us to put forward new definitions.

5. Conclusion

The previous sections should allow readers to judge for themselves the contribution of the empirical bases of the following evaluative definitions of the two factors (the "big two", as they are sometimes called):

- A person's *social desirability* is his or her reputation for arousing positive (vs. negative) affects in others and for going along with (vs. going against) other people's motivations. It has at least two components, namely morality and sociability (or agreeableness);
- A person's *social utility* is his or her reputation for being able (vs. unable) to occupy different positions in social organizations, positions ranged from the least high to the highest. It has at least three components, ranging from the least valued to the most valued, namely effort, competence and ease;
- A person's reputation for being more or less desirable and more or less useful is the product of the social evaluative practices to which the person has been subjected. When an evaluation is communicated in the form of personality traits, these traits activate in memory the behaviors that can or should be adopted towards that target person, in other words, what could or should be done with him/her. There are good reasons to think that people internalize the main aspects of their reputation.

The above evaluative conception can be summed up in a basic idea whereby the concepts of naive psychology are not intended to describe human beeing from a psychological, scientific or quasi-scientific point of view, but instead to evaluate them as *social actors or agents*. The dimensional structure of implicit personality theories does not reflect the structure of human psychology, but rather the two main registers of social values that people realize (or should realize) through their behavior (e.g., depending on whether they are *hardworking* or *lazy*). We do not claim that people are stupid or irrational. The fact of not being centred on the intrinsic, descriptive properties of objects and people must not be considered as an indication of stupidity. On the contrary, we claim that people behave as fine analysts when they deal with things that are important to them, namely, the *value* of people and things, even if the *intrinsic nature* of those people and things is not their main preoccupation[9]. The register of the social values is not a register which is used by default. It is not established by imaginary whims. This register is made by realities. People refer to these realities to hire somebody, to pay him/her, to associate him/her with projects of work or leisure activities

[9] Moreover, if our subjects are perfectly capable of mobilizing their I.P.T. and to produce both dimensions of the social value of the persons when we incite them to psychologize by asking them to describe pet rabbits with personality traits (Dubois & Beauvois, 2011, study 2, see above) , equivalent subjects, placed in quite a different situation, a situation of purchase on the market (Dubois & Beauvois, 2011, study 3), recognize that nobody would pay a high price for a rabbit because it is intelligent. In this situation, the subjects deal with the social value of a rabbit, without psychologizing. They say that we can pay a high price for a rabbit if it is beautiful and if it is of pure race. What corresponds to the reality of the market.

and even to marry him/her. In numerous domains of the life and the social life (agriculture, crafts, interpersonal relations…), people learnt at first to handle this register of social realities without adopting a scientific way of thinking. Science came much later, when it came: at this beginning of XXI° century, it is not sure that science came in psychology of individual differences. Indeed, what is presented as individual differences in *personality* are in fact differences in the *social value* of people. We can even wonder if a scientific psychology of the individual differences will not have to give up the concept of "personality" which is maybe too much filled with evaluative perception of people.

We conclude with the two main advantages of this evaluative conception.

The evaluative conception does not rely on *any* of the assumptions about the validity of the psychology used by laypeople as a tool of descriptive or scientific knowledge, assumptions which, since the fifties, and despite Heider (1958), have often been criticized by social psychologists either directly or indirectly. In particular, this conception does not require naive psychologists (1) to be aware of the psychological nature of their own personality or that of their target, (2) to have spontaneous access to that nature, or (3) to speak about that nature as an intuitive scientist would speak (which they *never* do for other objects of knowledge, except obviously when the person who speaks is a scientist in the exercise of his/her work).

The evaluative conception considers people in terms of their concrete social existence. The research reported in this chapter supports the idea that the evaluative approach is indeed derived from a psychology that is possibly scientific, but definitely *social*. People are evaluated on a daily basis in social situations which involve them as *agents* or *social actors*. They are not evaluated as human beings. We do not need to rely on what is, for us, a theoretical fantasy, namely the existence of a universal subject who, in a social vacuum, attempts to pin down the authentic nature of objects (and more particularly of persons) by relying solely on his/her cognitive abilities which predispose him/her to be an intuitive scientist. When people judge a person, they always consider this person in the social relationships which determine the social values which serve as reference to their judgment: this person is either a pupil or a worker or a teacher, or an artist… However, the dominant thinking in academic psychology well and truly considers the person judging (the teacher) and the judged person (the pupil) as if they were two *homo sapiens sapiens*. In fact, they never are *homo sapiens sapiens* but they are persons inserted into social situations involving roles and particular objectives. In brief, they are actors or social agents. In addition, describing a *homo sapiens sapiens* is not the same as judging a social agent or actor. Recognizing that we evaluate actors or social agents and not human beings would lead to question important postulates of the research on the "personality". Among these postulates, the most important, which is also the basis of what social psychologists have called the fundamental error, is that people always express their psychological nature to explain what they do. Accept the idea that they express especially their position of actor or social agent led to more concrete and less essentialist theoretical views.

6. References

Abele, A.E., Cuddy, A.J.C., Judd, C.M. & Yzezbyt, V.Y. (2008, special issue). Fondamental Dimensions of Social Judgement, *European Journal of Social Psychology, 38(7),* 1063-1224, 0046-2772

Abele, A.E. & Wojciszke, B. (2007). Agency and Communion from the Perspective of Self vs. Others. *Journal of Personality and Social Psychology, 93(5)*, 751-763, 0022-3514

Asch, S.E. (1946). Forming Impressions of Personality. *Journal of Abnormal and Social Psychology*, 41(3), 258-290, 0096-851X

Bachelard, G. (1938). *La Formation de l'Esprit Scientifique,* Vrin, 978-2711611508, Paris

Bachelard, G. (1953). *Le Matérialisme Rationnel,* Presses Universitaires de France, 978-2130562856, Paris

Beauvois, J.-L. (1976). Problématique des Conduites Sociales d'Evaluation. *Connexions, 19(1)*, 7-30, 0337-3126

Beauvois, J.-L. (1982). Théories implicites de la personnalité, évaluation et reproduction idéologique. *L'Année Psychologique, 82*, 513-536

Beauvois, J.-L. (1984). *La Psychologie Quotidienne,* Presses Universitaires de France, 978-2130385837, Paris

Beauvois, J.-L. (1995). La Connaissance des Utilités Sociales. *Psychologie Française, 40(4)*, 375-387, 0033-2984

Beauvois, J.-L. (2011). *Les Influences Sournoises. Précis des Manipulations Ordinaires,* François Bourin, 978-2849412596, Paris

Beauvois, J.-L. & Dépret, E. (2008). What about Social Value? *European Journal of Psychology of Education, 23(4)*, 493- 500, 0256-2928

Beauvois, J.-L. & Dubois, N. (1992). Traits as Evaluative Categories. *CPC-European Bulletin of Cognitive Psychology, 12(3)*, 253-270, 0954-1446

Beauvois, J.-L. & Dubois, N. (2000). Affordances in Social Judgment: Experimental Proof of Why it is a Mistake to Ignore How Others Behave Towards a Target and Look Solely at How the Target Behaves. *Swiss Journal of Psychology, 59(1)*, 16-33, 1421-0185

Beauvois, J.-L. & Dubois, N. (2008). Deux Dimensions du Jugement Personnologique: Approche Evaluative vs Approche Psychologique. *Psychologia Sociala, 21*, 105-119, 0035-3892

Beauvois, J.-L. & Dubois, N. (2009). Lay Psychology and the Social Value of Persons. *Social and Personality Psychology Compass, 3(6)*, 1082-1095, 1751-9004

Beauvois, J.-L., Dubois, N., Mira, L. & Monteil, J.-M. (1996). Evaluative Knowledge and Person Memory. *CPC: Current Psychology of Cognition, 15(1)*, 29-47, 0249-9185

Beauvois, J.-L., Dubois, N. & Tarquinio, C. (1994). *Personology and Evaluative Knowledge in Social Context.* E.A.E.S.P. Third European Conference on Social Cognition, Blois, France, April

Brambilla, M, Rusconi, P, Sacchi, S. & Cherubini, P. (2011). The Primary Role of Morality (vs. Sociability and Competence) in Information Gathering. *European Journal of Social Psychology, 41(2)*, 135-143, 1099-0992

Bruner, J. & Taguiri, R. (1954). The Perception of People, In: *Handbook of Social Psychology, vol. 2*, G. Lindzey, pp. 634-654, Addison-Wesley, 978-0195213768, Cambridge, MA

Cambon, L. (2004) La Désirabilité Sociale et l'Utilité Sociale des Professions et des Professionnels, In: *Perspectives cognitives et conduites sociales volume, vol. 9,* J.L. Beauvois, R.V. Joule, & J.M. Monteil, pp. 187-212, Presses Universitaires de Rennes, 978-2868479471, Rennes

Cambon, L. (2006). La Fonction Evaluative de la Personnologie. Vers la Mise en Evidence de Deux Dimensions de la Valeur: la Désirabilité Sociale et l'Utilité Sociale. *Psychologie Française, 51(3)*, 285-305, 0033-2984

Cambon, L. (2007). *Désirabilité et Utilité Sociales: Deux Dimensions du Jugement Social.* Paper presented at the meeting "35 ans de psychologie sociale avec Jean-Léon Beauvois", Paris, France, April

Cambon, L., Djouari, A. & Beauvois, J.-L. (2006). Social Judgement Norms and Social Utility: When it is More Valuable to be Useful than Desirable. *Swiss Journal of Psychology, 65(3)*, 167-180, 1421-0185

Dubois, N. (2003). *A Sociocognitive Approach to Social Norms*, Routledge, 978-0415257268, London

Dubois, N. (2005). Normes Sociales de Jugement et Valeur: Ancrage sur l'Utilité et Ancrage sur la Désirabilité. *Revue Internationale de Psychologie Sociale, 18(3)*, 43-79, 0992-986X

Dubois, N. (2006). La Valeur Sociale des Personnes. In: *Bilan et Perspectives en Psychologie Sociale, vol. 1*, R.V. Joule & P. Huguet, pp. 81-115, Presses Universitaires de Grenoble, 978-2706113741, Grenoble

Dubois, N. (2010a). Theory of the Social Value of Persons Applied to Organizations: Typologies of "Good" Leaders and Recruitment. *European Review of Applied Psychology, 60(4)*, 255-266, 1162-9088

Dubois, N. (2010b). *L'utilité Sociale dans les Organisations.* Paper presented at the 8th Congrès International de Psychologie Sociale en Langue Française, Nice, France, August

Dubois, N., & Aubert, E. (2010). Valeur Sociale des Personnes: Deux Informations Valent-Elles Mieux qu'Une ? *International Review of Social Psychology, 23(1)*, 57-92, 0992-986X

Dubois, N. & Beauvois, J.-L. (2001). Désirabilité et Utilité, Deux Composantes de la Valeur des Personnes dans l'Evaluation Sociale. *L'Orientation Scolaire et Professionnelle, 30(3)*, 391-405, 0249-6739

Dubois, N. & Beauvois, J.-L. (2005). Normativeness and Individualism. *European Journal of Social Psychology, 35(1)*, 123-146, 1099-0992

Dubois, N. & Beauvois, J.-L. (2011). Are Some Rabbits More Competent and Warm Than Others? The Lay Epistemologist is Interested in Object Value but not in Descriptive Parameters. *Swiss Journal of Psychology, 70(2)*, 63-73, 1421-0185

Heider, F. (1958). *The Psychology of Interpersonal Relations*, John Wiley & Sons, 978-0471368335, New York

Fiske, S., Cuddy, A.J.C. & Glick, P. (2007). Universal Dimensions of Social Perception: Warmth, then Competence. *Trends in Cognitive Science, 11(2)*, 77-83; 1364-6613

Judd, C.M., James-Hawkins, L., Yzebyt, V. & Kashima, Y. (2005). Fundamental Dimensions of Social Judgment: Understanding the Relations Between Judgments of Competence and Warmth. *Journal of Personality and Social Psychology, 89(6)*, 899-913, 0022-3514

Kervyn, N., Yzerbyt, V. & Judd, C.M. (2011). When Compensation Guides Inferences: Indirect and Implicit Measures of the Compensation Effect. *European Journal of Social Psychology, 41(2)*, 144-151, 1099-0992

Kim, M.P. & Rosenberg, S. (1980). Comparison of Two Structural Models of Implicit Personality Theory. *Journal of Personality and Social Psychology, 38(3)*, 375-389, 0022-3514

Kluckhohn, C. (1954). Culture and Behaviour, In: *Handbook of Social Psychology, vol 2,* G. Lindzey, pp. 921-976, Addison-Wesley, 978-0470137475 Cambridge, MA

Labourin, M.C. & Lecourvoisier, A. (1986). Le Rôle des Traits Centraux dans la Formation des Impressions. *Cahiers de Psychologie Cognitive, 6(1)*, 95-102, 0249-9185

Le Barbenchon, E. & Milhabet, I. (2005). L'Optimisme: Réponse Désirable et/ou Socialement Utile? *Revue Internationale de Psychologie Sociale, 18(3)*, 153-181, 0992-986X

Mignon, A. & Mollaret, P. (2002). Applying the affordance conception of traits: a person perception study. *Personality and Social Psychology Bulletin, 28(10)*, 1327-1334, 0146-1672

Milhabet, I. (2004). Que Reste-t-il en Mémoire des Comportements Adoptés à l'égard d'Autrui? Double Connaissance Personnologique et Effet d'Inconsistance, In: *Perspectives Cognitives et Conduites Sociales, vol 9*, J.-L. Beauvois, R.-V. Joule, & J.-M. Monteil, pp. 245-267, Presses Universitaires de Rennes, 978-2868479471, Rennes.

Mollaret, P. & Mignon, A. (2006). Vers une Approche Psychosociale du Jugement de "Personnalité". *Psychologie Française, 51(3)*, 307-325, 0033-2984

Mollaret, P & Miraucourt, D. (n.d). Aisance, Compétence, Effort : Trois Registres Distincts de la Valeur Sociale des Personnes. Laboratoire de psychologie Appliquée, Université de Reims

Montmollin, M. de (1972). *Les Psychopîtres*, Presses Universitaires de France, B004W5ZH8Y, Paris

Osgood, C.E. (1962). Studies of the Generality of Affective Meaning Systems. *American Psychologist, 17(1)*, 10-28, 0003-066X

Osgood, C. E., Suci, G. J. & Tannenbaum, P. H. (1957). *The Measurement of Meaning*, University of Illinois Press, 978-0252745393, Urbana

Passini, F. T. & Norman, W. T. (1966). A Universal Conception of Personality Structure. *Journal of Personality and Social Psychology, 4(1)*, 44-49, 0022-3514

Peeters, G. (1992). Evaluative Meanings of Adjectives in Vitro and in Context: Some Theoretical Implications and Practical Consequences of Positive-Negative Asymmetry and Behavioral-Adaptative Concepts of Evaluation. *Psychologica Belgica, 32,* 211-231, 0033-2879

Rosenberg, S. & Sedlak, A. (1972). Structural Representations of Implicit Personality Theory. In: *Advances in Experimental Social Psychology, vol. 6,* L. Berkowitz, pp. 235-297, Academic Press, 978-0120152063, New York

Schiffler, F., Dubois, N. & Mollaret, P. (2010). Modes de Connaissances des Objets Sociaux: Leur Induction et Leur Généralisation. Paper presented at the 8th Congrès International de Psychologie Sociale en Langue Française, Nice, France, August

Schneider, D. J. (1973). Implicit Personality Theory: A Review. *Psychological Bulletin, 79(5)*, 294-309. 0033-2909

Shweder, R.A. & D'Andrade, R.G. (1979). Accurate Reflection or Systematic Distorsion? *Journal of Personality and Social Psychology, 37(6)*, 1075-1084, 0022-3514

Srull, P.K. & Wyer, R.S. (1989). Person Memory and Judgment. *Psychological Review, 96(1)*, 58-63, 0033-295X

Suitner, C. & Maass, A. (2008). The Role of Valence in the Perception of Agency and Communion. *European Journal of Social Psychology, 38(7)*, 1073-1082, 1099-0992

Tiffin, J. & McCormick, E.J. (1965). *Industrial Psychology*, Prentice-Hall, 978-0041500578, Englewood Cliffs, NJ

Wojciszke, B. (1994). Multiple Meanings of Behavior: Construing Actions in Terms of Competence and Morality. *Journal of Personality and Social Psychology, 67(2)*, 222-232, 0022-3514

Wojciszke, B. (2005). Morality and Competence in Person and Self Perception. *European Review of Social Psychology, 1(2)6*, 155-188, 1046-3283

Yzerbyt, V.Y., Kervyn, N. & Judd, C. (2008). Compensation Versus Halo: The Unique Relation Between the Fundamental Dimensions of Social Judgment. *Personality and Social Psychology Bulletin, 34(8)*, 1110-1123, 0146-1672

Zuckier, H. (1986). The Paradigmatic and Narrative Models in Goal-Guided Inference, In: *Handbook of Motivation and Cognition: Foundations of Social Behaviour, vol. 1*, M. Sorrentino & E.T. Higgins, pp 465-502, Guilford Press, 978-0898624328, New York